The Dartmouth Atlas of Health Care 1998

The Center for the
Evaluative Clinical Sciences

Dartmouth Medical School

AHA books are published by American Hospital Publishing, Inc., an American Hospital Association company

Library of Congress Cataloging-in-Publication Data

Dartmouth Medical School. Center for the Evaluative Clinical Sciences.
    The Dartmouth atlas of health care 1998 / the Center for the Evaluative Clinical Sciences, Dartmouth Medical School.
    p.   cm.
    ISBN 1-55648-217-5
    1. Medical care—United States—Marketing—Maps. 2. Health facilities—United States—Statistics. I. Title.
G1201.E5D3   1996   (G&M)
362.1'0973'022—dc2096-11510

                                                              CIP
                                                              MAP

Catalog no. 044400

𝔸ℍ𝔸 is a service mark of the American Hospital Association used under license by American Hospital Publishing, Inc.

The Dartmouth Atlas of Health Care in the United States

John E. Wennberg, M.D., M.P.H., *Principal Investigator and Series Editor*

Megan McAndrew Cooper, M.B.A., M.S., *Editor*

and other members of the Dartmouth Atlas of Health Care Working Group

John D. Birkmeyer, M.D.

Kristen K. Bronner, M.A.

Thomas A. Bubolz, Ph.D.

Elliott S. Fisher, M.D., M.P.H.

Alan M. Gittelsohn, Ph.D.

David C. Goodman, M.D., M.S.

Katherine W. Herbst, M.S.

Jack E. Mohr

James F. Poage, Ph.D.

Sandra M. Sharp, S.M.

Jonathan S. Skinner, Ph.D.

Thérèse A. Stukel, Ph.D.

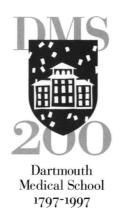

Dartmouth
Medical School
1797-1997

Dartmouth Medical School

The release of the 1998 Dartmouth Atlas of Health Care coincides with the celebration of Dartmouth Medical School's bicentennial. We take this opportunity to thank the many men and women of Dartmouth Medical School who have supported our work, and also to acknowledge the pioneering role in American medicine of the medical school's founder, Nathan Smith, M.D. Our work goes forward within the context of a curriculum that has honored for two hundred years the importance of excellent teaching, compassionate patient care, and significant research.

The Dartmouth Atlas of Health Care Working Group dedicates the 1998 edition of the Dartmouth Atlas of Health Care in the United States to the faculty, students, friends and supporters of the Dartmouth Medical School.

The research on which the Dartmouth Atlas of Health Care
is based was made possible by a grant from

The Robert Wood Johnson Foundation

The Center for the Evaluative Clinical Sciences
Dartmouth Medical School
Hanover, New Hampshire 03756
(603) 650-1820
http://www.dartmouth.edu/~atlas/

Published in cooperation with The Center for Health Care Leadership
of the American Hospital Association

American Hospital Publishing, Inc.
Chicago, Illinois

Table of Contents

Maps

Figures

Tables

CHAPTER ONE
Overview and Introduction

Overview and Introduction

The 1998 edition of the Dartmouth Atlas of Health Care in the United States is organized into seven chapters, three appendices; and an endnote which includes references. The Appendix on Methods provides a detailed description of the methods used in the Atlas. The Appendix on the Geography of Medical Care in the United States provides reference maps that describe the boundaries of the 306 hospital referral regions in the United States. The Appendix on the Physician Workforce provides additional information on the supply of specialists in the United States.

Overview

The Atlas shows once again that in health care, geography is destiny. The amount of care consumed by Americans is highly dependent on where they live — on the capacity of the health care system where they live, and on the practice styles of local physicians. Variations in the intensity of use of hospitals, the striking differences in the way terminal care is delivered, and the idiosyncratic patterns of elective surgery raise significant questions about the outcomes and value of health care. The fundamental questions posed by the Atlas are Which rate is right? How much is enough? and What is Fair?

Chapter Two documents the wide variations in Medicare spending and in the supply of acute care hospital resources and physicians among the nation's hospital referral regions. In Chapter Three, the Atlas examines the patterns of hospitalization for several medical conditions in order to demonstrate the relationship between rates of admissions to hospitals, physicians' practice styles, and hospital capacity. While the incidence of illness determines the rates of hospitalizations for a few conditions (such as hip fractures), hospitalization rates for most medical conditions, including heart failure, pneumonia and gastroenteritis, vary substantially among regions. In Chapter Three, we examine the close correlation between the incidence of hospitalization for these "high variation" conditions and the numbers of hospital beds per thousand residents.

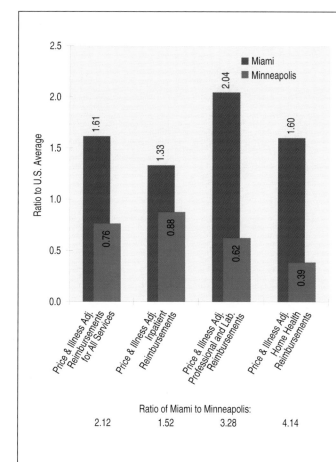

How Much is Enough?
Medicare Spending in Miami and Minneapolis

Medicare Spending, adjusted for illness and price, is substantially higher for the Medicare population living in the Miami hospital referral region than for those living in Minneapolis. On a per capita basis, overall spending for Miami residents is more than twice that for residents of Minneapolis. Miami is well above the national average, and Minneapolis is well below it. Home health payments for residents of Miami are more than four times higher than for residents of Minneapolis; payments for physician services and diagnostic laboratory services are more than three times higher; and 52% more is spent on inpatient care.

Figure 1.1. Age, Sex, Race, Illness and Price Adjusted Medicare Spending for Medicare Residents Living in the Miami and Minneapolis Hospital Referral Regions (1995)
The figure gives the ratio of rates of age, sex, race, illness and price adjusted spending for Medicare residents of Miami and Minneapolis to the national average and the ratio of spending for Miami residents to spending for Minneapolis residents.

Likewise, the amount and intensity of hospital care that Americans receive during the last six months of their lives varies remarkably from region to region, and also correlates with hospital capacity. Chapter Four examines a number of measures of the variations in the intensity of resources deployed during the last six months of life, including the average number of days in acute care hospitals, the average number of days in intensive care, and levels of expenditures.

Although the rates for most surgical procedures also vary substantially among regions, hospital capacity is not the most important determining factor in surgical variations. Procedures such as coronary artery bypass grafting, back surgery, and prostatectomy for benign and cancerous prostate disease vary in idiosyncratic ways. A given region may have high rates for one of these procedures, but low rates for another, resulting in "surgical signatures." Chapter Five provides a clinical explana-

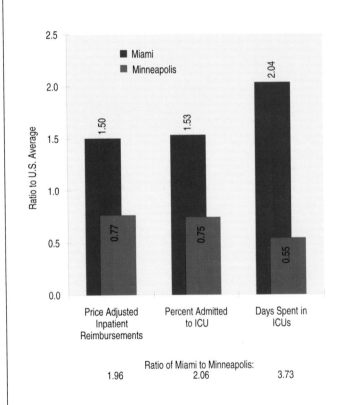

How Much is Enough?
The Likelihood of Hospitalization During the Last Six Months of Life in Miami and Minneapolis

Miami residents are much more likely to be admitted to hospitals as they near death than the national average; Minneapolis residents are much less likely than average to be admitted to hospitals. Price adjusted spending for inpatient care during the last six months of life is nearly twice as much per death in the Miami region ($14,212) than spending per death in Minneapolis ($7,246). During this period of their lives, residents of Miami receive much more care in intensive care units (ICUs): 45.7% were admitted to the ICU one or more times, compared to 23.1% of Minneapolis residents. During the last six months of life, Miami residents spent an average of 4.8 days in ICUs, more than twice the national average; Minneapolis residents spent an average of only 1.6 days, about half the national average.

Figure 1.2. Acute Hospital Care During the Last Six Months of Life Among Medicare Residents of the Miami and Minneapolis Hospital Referral Regions (1995)
The figure compares the rates of hospitalizations during the last six months of life among Medicare residents of Miami and Minneapolis to the national average, and gives the ratio of Miami to Minneapolis. Included are age, sex, race, illness and price adjusted spending for acute hospital care, the percent of Medicare enrollees experiencing one or more admissions to an intensive care unit and the average number of days spent in an ICU during the last six months of life.

tion for the surgical signature phenomenon, showing that they do not result from differences in patient demand, but instead result from scientific uncertainty and the failure of physicians — and, increasingly, health plans — to involve patients in a systematic and meaningful way in the surgical decision making process.

The role of illness in determining the allocation of resources and the use of medical care is examined in Chapter Six. While sick people do indeed use health services more often than the less sick, the rates of use of health care for all members of society — the sick and the not so sick — are higher in regions with more resources and more spending. Predicted demand (based on measures of illness) explains only a small part of the higher than average hospitalization rates in regions with higher than average per capita supplies of hospital beds. The need for medical care, as estimated by an index of community health, has very little to do with the level of Medicare spending.

The information in this Atlas points to the need for reform. The failure of illness rates to explain much of the regional variation in resources and utilization points once again to the questions of fairness and value. The subliminal effect of hospital capacity on the admission "threshold" — on the decision whether or not to admit a patient — determines the rates of hospitalizations in regions and the intensity of care in the last six months of life. This raises the question of whether more is better: are the benefits of greater use of hospital and intensity of care worth the associated risks and costs?

The "surgical signature" phenomenon points to the need to improve the scientific basis of medicine and to reform the way treatment choices are made so that the choice among treatment options primarily reflects the patient's, rather than the physician's or the health plan's, priorities and preferences.

Chapter Seven is a concluding essay that focuses on the debate over what should be done to address unwanted variations in health care delivery. The chapter deals with

Which Rate is Right? The "Surgical Signatures" of Miami and Minneapolis

Miami residents and Minneapolis residents have approximately the same overall rates of surgery, but surgical resources are allocated very differently within each region, and the rates are often very different from the national average — sometimes well above the average, sometimes well below it. The rates of revascularization procedures used to treat coronary artery disease (coronary bypass surgery and percutaneous transluminal coronary angioplasty) and lower extremity bypass operations are higher among residents of Miami than among residents of Minneapolis. Rates of prostate cancer surgery and knee replacements are higher among Medicare residents of Minneapolis than among residents of Miami. Rates of carotid endarterectomy are well below the national average in both hospital referral regions.

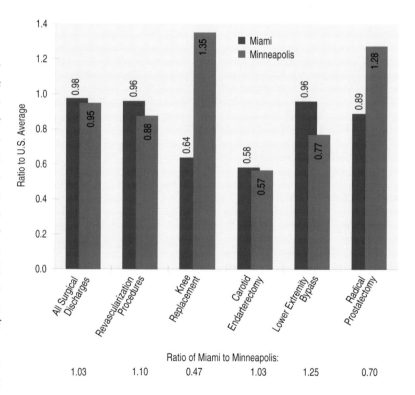

Figure 1. 3. Age, Sex and Race Adjusted Surgical Rates Among Medicare Residents of the Miami and Minneapolis Hospital Referral Regions (1994-95)

The figure compares rates of surgery among residents of Miami and Minneapolis to the national average for all surgical discharges and for selected procedures. The rate of revascularization procedures is the combined rates of coronary bypass surgery and percutaneous transluminal coronary angioplasty.

Medicare fairness and the equity implications of current Medicare formulas for re-imbursing managed care health plans. In brief, the policy problem is that Medicare's method of determining payment for capitated care is calculated at the county level (the AAPCC or average adjusted per capita costs). It reflects historical patterns of spending under fee-for-service health care delivery systems in local markets. One result is that differences in spending that cannot be attributed to differences in illness or in prices create unfair subsidies, which are in some cases substantial. For example, on a price and illness adjusted basis, managed care companies enrolling a resident of the Miami hospital referral region received $8,117 in 1997; managed care companies enrolling residents of the Minneapolis region received only $4,478 per enrollee. The higher spending for the residents of Miami is funded by taxes collected from residents of all hospital referral regions, including Minneapolis and other regions where Medicare spending is below the national average.

An unintended consequence of the federal government's AAPCC-based reimbursement policy is that managed health plans being reimbursed at Miami's rate could provide benefits at a reasonable level (such as the level currently provided in Minneapolis) and still have money available to expand the benefit package to include such additional services as prescription drugs, hearing aids and exercise programs. In Chapter Seven, we estimate that managed care companies providing services for residents of Miami could realize a surplus of more than $3,400 per enrollee for distribution as additional benefits, or retain that amount as profit, simply by achieving the efficiencies of fee-for-service medicine in Minneapolis.

In a statement contained in The 1998 Budget Resolution, the United States Senate recognized that while "all Americans pay the same payroll tax of 2.9 percent to the Medicare trust funds and they deserve the same choices and services regardless of where they retire," some regions "receive 2.5 times more in Medicare reimbursements than others." In addressing the issue of fairness the Congress inevitably faces the questions, Which rate is right? and How much is enough? In its "Sense of the Senate Resolution," the Senate appears to implicitly accept the national average as the "right" rate. The statement calls on the Finance Committee to implement policy to reduce the geographic variation in risk plan payment rates by raising "the lower payment areas closer to the average while taking into account actual differences in input costs."

But which rate is right? How much is enough? The national average, whether for coronary bypass grafting, the use of hospitals for medical conditions, the amount of money spent in the last six months of life, or overall Medicare spending, has no normative value. It is simply the average of the many different ways of practicing medicine documented in the Atlas, as for example the patterns of practice and Medicare spending seen in Minneapolis and Miami (Figures 1.1, 1.2 and 1.3).

Ideally, resource allocation decisions would be guided at the patient level by need, by knowledge of outcomes, and by the tradeoffs patients make between the costs, risks and benefits of care. At the population level, resource allocation decisions would be made based on society's beliefs about cost effectiveness and social justice. The Medicare program's spending would reflect these goals of efficiency, effectiveness and equity.

In Chapter Seven, we propose a two-part strategy to move the nation closer to this ideal. The first part of the strategy is a patient-level approach to the question of Which rate is right? It is based on outcomes research and the creation of the opportunity for patients to participate actively in the choice among treatments — for example, the choice between lumpectomy and mastectomy for breast cancer, and the choice between surgery and medical management for coronary artery disease. Choices among these options involve significant tradeoffs that only patients are qualified to make (Chapter Five). When patients participate in medical decisions (shared decision making) local rates reflect what informed patients actually want. Areas with such patient-driven rates might well have lower rates of surgery than the current national average. Studies of shared decision making suggest that the demand for invasive treatment by fully informed patients is actually less than the amount now being provided in most markets in the United States.

The second part of the strategy is a macro-level approach, one based on answering the question How much is enough? The strategy involves "benchmarking;" that is, comparing regions with high levels of resource allocation and spending to areas where resources and spending are more constrained. By using benchmarking, the outcomes question can be approached from the perspective of the population living in such regions. What is the evidence that greater investments in resources improve population health? Other research has found no evidence that mortality rates are lower, after adjustment for differences in demographics and illness, in regions with higher levels of spending for acute hospital care. We argue in Chapter Seven that benchmarks based on the experience of low rate regions do not represent

health care rationing — services recognized as necessary for improving life expectancy and well being are not being withheld in those regions.

The importance for health policy of coming to terms with the questions of Which rate is right? and How much is enough? is clearly important in terms of the solvency of the Medicare trust fund. If, on a price and illness adjusted basis, the level of Medicare spending for all hospital referral regions with higher rates were brought down to the level of spending in the Minneapolis region, the impending bankruptcy of the Medicare program (currently predicted for the year 2,005) would be averted (Figure 1.4).

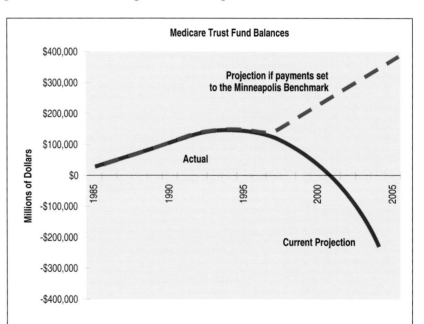

Figure 1.4. Projected Medicare Trust Fund Balances Under Current Levels of Spending and Under Spending Reduced to the Levels of Expenditures per Enrollee in the Minneapolis Hospital Referral Region (1995-2005)

The lower curve, labeled "Actual" and "Current Projection," shows the actual and projected balances of the combined Part A (hospital) and Part B (physician services) Medicare Trust Fund using intermediate assumptions. The upper curve shows the projected balances of the Medicare Trust Fund under the assumption that all hospital referral regions with price- and illness-adjusted per enrollee Medicare spending above the amount in Minneapolis adjust their spending downward in 1998 to the level of Minneapolis. Medicare spending then continues to grow through 2005 using the Trust Fund intermediate assumptions. (Source: Skinner, J. and Fisher, E., "Regional Disparities in Medicare Expenditures: An Opportunity for Reform" National Tax Journal (1997).

The nature of the relationship between supply and utilization; the lack of evidence that more is better in improving life expectancy; and the finding that fully informed patients actually want less invasive care than they are currently receiving, all suggest that from the point of view of both patients and populations, price and illness adjusted spending at the level of fee-for-service care in Minneapolis is a reasonable goal for all Americans. Indeed, achieving on a national basis the health care delivery efficiencies demonstrated in this region could help resolve a pressing issue of fairness: it would generate savings to address the very real problems in social justice posed by the nation's uninsured.

The Geography of Health Care in the United States

Most of the tools used to measure and explore variation in this edition of the Atlas will be familiar to most readers. We have again based our measurements on the experience of populations — how health care is used by defined populations, rather than the physical location of health care resources. This methodology, which is generally known as small area analysis, is at the core of our work. Readers who are unfamiliar with the strategies of studying population-based rates of resource distribution and utilization are urged to read the Appendix on Methods. The endnote provides references for further reading.

The first task of the Atlas project, undertaken in 1993, was to establish the geographic boundaries of naturally occurring health care markets in the United States. Based on a study of where Medicare patients were hospitalized, 3,436 geographic hospital service areas were defined. The hospital service areas were then grouped into 306 hospital referral regions on the basis of where Medicare patients were hospitalized for major cardiovascular surgical procedures and neurosurgery, markers for regionalization. The Appendix on the Geography of Medical Care in the United States, which is reprinted in part from the first edition of the Atlas, describes how this was done, and contains a series of maps that detail each hospital referral region in the United States. One important finding was that most hospital service areas and hospital referral regions, as defined by where patients actually receive their care, correspond poorly to political configurations, such as counties, which have traditionally been used to measure health care resources and utilization.

About Rates in the Atlas

In order to make comparisons easier, all rates in the Atlas are expressed in terms that result in at least one digit to the left of the decimal point (e.g., 1.6 cardiologists per hundred thousand residents, 3.9 hospital beds per thousand residents). In order to achieve this result, different denominators were used in calculating rates.

The levels of supply of hospital beds and hospital full time equivalent employees are expressed as beds and employees per thousand residents of the hospital referral region, based on American Hospital Association and Medicare data.

Reimbursements are expressed as dollars per capita, or per resident of the hospital referral region, based on Medicare claims data and census calculations.

The numbers of physicians providing services to residents of hospital referral regions are expressed as physicians per hundred thousand residents, based on American Medical Association and American Osteopathic Association data and census calculations.

The numbers of surgical and diagnostic procedures performed are expressed as procedures per thousand Medicare enrollees in the hospital referral region, or as procedures per thousand male or female Medicare enrollees in the region (for procedures like prostatectomy or mastectomy that apply only to one sex) based on Medicare claims data.

Patient day rates are expressed as total inpatient days per thousand Medicare enrollees.

Making Fair Comparisons Between Regions

Some areas of the country have greater needs for health care services and resources than others; for example, in some communities in Florida, as many as 60% of residents are over 65. Other parts of the country — including some with large college populations, or ski resorts — have much larger proportions of younger people. To ensure fair comparisons between areas, all rates in the Atlas have been adjusted to remove the differences that might be due to the different age and sex composition of local populations. This adjustment avoids identifying some areas as having high rates of utilization simply because of their larger proportions of elderly residents. When data were available, rates have also been adjusted for differences in race.

This edition of the Atlas provides an important new method for adjusting for differences in illness based on a community health index. The index is used to adjust for differences in mortality and for the incidence of certain diseases, such as coronary artery disease and stroke.

Some areas, such as major urban centers, have higher costs of living than others. Such areas are likely to have high health care expenditures because the costs of personnel, real estate, and supplies are higher, and not necessarily because they are providing more services. Adjusting for such variation provides a more comparable measure of differences in real health care spending that is not simply due to differences in costs of living among areas. Medicare reimbursement rates were adjusted to take into account the differences between hospital service areas in costs of living.

The methods used to adjust for age, sex, race, illness and price of medical care are detailed in the Appendix on Methods.

About the Dartmouth Atlas on CD-ROM

A sophisticated CD-ROM data viewer has been developed which makes it possible to query, manipulate, and display the Dartmouth Atlas data base using point-and-click techniques. The viewer contains both the hospital referral region and hospital service area levels of data used to create the Dartmouth Atlas. For more information about the CD-ROM, contact AHA Order Services at 1-800-242-2626.

Communicating With Us About the Atlas

Our Atlas Home Page on the World Wide Web contains Atlas information, including a summary of Dartmouth-related research and electronic copies of some hard-to-find references. Please send us your comments on the Atlas, particularly suggestions on how to improve it in the future.

We are at http://www.dartmouth.edu/~atlas.

Variations in Hospital Resources, Medicare Spending and the Physician Workforce

This chapter provides measures of the allocation of hospital resources, Medicare reimbursements, and the physician workforce to the populations living in the nation's 306 hospital referral regions. The estimates have been adjusted for differences in age and sex, and, in the case of reimbursements, regional differences in prices. The allocation method adjusts for patient migration to hospitals and physicians located outside of the hospital referral region where the patient resides. (See the Appendix on Methods.)

Acute Care Hospital Resources

The dramatic differences in levels of acute care hospital resources that were documented in the 1996 edition of the Dartmouth Atlas of Health Care (data for 1992-93) are demonstrated in this section to have persisted through 1994-95, although the health care industry was undergoing a period of profound change. The numbers of acute care hospital beds, intensive care hospital beds, hospital employees, and registered nurses employed by hospitals varied substantially among regions, and in many cases within states. Generally the supply of hospital resources was higher in the East, South, and Midwest than in the West and on the West Coast; but the idiosyncratic nature of the distribution of resources remained a constant attribute of the American health care system.

Data from the American Hospital Association and the Medicare Program were used to estimate the numbers of staffed acute care hospital beds, full time equivalent hospital employees, and registered nurses employed in acute care hospitals allocated to care for the population of each region.

Acute Care Hospital Beds

There were more than 779,000 acute care hospital beds in the United States in 1995, an average of 3.0 beds per thousand residents. In 1993, there were more than 827,000 acute care hospital beds, an average of 3.3 per thousand residents. Reduction in hospital bed capacity per thousand residents was observed in hospital referral regions with both high and low rates of allocated beds. The supply of beds in the Bronx, New York, for example, fell from 4.9 per thousand to 4.8; but the supply in San Jose, California, fell from 2.1 in 1993 to 1.7 in 1995, an even larger decrease. The numbers of hospital beds per thousand residents of hospital referral regions in 1995, after adjusting for differences in age and sex, varied by a factor of about 3, from fewer than 1.6 to 5.0 per thousand residents.

Among the hospital referral regions with large populations, those with the highest numbers of hospital beds per thousand residents included the Bronx, New York (4.8); Newark, New Jersey (4.7); Jackson, Mississippi (4.6); and Chicago (4.4).

Regions with more than one million residents that had comparatively low numbers of hospital beds per thousand residents were San Jose, California (1.7); Seattle, Washington (1.8); Austin, Texas (1.8); Portland, Oregon (1.9); and Sacramento, California (1.9).

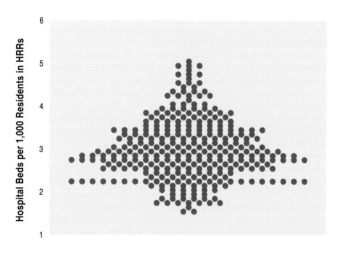

Figure 2.1. Acute Care Hospital Beds Allocated to Hospital Referral Regions (1995)

The number of hospital beds per thousand residents, after adjusting for differences in the age and sex of the local population, ranged from fewer than 1.6 to more than 5.0. Each point represents one of the 306 hospital referral regions in the United States.

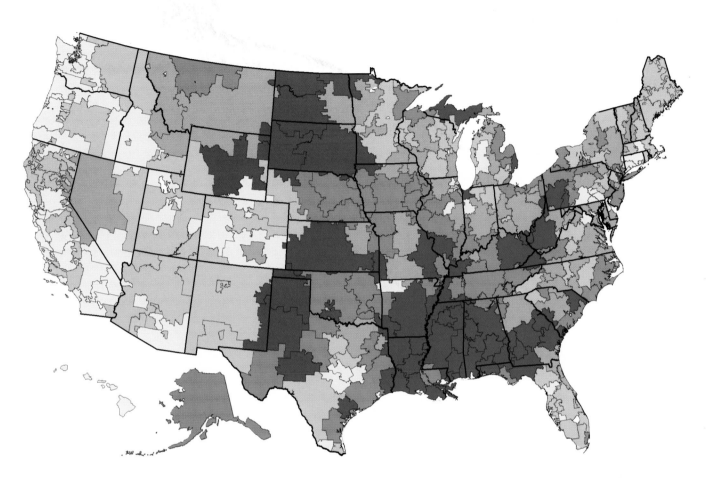

Map 2.1. Acute Care Hospital Beds

The Great Plains states, the Midwest, parts of Texas and much of the South had higher supplies of hospital beds than most states in the West, on the West Coast, or in the Northeast.

Acute Care Hospital Beds per 1,000 Residents
by Hospital Referral Region (1995)

- 3.55 to 5.05 (62)
- 3.08 to <3.55 (63)
- 2.78 to <3.08 (55)
- 2.38 to <2.78 (64)
- 1.58 to <2.38 (62)
- Not Populated

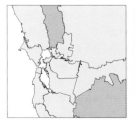

San Francisco

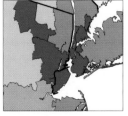

Chicago

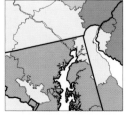

New York

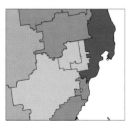

Washington-Baltimore

Detroit

Acute Care Hospital Employees

There were more than 3.58 million workers employed in acute care hospitals in the United States in 1995. This represented a slight increase from the 3.56 million hospital employees in 1993, in spite of the fact that the number of acute care beds declined in the same period. The numbers of full time equivalent hospital employees per thousand residents, after adjusting for differences in population age and sex, varied by a factor of about 4.0, from fewer than 7.5 to almost 28.

Among large hospital referral regions, the numbers of full-time equivalent hospital employees allocated to local populations were exceptionally high in the Bronx, New York (27.6); Chicago (21.8); Manhattan (21.6); New Orleans (21.3); and Newark, New Jersey (19.6).

The number of full-time equivalent hospital employees allocated to the residents of the San Diego hospital referral region (8.1) was less than one-third the number allocated to residents of the Bronx. Other large hospital referral regions with relatively low numbers of allocated full-time equivalent hospital employees were Arlington, Virginia (8.2); Austin, Texas (8.4); Orange County, California (8.7); and San Jose, California (8.7).

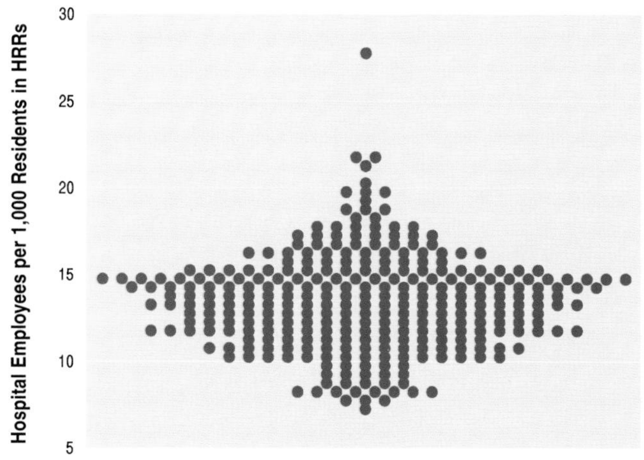

Figure 2.2. Hospital Employees Allocated to Hospital Referral Regions (1995)

The number of full time equivalent hospital employees per thousand residents, after adjusting for differences in the age and sex of the local population, ranged from fewer than 7.5 to more than 27. Each point represents one of the 306 hospital referral regions in the United States.

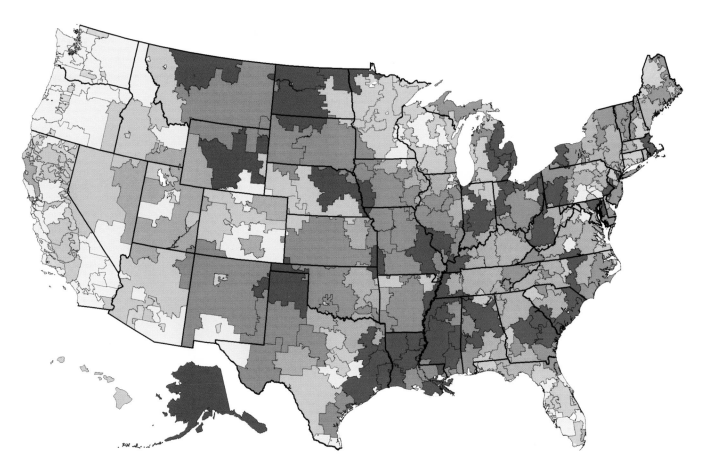

Map 2.2. Acute Care Hospital Employees

There were relatively large supplies of hospital employees per thousand residents in parts of the Great Plains and Mountain states, the Midwest, the South, and parts of Texas; some areas in the Southeast and Northeast also had large workforces devoted to acute care. The West Coast and the Western states generally had smaller per capita workforces than other areas of the country.

**Hospital Employees
per 1,000 Residents**

by Hospital Referral Region (1995)

■	15.43 to 27.64 (60)
■	14.14 to <15.43 (61)
■	12.72 to <14.14 (62)
□	11.14 to <12.72 (60)
□	7.26 to <11.14 (63)
■	Not Populated

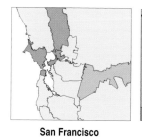

San Francisco

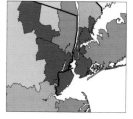

Chicago

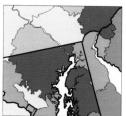

New York

Washington-Baltimore

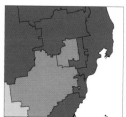

Detroit

Registered Nurses Employed in Acute Care Hospitals

There were more than 882,000 full time equivalent registered nurses employed in acute care hospitals in the United States in 1995. The numbers of hospital-based registered nurses per thousand residents, after adjusting for differences in age and sex of the local populations, varied by a factor of 2.7, from 1.9 per thousand allocated to residents of the Austin, Texas hospital referral region, to 5.1 per thousand allocated to residents of the hospital referral region in the Bronx, New York.

Large hospital referral regions with relatively high numbers of registered nurses employed by acute care hospitals included, in addition to the Bronx, Chicago (5.1); New Orleans (4.8); Detroit (4.7); Manhattan (4.7); Newark, New Jersey (4.5); Toledo, Ohio (4.4); and Dayton, Ohio (4.3).

Among large hospital referral regions with lower numbers of hospital-based registered nurses allocated to the population of the hospital referral regions were, in addition to Austin, Contra Costa County, California (2.1); Arlington, Virginia (2.2); San Jose, California (2.3); and Orange County, California (2.4).

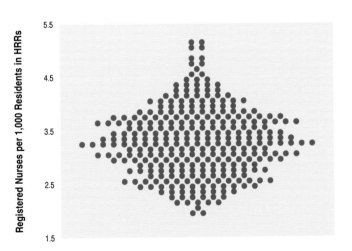

Figure 2.3. Hospital-Based Registered Nurses Allocated to Hospital Referral Regions (1995)

The acute care hospital-employed registered nurse workforce varied from 1.9 per thousand residents to 5.1. Each point represents one of the 306 hospital referral regions in the United States.

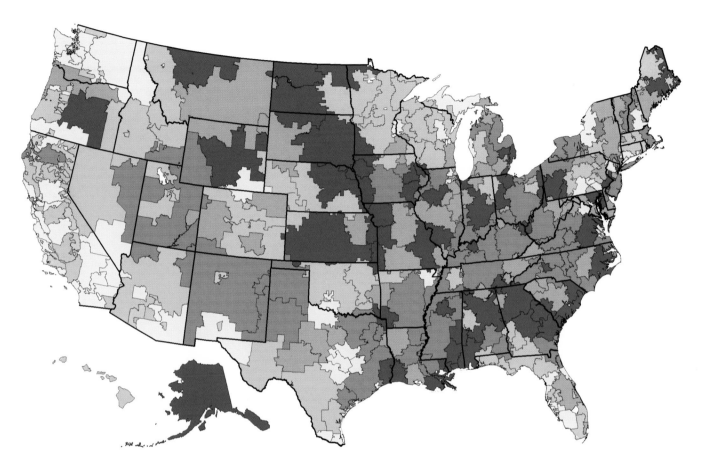

Map 2.3. Registered Nurses Employed in Acute Care Hospitals

The distribution of the registered nurse workforce resembled that of acute care hospital employees, with some exceptions, including central Oregon, parts of Maine, and some parts of Nevada. The West Coast generally had lower numbers of registered nurses per thousand residents than other areas of the country.

**Registered Nurses
per 1,000 Residents**
by Hospital Referral Region (1995)

■	3.80 to 5.13 (61)
■	3.44 to <3.80 (61)
■	3.13 to <3.44 (59)
■	2.75 to <3.13 (63)
□	1.92 to <2.75 (62)
■	Not Populated

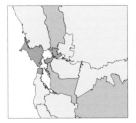

San Francisco

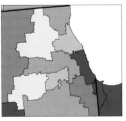

Chicago

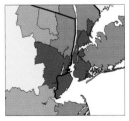

New York

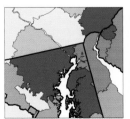

Washington-Baltimore

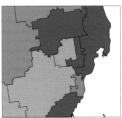

Detroit

Medicare Spending

In 1995, most Americans over the age of 65 were enrolled in the Medicare program. Most received their care from "traditional" Medicare — that is, from providers who charged on a fee-for-service basis, either as independent practitioners or as members of health maintenance organizations that were not capitated. In 1995, according to HCFA records, $163.1 billion — over 92.5% of Medicare outlays for people over 65 — was reimbursed on a fee-for-service basis.

There were large differences in these reimbursements between hospital referral regions. Total program outlays per capita varied by a factor of about 3.0, even after adjusting for differences in prices among regions. Price adjusted reimbursements for acute hospital care varied more than 2.5-fold, professional and laboratory services by more than 4.7-fold, and home health services by a factor of more than 30.0. The uneven distribution of reimbursements raises the question of whether areas with lower levels of acute care hospital services might have been achieving their inpatient savings by substituting outpatient care, hospice care, or home health services. However, research shows very little evidence of substitution; the opposite is often the case. Regions with higher reimbursements for acute care hospital services tended also to have higher reimbursements for hospital-based outpatient care, as well as higher reimbursements for physician services and for home health services (see endnote).

Estimates of Medicare reimbursements are based on a 5% sample of the Medicare population as recorded in the Continuous Medicare History File. Fee-for-service reimbursements have been price adjusted to take into account differences in the cost of living among hospital referral regions.

Medicare Reimbursements for Noncapitated Medicare

In 1995, Medicare payments for Americans enrolled in both Medicare parts A and B over the age of 65 for services reimbursed on a fee-for-service basis (including non-risk bearing health maintenance organizations) amounted to about $163.6 billion. The average per enrollee reimbursement for those enrolled in both the Part A and Part B programs was $4,790. This represented a 22% increase over 1993 payments of $115.9 billion ($3,929 per enrollee). Price adjusted per enrollee reimbursements varied remarkably among hospital referral regions. The rate in the region with the highest rate of Medicare reimbursement was more than 2.9 times higher than the rate in the region with the lowest rate of reimbursements.

Among the hospital referral regions with the highest per capita Medicare reimbursements for all services were Miami ($7,955); New Orleans ($7,205); San Antonio, Texas ($6,434); Houston ($6,216); Nashville, Tennessee ($6,000); and Los Angeles ($5,900).

Among the large hospital referral regions with lower price adjusted Medicare reimbursements per capita were Honolulu ($3,332); Minneapolis ($3,528); Portland, Oregon ($3,680); Madison, Wisconsin ($3,812); and Arlington, Virginia ($3,871).

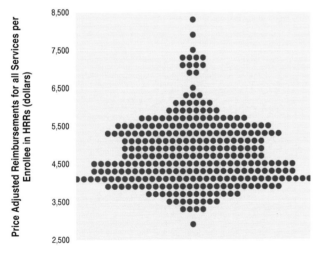

Figure 2.4. Price Adjusted Reimbursements for Noncapitated Medicare Among Hospital Referral Regions (1995)

Per enrollee reimbursements by the Medicare program for all services varied by a factor of 2.8, from less than $3,000 to more than $8,300. Each point represents one of the 306 hospital referral regions in the United States.

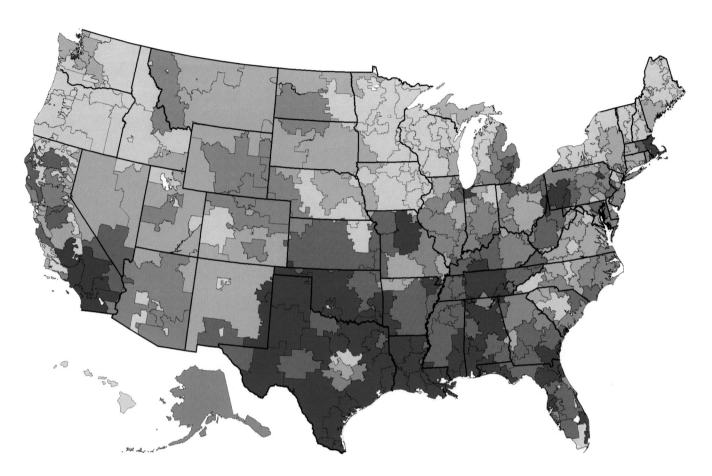

Map 2.4. Price Adjusted Reimbursements for Noncapitated Medicare

Total Medicare reimbursements were higher in the South, most of Texas, parts of the Midwest, Florida, and Southern California than in most of the Northeast, the Great Plains, and the Northwest.

Total Medicare Reimbursements per Medicare Enrollee
by Hospital Referral Region (1995)

- $5465 to 8385 (61)
- 4923 to < 5465 (60)
- 4451 to < 4923 (61)
- 4053 to < 4451 (62)
- 2928 to < 4053 (62)
- Not Populated

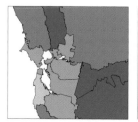

San Francisco

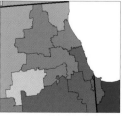

Chicago

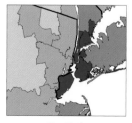

New York

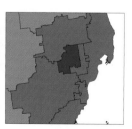

Washington-Baltimore

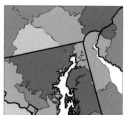

Detroit

Medicare Reimbursements for Inpatient Hospital Services

In 1995, Medicare reimbursements to hospitals for acute, short-stay care for Americans over age 65 whose care was paid for on a fee-for-service basis totaled $77.7 billion. The average per enrollee reimbursement for those enrolled in both Part A and Part B programs was $2,279, an increase of about 13% from 1993. These payments represented 47.5% of the Medicare program's total outlays for traditional Medicare. Price adjusted reimbursements to hospitals per Medicare enrollee were more than 2.5 times higher in the highest rate hospital referral region than in the lowest rate region.

Among the large hospital referral regions with the highest rates of per enrollee reimbursements for acute hospital care were Manhattan ($3,318); the Bronx, New York ($3,289); and New Orleans ($3,178). Other areas where per enrollee reimbursements for hospital care were high included Miami ($3,056); Chicago ($3,010); Houston ($2,894); Baltimore ($2,829); and Pittsburgh ($2,785).

Other large metropolitan hospital referral regions had relatively low per enrollee payments for acute hospital care; they included Honolulu ($1,656); Austin, Texas ($1,711); Fresno, California ($1,740); Salt Lake City, Utah ($1,747); and Portland, Oregon ($1,802).

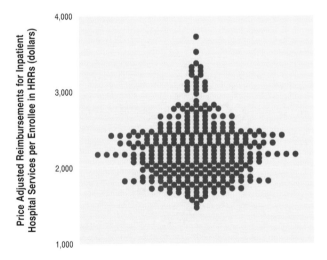

Figure 2.5. Price Adjusted Medicare Reimbursements for Inpatient Hospital Services Among Hospital Referral Regions (1995)

Per enrollee Medicare reimbursements for acute care hospital services varied by a factor of more than 2.5, from less than $1,500 to more than $3,700. Each point represents one of the 306 hospital referral regions in the United States.

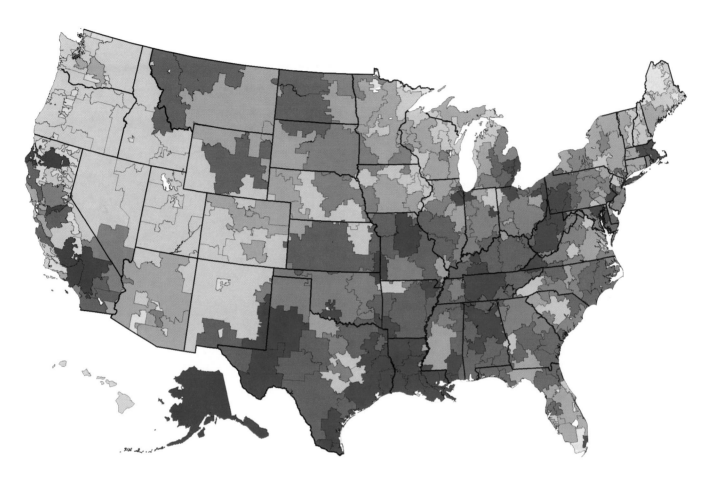

Map 2.5. Price Adjusted Medicare Reimbursements for Inpatient Hospital Services

Medicare reimbursements for inpatient hospital services were generally lower in the Western states, parts of the Great Lakes states, and parts of the Northeast than in the Midwest, South, Texas and California. Medicare spending for inpatient services varied widely even in contiguous areas, such as Western Texas and Eastern New Mexico.

Inpatient Hospital Services per Medicare Enrollee
by Hospital Referral Region (1995)

- $2516 to 3723 (61)
- 2321 to < 2516 (60)
- 2117 to < 2321 (61)
- 1893 to < 2117 (62)
- 1483 to < 1893 (62)
- Not Populated

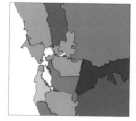

San Francisco

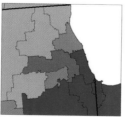

Chicago

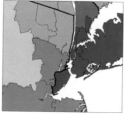

New York

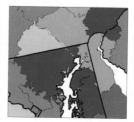

Washington-Baltimore

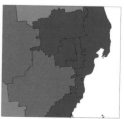

Detroit

Medicare Reimbursements for Professional and Laboratory Services

Professional services reimbursements include payments to surgeons and medical doctors for activities such as office consultations, vaccinations, and open heart surgery. Among the more common laboratory services are biopsy evaluations and blood tests. In 1995, reimbursements for professional and laboratory services for Americans over age 65 paid for on a fee-for-service basis totaled $33.2 billion. The average per enrollee reimbursement for those enrolled in both the Part A and Part B programs was $1,002, an increase of about 20% from 1993. These payments represented 20.3% of Medicare outlays for traditional Medicare.

With price adjusted reimbursements for professional and laboratory services of $2,141 per enrollee, Miami had the highest rate in the United States. Los Angeles ($1,488) was substantially lower than Miami, but was still more than 3.2 times higher than the lowest-rate region. Other regions with high per enrollee reimbursements included Orange County, California ($1,414); Takoma Park, Maryland ($1,345); Manhattan ($1,326); and Las Vegas, Nevada ($1,298).

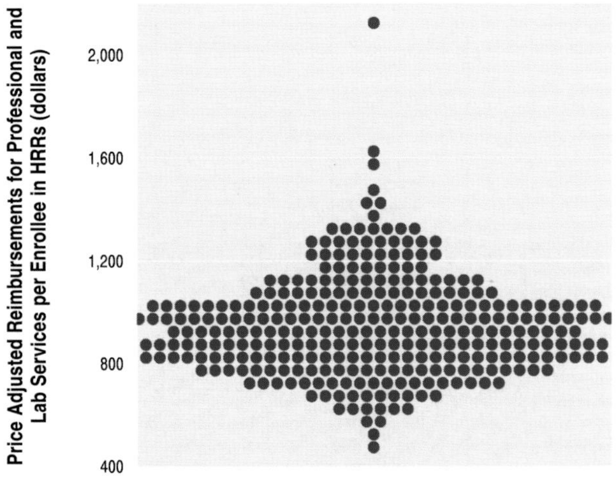

Among the large hospital referral regions with relatively low per capita reimbursements for professional and laboratory services were Minneapolis ($618); St. Paul, Minnesota ($623); Salt Lake City ($658); Portland, Oregon ($680); and Rochester, New York ($747).

Figure 2.6. Price Adjusted Part B Medicare Reimbursements for Professional and Laboratory Services Among Hospital Referral Regions (1995)
Reimbursements for professional and laboratory services varied by a factor of more than 4.7, from $454 per Medicare enrollee to $2,141. Each point represents one of the 306 hospital referral regions in the United States.

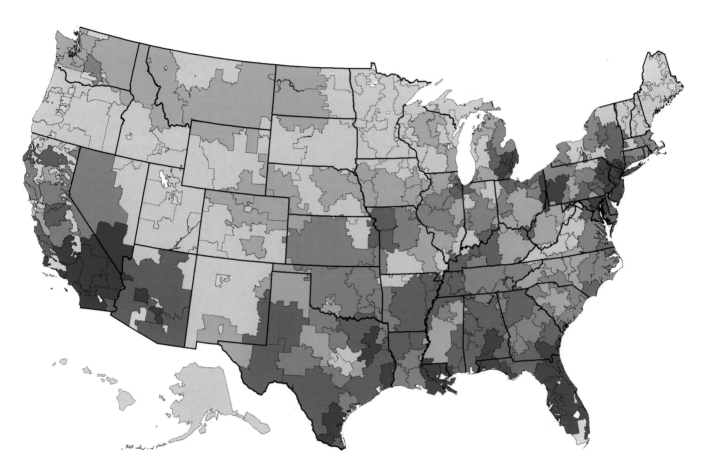

Map 2.6. Price Adjusted Medicare Reimbursements for Professional and Laboratory Services

Reimbursements for fee-for-service professional and laboratory services were highest in the South and on the West Coast; parts of the Midwest and most of Florida and the Middle Atlantic States also had high reimbursements. Some areas, including Texas and Missouri, had wide variations among hospital referral regions within the state.

Professional and Laboratory Services per Medicare Enrollee
by Hospital Referral Region (1995)

- $1081 to   2141 (63)
- 975 to < 1081 (59)
- 877 to < 975 (62)
- 794 to < 877 (57)
- 454 to < 794 (65)
- Not Populated

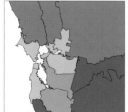

San Francisco

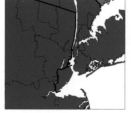

Chicago

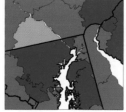

New York

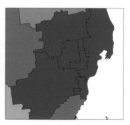

Washington-Baltimore

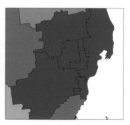

Detroit

Medicare Reimbursements for Outpatient Services

In 1995, Medicare reimbursements for the use of outpatient services paid for on a fee-for-service basis totaled $15.2 billion. The average per enrollee reimbursement for those enrolled in both the Part A and Part B programs was $396, an increase of about 13% from 1993. These reimbursements represented 15.8% of total outlays for traditional Medicare.

Price adjusted reimbursements varied by a factor of 3 between the lowest rate hospital referral region and the highest rate region. Among the hospital referral regions with the highest rates of price adjusted Medicare reimbursements for outpatient services per enrollee were Miami ($583); Wichita, Kansas ($541); Ann Arbor, Michigan ($540); Baltimore, Maryland ($513); and Albuquerque, New Mexico ($509).

Among the hospital referral regions with relatively low per enrollee rates of reimbursement for outpatient services in 1995 were Las Vegas, Nevada ($219); New Brunswick, New Jersey ($236); Mesa, Arizona ($255); Newark, New Jersey ($281); San Jose, California ($283); White Plains, New York ($285); Richmond, Virginia ($316); and Albany, New York ($320).

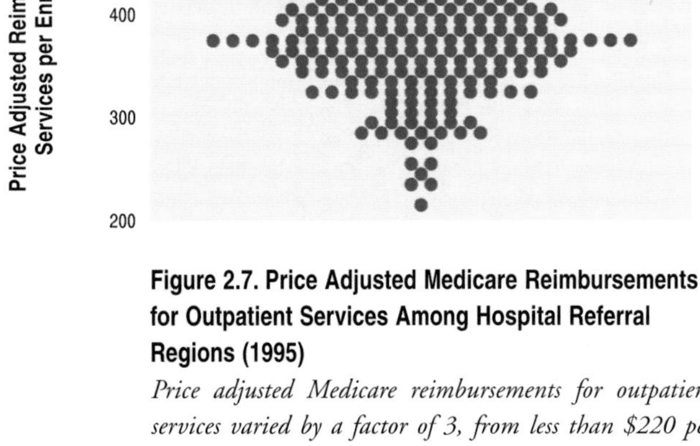

Figure 2.7. Price Adjusted Medicare Reimbursements for Outpatient Services Among Hospital Referral Regions (1995)

Price adjusted Medicare reimbursements for outpatient services varied by a factor of 3, from less than $220 per enrollee to more than $670. Each point represents one of the 306 hospital referral regions in the United States.

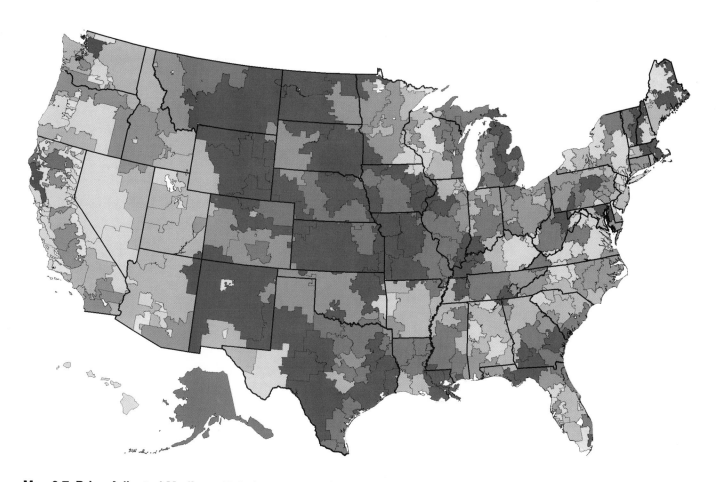

Map 2.7. Price Adjusted Medicare Reimbursements for Outpatient Services

Medicare reimbursements for outpatient services were sharply higher in the Midwest, the Mountain states, the Great Plains states, and the Southwest than in the Northeast, Southeast, and West. There were wide differences in reimbursements in some contiguous areas of the Northeast and in the Great Lakes states.

Outpatient Services per Medicare Enrollee
by Hospital Referral Region (1995)

- $480 to   674 (61)
- 431 to < 480 (61)
- 389 to < 431 (59)
- 351 to < 389 (63)
- 218 to < 351 (62)
- Not Populated

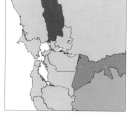

San Francisco

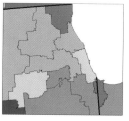

Chicago

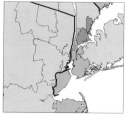

New York

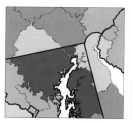

Washington-Baltimore

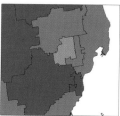

Detroit

Medicare Reimbursements for Home Health Services

In 1995, Medicare reimbursements for home health care services for enrollees over age 65 paid for on a fee-for-service basis totaled $15.6 billion. The average per enrollee reimbursement for those enrolled in both the Part A and Part B programs was $495. These reimbursements represented 9.5% of noncapitated Medicare program outlays. Variations in the levels of Medicare reimbursements for home health care services were extreme. The highest price adjusted reimbursement rate per Medicare enrollee was almost 30 times higher than reimbursements in the region with the lowest rate. In general, the rate of reimbursements for home health services grew substantially between 1993 and 1995.

The per capita reimbursement for Medicare enrollees in the Chattanooga, Tennessee hospital referral region in 1993 was 25% higher than the next highest region. By 1995, although Chattanooga's rate ($1,522) was 18% higher than in 1993, Chattanooga's rate was no longer the highest in the country. Per capita reimbursements were higher in Baton Rouge, Louisiana ($1,948) and several other areas in the South. Other hospital referral regions with high reimbursement rates for home health care included New Orleans ($1,320); Nashville, Tennessee ($1,258); and Knoxville, Tennessee ($1,181).

Among the hospital referral regions with the lowest per capita rates of reimbursement were Sioux Falls, South Dakota ($159); Minneapolis ($169); and Milwaukee, Wisconsin ($175).

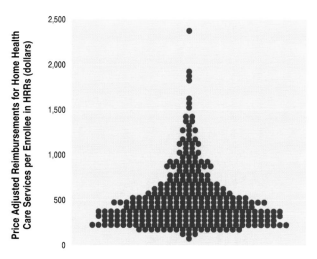

Figure 2.8. Price Adjusted Medicare Reimbursements for Home Health Care Services Among Hospital Referral Regions (1995)

Price adjusted Medicare reimbursements for home health care services varied by a factor of almost 30, from $83 per enrollee to almost $2,400. Each point represents one of the 306 hospital referral regions in the United States.

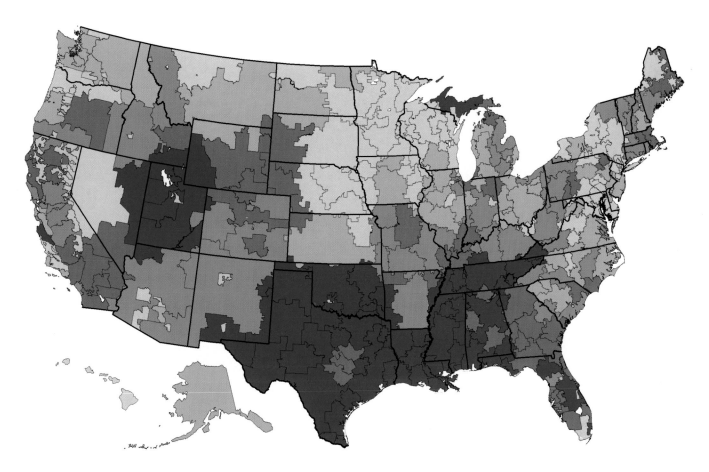

Map 2.8. Price Adjusted Medicare Reimbursements for Home Health Care Services

Per-enrollee reimbursements for home health services were far higher in the South than in the Great Plains and in most of the East. Texas, Louisiana, Mississippi, Alabama, and Tennessee, as well as most of Florida, were almost uniformly in the highest quintile of reimbursements for home health.

Home Health Services per Medicare Enrollee
by Hospital Referral Region (1995)

- $737 to 2381 (61)
- 498 to < 737 (60)
- 375 to < 498 (62)
- 268 to < 375 (61)
- 83 to < 268 (62)
- Not Populated

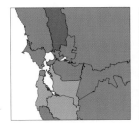

San Francisco

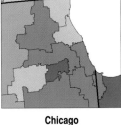

Chicago

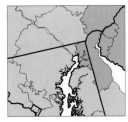

New York

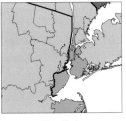

Washington-Baltimore

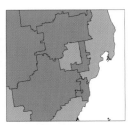

Detroit

The Physician Workforce

This section examines the physician workforce in the nation's 306 hospital referral regions. The data come from the American Medical Association, the American Osteopathic Association, and the Medicare program, and are for 1996. A clinically active physician is defined as one who reported that he or she spent at least 20 hours a week in patient care. The population count is the Claritas® estimate for 1995.

The estimates of the number of physicians allocated to populations per 100,000 residents take into account patient migration across the boundaries of the regions, using a method similar to that used for hospital beds. For example, medical specialists and primary care physicians were allocated on the basis of medical admissions.

The estimates have been adjusted for differences in the age and sex of the population. (See the Appendix on Methods.)

The Physician Workforce Active in Patient Care

In 1970, there were 235,241 physicians active in patient care in the United States. By 1993, the number had increased to 469,603, an increase that was largely attributable to growth in medical schools, an increase in class sizes, and policies that encouraged international medical graduates to enter the professional workforce in the United States. In 1996, there were 495,510 physicians in active practice, an increase of 5.5% from 1993.

The distribution of the physician workforce did not change in any dramatic way between 1993 and 1996; there was some growth in the number of physicians per hundred thousand residents of parts of the Western and Mountain states, but for the most part the workforce remained concentrated in urban areas.

Among the hospital referral regions with the highest total numbers of active physicians per hundred thousand residents in 1996 were White Plains, New York (333.5); Hackensack, New Jersey (299.6); Royal Oak, Michigan (288.5); San Francisco (282.2); and Takoma Park, Maryland (277.8). Some regions of the United States had fewer than half as many physicians per hundred thousand residents; the McAllen, Texas hospital referral region had the lowest supply (88.2). Other regions with fewer than average physicians per hundred thousand residents included Provo, Utah (131.5); San Bernardino, California (144.7); Wichita, Kansas (147.5); and Dayton, Ohio (147.7).

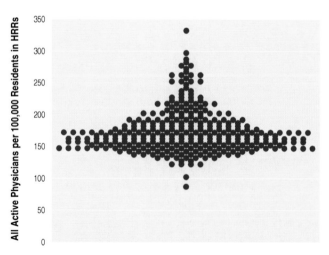

Figure 2.9. Physicians Allocated to Hospital Referral Regions (1996)

The number of physicians in active practice per hundred thousand residents, after adjusting for differences in age and sex of the local population, ranged from fewer than 90 to more than 330. Each point represents one of the 306 hospital referral regions in the United States.

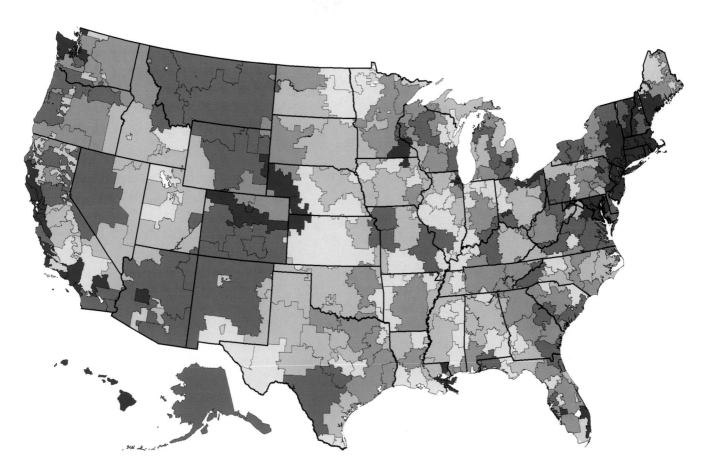

Map 2.9. The Physician Workforce

In 1996, there were higher than average numbers of physicians per hundred thousand residents of the East and West Coasts, parts of the Mountain and Southwestern States, and in the Pacific Northwest. Some regions with very high supplies of physicians were contiguous with areas that had much lower supplies, as in Nebraska, New Mexico, and Idaho.

Physician Workforce Active in Patient Care per 100,000 Residents
by Hospital Referral Region (1995)

- 195.6 to 333.5 (60)
- 174.1 to <195.6 (62)
- 161.2 to <174.1 (61)
- 148.6 to <161.2 (61)
- 88.1 to <148.6 (62)
- Not Populated

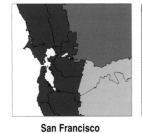

San Francisco

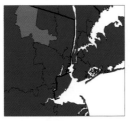

Chicago

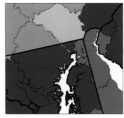

New York

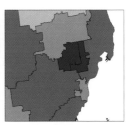

Washington-Baltimore

Detroit

Physicians in Primary Care

The number of active physicians in primary care practice increased by 62% between 1970 and 1993, and by 3.9% between 1993 and 1996. The proportion of physicians who were in primary care, 35% of the workforce, did not change between 1993 and 1996. Among hospital referral regions, the supply of physicians clinically active in primary care in 1966 varied from 33.8 in McAllen, Texas, to 105.1 in White Plains, New York; the national average among hospital referral regions was 65.0 per hundred thousand residents.

Among hospital referral regions with the highest number of primary care physicians per hundred thousand residents were Royal Oak, Michigan (102.9); San Francisco (102.1); Hackensack, New Jersey (99.9); Evanston, Illinois (98.1); Philadelphia (89.4); and Napa, California (89.0).

Few hospital referral regions with large populations had lower than average supplies of physicians in primary care; the exceptions included El Paso, Texas (41.6); Las Vegas, Nevada (47.4); Shreveport, Louisiana (47.9); Fort Wayne, Indiana (48.2); and Salt Lake City (48.3).

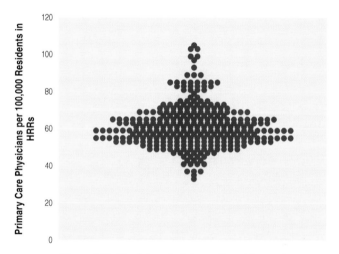

Figure 2.10. Physicians in Primary Care Allocated to Hospital Referral Regions in the United States (1996)

The number of primary care physicians in active practice per hundred thousand residents, after adjusting for differences in age and sex of the local population, ranged from fewer than 34 to more than 105. Each point represents one of the 306 hospital referral regions in the United States.

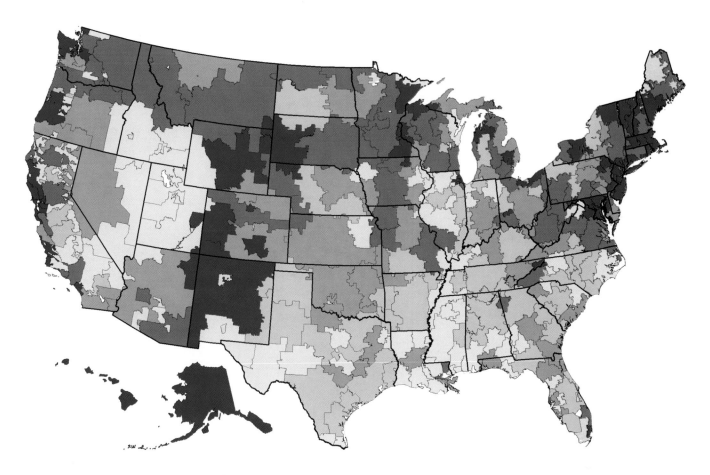

Map 2.10. Physicians in Primary Care

In 1996, the numbers of primary care physicians per hundred thousand residents were greatest in the Northeast, the Mountain States, the Pacific Northwest, northern California, Alaska and Hawaii. There were relatively few primary care physicians in the Southeastern United States, Texas, southern Idaho, western Wyoming, Utah, and eastern Nevada.

Primary Care Physicians per 100,000 Residents
by Hospital Referral Region (1995)

- 69.2 to 105.1 (61)
- 63.0 to <69.2 (60)
- 57.9 to <63.0 (63)
- 53.2 to <57.9 (59)
- 33.7 to <53.2 (63)
- Not Populated

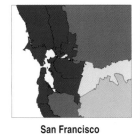
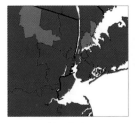
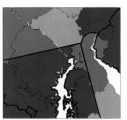
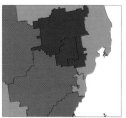

San Francisco   **Chicago**   **New York**   **Washington-Baltimore**   **Detroit**

Specialist Physicians

In 1970, there were 130,784 clinically active physicians who were identified as specialists; by 1993 the number had increased to 302,511, representing about 65% of the physician workforce. Between 1993 and 1996, the number of specialists (medical and surgical) increased 6.6%, in spite of growing efforts to encourage medical graduates to enter primary care. The population ratio increased by about 1%, from 121.7 specialists per hundred thousand in 1993 to 122.9 in 1996.

Among the areas with the highest numbers of specialists per hundred thousand residents were White Plains, New York (227.0); Hackensack, New Jersey (198.3); Royal Oak, Michigan (185.2); Takoma Park, Maryland (184.7); Washington, D.C. (182.7); and Metairie, Louisiana (181.8). The per capita number of specialists serving the population of White Plains was about 85% higher than the national average of 122.9.

The number of specialists allocated to the McAllen, Texas hospital referral region (53.3) actually declined slightly between 1993 and 1996. Other areas with lower than average numbers of specialists included Fort Wayne, Indiana (82.4); Wichita, Kansas (84.9); Springfield, Illinois (87.3); and Springfield, Missouri (87.6).

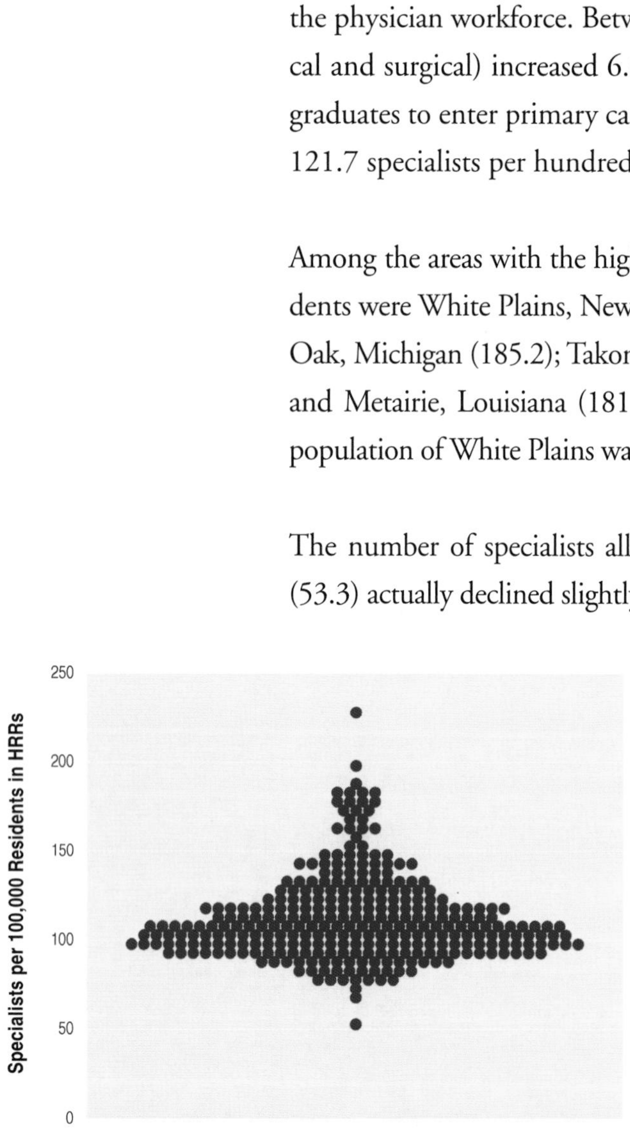

Figure 2.11. Specialist Physicians Allocated to Hospital Referral Regions (1996)

The number of specialist physicians per hundred thousand residents, after adjusting for differences in age and sex of the local population, ranged from about 50 to more than 225. Each point represents one of the 306 hospital referral regions in the United States.

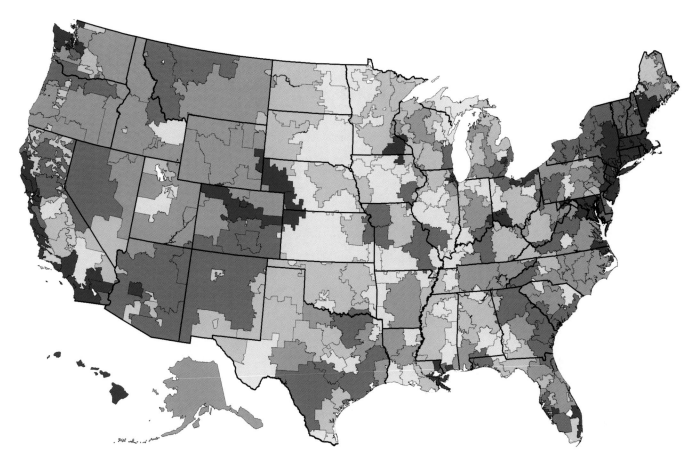

Map 2.11. Specialist Physicians

In 1996, the supply of specialists per hundred thousand residents was highest on the East and West Coasts and lowest in the Midwest, the East South Central States, and the Upper Midwest. The Northeast and California also had very high supplies of specialists.

Specialist Physicians per 100,000 Residents

by Hospital Referral Region (1995)

■	126.7 to 227.0 (62)
■	112.5 to <126.7 (59)
■	102.7 to <112.5 (62)
■	94.5 to <102.7 (59)
□	53.2 to <94.5 (64)
■	Not Populated

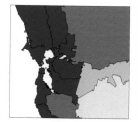

San Francisco

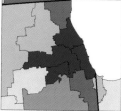

Chicago

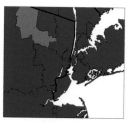

New York

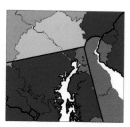

Washington-Baltimore

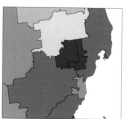

Detroit

Chapter Two Table   All measures of allocated hospital resources are expressed in rates per thousand residents. Reimbursements are expressed in rates per person, and are adjusted for regional differences in prices and race. The physician supply is expressed in rates per hundred thousand residents. All rates are adjusted for differences in the age and sex composition of the population. Estimates of allocated hospital employees and registered nurses are expressed as full time equivalents (FTEs). Medicare data exclude enrollees who were members of risk bearing health maintenance organizations.

See the Appendix on Methods for details on the methods used for allocating resources, estimating populations and adjusting rates, and for other details concerning the rates in these tables.

CHAPTER TWO TABLE

Acute Care Hospital Resources (1995), Price Adjusted Medicare Reimbursements (1995) and The Physician Workforce Allocated to Hospital Referral Regions (1996)

Hospital Referral Region	Medicare Enrollees (1995)	Total Population (1995)	Acute Care Beds	Hospital Employees	Hospital-based Registered Nurses	Price Adjusted Reimbursements for Non-Capitated Medicare	Price Adjusted Reimbursements for Inpatient Hospital Services	Price Adjusted Reimbursements for Professional and Lab. Services	Price Adjusted Reimbursements for Outpatient Services	Price Adjusted Reimbursements for Home Health Services	All Physicians	Physicians in Primary Care	Specialist Physicians
Alabama													
Birmingham	264,920	2,067,166	4.2	16.1	4.3	5,650	2,765	1,051	387	769	157.5	54.9	101.8
Dothan	44,420	341,377	3.8	14.1	3.6	5,390	2,342	1,016	388	901	145.6	53.0	91.6
Huntsville	51,660	512,335	3.3	12.6	3.4	4,842	2,326	927	338	635	145.2	54.3	90.0
Mobile	80,880	735,828	3.8	14.8	3.9	5,606	2,449	1,018	394	1,061	164.1	51.3	111.8
Montgomery	46,840	420,205	3.6	12.9	3.5	5,153	2,349	1,109	248	658	142.7	49.6	92.3
Tuscaloosa	27,660	233,184	3.6	14.8	2.9	5,103	2,455	1,005	322	730	156.4	56.6	98.7
Alaska													
Anchorage	26,620	615,424	3.2	16.9	4.1	4,739	2,802	763	442	321	186.9	73.0	112.2
Arizona													
Mesa	51,640	759,053	1.7	8.0	2.3	4,717	2,159	1,117	255	313	151.2	53.0	97.2
Phoenix	178,580	2,230,182	2.4	11.4	2.8	4,763	2,044	1,056	377	429	177.9	59.5	117.5
Sun City	45,580	162,537	2.1	7.9	2.1	3,950	1,663	1,254	256	207	201.0	64.3	135.7
Tucson	72,620	935,802	2.1	10.3	2.5	4,856	2,068	983	426	381	179.9	63.3	115.7
Arkansas													
Fort Smith	44,660	316,211	3.5	13.1	3.2	6,026	2,417	955	338	1,441	145.9	57.7	86.9
Jonesboro	29,360	207,464	3.4	11.5	2.6	5,766	2,805	1,007	466	536	133.3	53.9	78.7
Little Rock	189,560	1,378,605	3.7	14.9	3.6	5,137	2,430	976	372	492	163.9	57.7	105.2
Springdale	45,460	344,873	2.3	12.3	2.9	4,328	1,835	786	371	502	146.0	58.4	86.5
Texarkana	33,960	251,418	4.4	15.0	3.9	6,143	2,686	916	425	984	137.7	53.4	83.3
California													
Orange Co.	127,960	2,732,562	2.3	8.7	2.4	5,564	2,288	1,414	355	439	211.8	73.1	137.9
Bakersfield	58,280	841,548	2.3	11.8	2.9	5,826	2,531	1,290	395	544	145.9	49.5	95.5
Chico	33,920	263,211	2.4	12.6	2.8	4,452	1,879	866	408	553	171.9	55.3	115.6
Contra Costa Co.	56,760	862,123	1.7	8.1	2.1	4,204	2,005	774	318	384	214.9	69.2	144.6
Fresno	75,840	974,617	2.1	11.8	2.7	4,164	1,740	953	420	379	152.4	54.6	96.7
Los Angeles	448,600	9,230,785	2.7	11.1	2.8	5,900	2,678	1,488	369	502	197.6	64.9	131.9
Modesto	56,760	717,600	2.5	10.7	3.0	5,209	2,327	1,038	367	472	148.9	54.3	93.5
Napa	35,220	250,705	2.6	13.3	2.9	5,365	2,435	943	526	579	243.9	89.0	154.2
Alameda Co.	93,540	1,348,508	2.1	10.8	3.0	4,444	2,311	827	290	314	223.9	82.2	141.1
Palm Spr/Rancho Mir	28,960	248,351	2.2	9.1	2.3	5,982	2,343	1,550	392	608	197.5	55.5	141.0
Redding	42,160	314,477	2.4	11.7	3.5	5,142	2,550	1,045	447	500	185.8	68.4	116.4
Sacramento	168,680	1,987,776	1.9	9.5	2.4	4,523	2,167	901	318	437	184.2	64.9	118.3
Salinas	30,820	337,282	1.9	10.6	2.5	5,263	2,396	1,008	343	751	192.5	60.4	131.4
San Bernardino	83,660	2,306,438	2.2	9.1	2.7	5,868	2,580	1,228	353	568	144.7	49.8	93.9
San Diego	156,340	3,006,551	1.9	8.1	2.4	5,685	2,452	1,225	396	616	194.1	61.1	132.1
San Francisco	104,260	1,323,898	2.3	13.7	3.2	4,085	2,023	756	329	389	282.2	102.1	180.0
San Jose	86,520	1,525,072	1.7	8.7	2.3	4,140	2,041	826	283	303	196.2	69.2	126.1
San Luis Obispo	21,260	213,259	2.1	7.3	2.4	3,919	1,838	1,049	296	165	227.7	77.6	149.3
San Mateo Co.	54,680	761,040	1.9	10.7	2.3	3,603	1,830	737	295	314	234.7	72.3	161.2
Santa Barbara	30,360	393,410	1.8	7.6	2.0	4,130	1,780	1,131	301	271	215.2	73.3	140.9

Hospital Referral Region	Medicare Enrollees (1995)	Total Population (1995)	Acute Care Beds	Hospital Employees	Hospital-based Registered Nurses	Price Adjusted Reimbursements for Non-Capitated Medicare	Price Adjusted Reimbursements for Inpatient Hospital Services	Price Adjusted Reimbursements for Professional and Lab. Services	Price Adjusted Reimbursements for Outpatient Services	Price Adjusted Reimbursements for Home Health Services	All Physicians	Physicians in Primary Care	Specialist Physicians
Santa Cruz	21,400	245,459	1.7	7.7	2.0	4,472	2,131	1,042	237	476	223.6	73.9	149.0
Santa Rosa	37,800	419,080	1.8	8.4	2.3	4,461	1,907	890	271	480	228.2	84.1	143.0
Stockton	36,180	452,439	2.3	11.7	2.7	5,264	2,584	1,019	429	394	149.8	50.3	98.8
Ventura	41,920	744,436	2.0	9.0	2.5	4,735	1,966	1,288	373	364	203.5	68.4	134.2
Colorado													
Boulder	14,220	238,607	1.6	10.1	2.8	4,408	1,946	722	372	475	231.8	85.0	145.7
Colorado Springs	57,580	643,355	2.3	11.0	3.0	4,074	1,667	725	426	413	174.9	59.0	115.0
Denver	145,020	2,124,949	2.4	11.9	3.0	4,830	1,985	859	481	563	203.2	69.1	133.1
Fort Collins	24,540	261,453	2.0	10.9	2.5	4,502	1,747	830	509	561	169.4	61.8	106.5
Grand Junction	29,380	237,226	2.1	12.0	3.3	3,756	1,851	454	391	411	182.1	71.3	109.7
Greeley	28,680	257,786	2.7	12.8	3.4	4,721	2,060	829	462	443	169.4	62.6	105.7
Pueblo	17,720	140,345	2.9	13.8	3.2	4,905	2,057	829	449	695	193.4	70.9	121.5
Connecticut													
Bridgeport	83,600	627,917	2.2	10.5	2.5	4,395	1,980	1,036	360	557	258.8	83.2	174.4
Hartford	187,880	1,384,445	2.1	12.0	2.9	4,282	1,933	897	413	452	217.8	68.3	148.2
New Haven	171,220	1,352,454	2.2	11.8	2.7	4,396	2,000	999	395	451	236.8	74.6	161.0
Delaware													
Wilmington	74,880	672,137	2.3	14.1	3.7	4,110	1,942	1,057	340	291	186.9	65.5	120.4
District of Columbia													
Washington	203,960	2,254,795	2.8	14.1	3.3	4,330	2,189	1,081	386	204	268.6	84.5	182.7
Florida													
Bradenton	46,860	210,696	2.5	8.3	2.3	4,671	1,836	1,168	330	501	163.4	48.3	114.1
Clearwater	89,560	468,567	2.6	8.7	2.3	5,586	2,171	1,365	337	649	190.7	63.9	125.7
Fort Lauderdale	313,740	2,147,234	2.7	10.0	2.8	5,500	2,006	1,616	456	639	215.4	68.4	145.8
Fort Myers	168,540	717,985	2.6	10.7	2.6	5,311	2,111	1,333	384	677	171.4	54.5	115.9
Gainesville	47,640	445,145	2.7	12.1	3.0	5,746	2,467	1,085	413	875	170.1	61.8	107.3
Hudson	83,640	310,353	2.6	9.4	2.2	5,638	2,312	1,411	338	706	166.2	55.0	110.1
Jacksonville	117,200	1,240,525	3.1	14.6	3.7	5,533	2,353	1,244	449	635	181.0	59.9	120.2
Lakeland	42,700	302,262	2.7	11.2	2.8	5,241	2,404	1,176	291	521	146.7	48.8	97.2
Miami	214,520	2,513,109	3.2	12.8	3.3	7,955	3,056	2,141	583	830	229.7	83.0	146.3
Ocala	81,220	341,901	2.2	9.8	2.4	5,032	2,066	1,187	328	490	147.1	45.6	100.5
Orlando	349,420	2,535,044	2.7	12.4	3.1	5,351	2,103	1,255	360	738	162.8	54.0	107.9
Ormond Beach	44,900	290,820	2.9	10.5	2.5	4,848	1,850	1,112	473	635	160.2	54.9	104.4
Panama City	22,560	179,736	3.3	12.8	2.9	6,288	2,419	1,218	500	931	148.2	45.2	102.5
Pensacola	71,500	647,155	3.6	12.7	3.1	5,689	2,419	1,084	397	936	174.3	58.5	114.8
Sarasota	95,980	339,490	2.3	10.0	2.7	5,115	1,997	1,325	358	697	205.4	61.4	142.4
St Petersburg	66,980	402,889	3.0	12.3	3.1	5,859	2,321	1,349	476	674	202.9	69.0	132.9
Tallahassee	69,920	672,896	3.6	14.1	3.1	5,161	2,097	1,018	481	571	155.8	57.7	97.1
Tampa	86,240	933,943	2.8	12.5	2.9	5,720	2,338	1,273	411	624	181.4	60.0	120.4
Georgia													
Albany	20,980	208,867	3.9	14.9	3.1	4,962	2,436	907	507	656	124.1	40.6	83.1
Atlanta	352,220	4,200,842	2.9	13.3	3.9	4,822	2,310	1,016	355	584	173.0	56.6	115.5
Augusta	62,940	594,919	3.8	17.4	3.9	4,750	2,280	925	429	490	179.0	56.6	121.6
Columbus	33,420	316,092	4.3	12.7	2.9	4,183	1,724	897	370	539	144.7	52.0	91.8
Macon	69,460	633,839	3.9	16.3	3.9	5,119	2,398	969	440	657	167.5	58.3	108.2
Rome	30,300	231,352	3.3	13.4	3.3	4,977	2,305	935	403	797	159.9	63.2	95.7

Hospital Referral Region	Medicare Enrollees (1995)	Total Population (1995)	Acute Care Beds	Hospital Employees	Hospital-based Registered Nurses	Price Adjusted Reimbursements for Non-Capitated Medicare	Price Adjusted Reimbursements for Inpatient Hospital Services	Price Adjusted Reimbursements for Professional and Lab. Services	Price Adjusted Reimbursements for Outpatient Services	Price Adjusted Reimbursements for Home Health Services	All Physicians	Physicians in Primary Care	Specialist Physicians
Savannah	69,860	656,550	3.6	16.3	4.3	5,253	2,431	1,078	511	693	169.9	54.2	115.1
Hawaii													
Honolulu	86,860	1,190,170	2.0	11.2	2.8	3,332	1,656	752	343	187	208.7	75.8	132.0
Idaho													
Boise	69,800	605,996	2.2	11.2	3.0	3,980	1,768	752	421	403	156.8	51.0	105.0
Idaho Falls	17,220	181,481	2.8	10.0	2.8	3,776	1,565	701	375	574	127.6	37.9	89.6
Illinois													
Aurora	16,920	200,393	2.5	11.0	2.4	3,755	2,042	745	283	264	136.9	45.1	91.3
Blue Island	90,560	855,979	2.9	14.4	3.5	5,302	2,724	1,044	390	443	184.7	67.0	116.7
Chicago	221,300	2,590,942	4.4	21.8	5.1	5,280	3,010	988	333	414	225.4	84.5	140.2
Elgin	41,400	617,504	2.1	10.2	2.5	4,498	2,104	913	361	440	150.7	51.8	98.1
Evanston	111,200	908,751	2.4	13.3	3.0	4,534	2,298	1,050	359	265	276.1	98.1	177.4
Hinsdale	31,620	394,729	1.9	10.3	2.8	4,923	2,292	982	416	507	253.5	89.0	163.8
Joliet	46,680	461,271	3.5	14.8	3.4	5,116	2,712	1,009	420	427	166.6	54.7	111.0
Melrose Park	128,440	1,261,491	2.6	13.9	3.3	4,695	2,361	938	361	380	223.2	81.2	141.2
Peoria	95,480	606,294	3.1	15.4	4.1	4,567	2,172	905	504	356	148.0	53.3	93.7
Rockford	82,740	655,790	2.9	13.6	3.8	4,096	2,034	876	369	307	154.9	52.8	101.3
Springfield	123,540	828,552	3.3	15.0	3.3	4,532	2,368	895	439	333	140.3	52.0	87.3
Urbana	54,800	425,820	3.0	13.4	3.2	4,267	2,064	870	423	299	159.5	56.5	102.1
Bloomington	19,520	174,433	2.4	14.4	3.2	3,930	1,933	903	473	248	143.7	50.2	92.7
Indiana													
Evansville	96,560	658,585	3.5	14.8	3.7	4,737	2,178	787	489	531	143.4	53.8	88.5
Fort Wayne	98,700	791,565	2.7	12.4	3.1	3,938	1,637	787	389	508	131.5	48.2	82.4
Gary	54,860	498,010	4.3	16.2	4.1	5,852	3,219	1,076	407	626	146.0	50.6	94.5
Indianapolis	283,160	2,448,580	2.9	16.1	3.8	4,717	2,233	882	464	398	170.4	58.9	110.6
Lafayette	22,320	208,245	2.3	12.1	3.3	4,253	2,179	725	357	356	141.8	46.4	94.6
Muncie	21,700	169,763	2.8	13.1	3.2	4,783	2,678	860	380	202	160.8	59.0	101.0
Munster	38,760	306,380	4.3	18.0	5.0	5,397	2,843	1,039	434	497	159.6	58.4	100.3
South Bend	80,100	640,771	2.7	11.8	3.3	4,204	2,074	813	380	354	147.0	55.9	90.1
Terre Haute	25,100	179,192	3.1	16.3	3.7	4,739	2,195	968	389	493	153.2	55.2	96.8
Iowa													
Cedar Rapids	33,380	263,391	3.5	13.8	4.0	3,511	1,696	805	521	118	143.3	51.3	91.1
Davenport	68,960	496,950	3.3	14.1	3.5	3,946	1,834	808	481	303	155.0	52.9	101.3
Des Moines	137,620	955,106	3.4	15.2	3.5	3,974	1,973	843	476	276	155.9	63.3	91.6
Dubuque	21,380	148,398	3.3	13.3	4.1	3,524	1,886	599	447	255	152.4	48.9	102.7
Iowa City	40,820	318,164	3.3	15.2	4.1	4,038	1,989	808	594	250	174.0	58.5	114.5
Mason City	27,160	141,892	3.0	13.6	3.1	3,896	1,735	701	555	353	147.0	64.1	81.8
Sioux City	39,620	260,316	3.1	14.6	4.2	3,691	1,675	806	442	192	127.7	52.4	74.0
Waterloo	31,800	206,613	3.3	14.5	3.6	3,627	1,751	690	532	178	149.5	60.2	88.4
Kansas													
Topeka	54,880	432,709	2.8	13.8	3.4	3,823	1,804	757	442	248	154.0	52.1	101.1
Wichita	174,560	1,196,236	3.7	15.0	3.9	4,960	2,437	966	541	297	147.5	61.2	84.9
Kentucky													
Covington	35,560	339,291	2.9	12.8	3.3	4,430	2,114	841	398	325	159.1	58.7	99.4
Lexington	152,400	1,359,503	3.6	13.9	3.6	4,872	2,513	862	349	455	153.0	57.4	94.5
Louisville	184,080	1,527,661	3.3	14.1	3.7	5,105	2,482	1,021	361	460	176.0	59.6	115.5

Hospital Referral Region	Medicare Enrollees (1995)	Total Population (1995)	Acute Care Beds	Hospital Employees	Hospital-based Registered Nurses	Price Adjusted Reimbursements for Non-Capitated Medicare	Price Adjusted Reimbursements for Inpatient Hospital Services	Price Adjusted Reimbursements for Professional and Lab. Services	Price Adjusted Reimbursements for Outpatient Services	Price Adjusted Reimbursements for Home Health Services	All Physicians	Physicians in Primary Care	Specialist Physicians
Owensboro	17,840	135,989	2.9	13.3	4.0	5,146	2,574	1,072	485	420	134.8	40.9	93.2
Paducah	55,220	354,665	3.9	15.5	3.8	5,131	2,408	1,043	489	523	141.5	50.2	90.3
Louisiana													
Alexandria	32,780	274,229	4.4	17.4	3.7	7,178	3,526	973	479	1,233	164.1	59.5	103.5
Baton Rouge	66,340	775,757	3.5	15.1	3.7	7,227	2,651	1,099	521	1,948	152.5	52.7	99.0
Houma	23,580	251,883	3.9	17.9	4.0	6,959	3,205	1,186	559	1,399	132.2	37.0	95.3
Lafayette	58,240	560,865	4.2	15.3	3.3	5,739	2,646	932	360	939	141.3	48.2	92.3
Lake Charles	24,400	255,156	4.5	19.1	3.9	6,032	3,070	934	371	766	138.7	43.9	94.0
Metairie	40,740	416,838	4.1	17.5	4.3	7,013	3,062	1,233	621	1,376	251.8	68.5	181.8
Monroe	33,080	271,786	5.0	18.8	3.6	7,385	3,014	995	457	1,824	137.4	49.9	86.5
New Orleans	79,100	834,289	5.0	21.3	4.8	7,205	3,178	1,215	492	1,320	220.4	59.4	159.6
Shreveport	82,800	657,767	3.9	17.6	3.3	6,167	3,250	994	461	742	157.4	47.9	108.6
Slidell	15,600	160,715	3.7	15.4	4.2	7,019	3,377	1,137	480	1,118	164.9	46.7	117.5
Maine													
Bangor	55,000	397,915	2.8	14.9	4.0	4,022	1,779	721	488	596	170.3	65.4	103.9
Portland	127,580	970,466	2.6	13.0	3.2	4,094	1,961	793	366	497	200.8	73.0	126.9
Maryland													
Baltimore	270,160	2,309,251	3.0	16.0	4.2	5,240	2,829	1,118	513	264	250.3	82.6	166.7
Salisbury	53,520	330,541	3.0	14.4	3.2	4,820	2,475	1,008	430	224	189.1	62.6	125.5
Takoma Park	61,700	818,509	2.3	10.4	2.6	4,697	2,254	1,345	360	181	277.8	92.2	184.7
Massachusetts													
Boston	536,340	4,456,609	2.6	16.1	3.5	5,564	2,587	975	490	668	260.4	84.7	174.7
Springfield	97,520	718,474	2.6	12.7	2.9	4,322	1,998	781	378	493	202.0	71.9	129.2
Worcester	67,820	721,916	2.3	12.1	3.0	5,377	2,570	907	517	547	215.6	81.2	133.5
Michigan													
Ann Arbor	129,920	1,263,300	2.6	14.2	3.2	5,079	2,508	1,123	540	381	189.7	66.3	122.4
Dearborn	72,500	517,047	3.5	16.8	3.8	5,372	2,771	1,216	484	381	174.0	60.9	112.2
Detroit	225,400	1,874,979	3.8	20.0	4.7	5,321	2,734	1,289	441	350	175.8	61.2	113.6
Flint	57,500	564,745	3.5	17.3	4.0	5,460	2,802	1,279	469	388	163.8	71.6	90.7
Grand Rapids	112,560	1,022,322	2.2	12.0	3.1	3,989	1,902	769	417	274	154.1	57.4	95.6
Kalamazoo	75,620	638,376	2.8	12.5	3.3	4,477	2,293	841	463	298	166.8	60.2	105.6
Lansing	62,540	655,609	2.9	17.3	3.7	4,858	2,448	1,010	514	434	174.9	68.0	105.9
Marquette	32,880	204,947	3.6	14.6	2.7	4,284	1,934	684	469	894	153.0	59.5	92.5
Muskegon	35,320	253,057	2.7	12.6	2.7	3,850	1,870	787	426	340	155.0	63.7	89.9
Petoskey	25,200	162,989	2.8	12.2	3.4	4,009	1,680	855	528	505	168.0	65.3	101.6
Pontiac	36,160	430,414	2.8	14.9	3.4	5,792	3,128	1,252	425	372	252.5	84.2	167.1
Royal Oak	80,860	667,417	2.6	16.9	4.0	5,452	2,658	1,341	457	424	288.5	102.9	185.2
Saginaw	92,200	644,015	3.3	16.4	3.5	4,489	2,235	919	490	414	155.7	59.9	94.8
St Joseph	19,780	147,378	3.0	14.3	3.4	4,611	2,170	929	524	536	164.1	58.1	105.0
Traverse City	31,660	192,826	2.7	15.1	3.6	3,938	1,839	868	479	372	180.1	70.1	109.1
Minnesota													
Duluth	54,520	333,442	3.1	11.9	2.8	3,369	1,843	538	354	227	167.0	69.4	96.5
Minneapolis	276,540	2,761,315	2.6	11.4	2.9	3,528	1,917	618	390	169	169.7	68.0	100.5
Rochester	54,480	373,148	2.9	10.6	3.2	3,881	2,234	751	321	112	205.0	70.4	133.6
St Cloud	24,380	215,944	2.8	12.2	3.0	3,539	1,860	719	359	195	150.3	64.6	83.9
St Paul	73,160	897,880	2.4	10.8	2.7	3,771	2,067	623	371	182	188.4	80.4	106.6

Hospital Referral Region	Medicare Enrollees (1995)	Total Population (1995)	Acute Care Beds	Hospital Employees	Hospital-based Registered Nurses	Price Adjusted Reimbursements for Non-Capitated Medicare	Price Adjusted Reimbursements for Inpatient Hospital Services	Price Adjusted Reimbursements for Professional and Lab. Services	Price Adjusted Reimbursements for Outpatient Services	Price Adjusted Reimbursements for Home Health Services	All Physicians	Physicians in Primary Care	Specialist Physicians
Mississippi													
Gulfport	18,880	190,269	4.0	15.2	4.3	7,023	3,147	1,063	500	1,300	173.7	46.1	126.7
Hattiesburg	30,960	269,497	4.7	17.8	4.2	5,595	2,569	1,042	461	850	137.7	42.6	94.5
Jackson	117,660	1,008,214	4.6	16.2	3.6	5,354	2,101	855	476	1,149	149.0	52.3	95.8
Meridian	25,840	196,424	4.7	20.2	5.0	5,574	2,420	1,007	385	934	140.1	54.3	84.5
Oxford	17,480	131,140	4.8	18.9	4.1	5,121	2,247	887	370	1,158	139.7	50.2	88.6
Tupelo	45,080	367,620	4.2	14.4	3.5	5,202	2,469	810	449	985	123.3	46.1	76.3
Missouri													
Cape Girardeau	36,760	256,947	3.1	14.6	3.3	4,383	2,015	763	477	518	136.8	48.4	87.4
Columbia	86,360	614,064	3.0	14.9	3.4	5,776	2,987	888	646	594	157.3	59.4	96.9
Joplin	49,340	323,324	3.6	17.4	4.2	5,432	2,778	909	525	443	150.2	58.4	90.6
Kansas City	231,380	2,115,460	3.1	15.0	3.9	5,205	2,393	1,005	487	469	180.1	65.1	114.1
Springfield	106,080	685,835	3.0	14.6	3.4	4,389	2,119	784	508	380	144.3	55.7	87.6
St Louis	404,240	3,202,811	3.6	15.6	3.8	4,809	2,422	873	449	401	182.3	63.5	117.9
Montana													
Billings	61,040	500,410	3.0	15.2	3.4	4,351	2,035	804	503	322	177.7	65.0	111.7
Great Falls	20,000	151,554	3.5	18.4	4.1	4,349	2,376	691	474	259	175.4	61.8	112.5
Missoula	41,000	322,927	2.8	12.1	3.0	4,809	2,479	833	406	450	191.7	64.3	126.5
Nebraska													
Lincoln	76,160	527,095	3.2	11.9	3.1	3,550	1,689	749	465	183	134.4	56.3	76.8
Omaha	150,640	1,151,585	3.4	15.9	3.9	4,328	2,244	813	498	238	160.2	58.6	100.6
Nevada													
Las Vegas	78,240	1,039,539	2.2	9.4	2.4	5,278	2,320	1,298	219	653	148.8	47.4	100.6
Reno	61,400	539,845	2.8	11.8	3.1	4,155	1,834	903	346	258	179.9	59.6	119.3
New Hampshire													
Lebanon	52,420	374,665	3.0	14.7	3.6	3,819	1,865	585	506	491	200.8	74.2	125.6
Manchester	81,120	747,835	2.4	11.8	2.6	3,583	1,766	748	343	271	186.3	64.4	120.9
New Jersey													
Camden	349,480	2,544,746	3.1	14.5	3.6	4,562	2,246	1,219	355	268	218.8	73.5	144.2
Hackensack	152,200	1,142,994	3.4	14.7	3.7	4,107	2,004	1,194	302	216	299.6	99.9	198.3
Morristown	104,380	930,015	2.7	11.4	2.5	3,914	1,884	1,110	285	223	249.2	83.7	164.3
New Brunswick	98,200	883,173	2.9	13.8	3.3	4,140	2,156	1,151	236	217	236.4	82.8	152.7
Newark	165,940	1,450,943	4.7	19.6	4.5	4,183	2,162	1,222	281	206	216.6	74.7	141.0
Paterson	40,080	378,389	3.7	15.6	3.2	4,123	2,084	1,166	284	159	189.2	69.0	119.2
Ridgewood	42,460	386,390	2.7	11.8	3.2	3,946	1,893	1,148	277	172	263.2	84.6	177.5
New Mexico													
Albuquerque	106,580	1,384,541	2.4	15.2	3.6	4,382	1,876	780	509	445	194.6	71.0	122.5
New York													
Albany	231,580	1,749,451	3.0	13.3	3.4	4,079	2,067	976	320	239	201.4	66.2	134.1
Binghamton	56,320	378,203	2.7	13.2	2.8	3,626	1,856	781	399	220	172.7	58.5	113.3
Bronx	95,280	1,205,120	4.8	27.6	5.1	5,473	3,289	1,183	399	231	201.1	66.7	133.5
Buffalo	202,440	1,445,723	3.4	15.6	3.7	3,997	2,063	923	350	241	189.9	67.1	121.9
Elmira	53,840	345,998	3.4	15.0	3.6	4,126	2,145	977	410	217	185.7	59.1	125.7
East Long Island	458,840	4,303,545	3.3	14.6	3.6	4,806	2,594	1,301	289	241	273.7	96.4	176.6
New York	422,100	4,574,772	4.3	21.6	4.7	5,649	3,318	1,326	355	305	260.5	84.6	175.0
Rochester	146,540	1,274,455	2.8	15.2	3.7	3,944	2,161	747	354	336	195.6	72.6	122.1

Hospital Referral Region	Medicare Enrollees (1995)	Total Population (1995)	Acute Care Beds	Hospital Employees	Hospital-based Registered Nurses	Price Adjusted Reimbursements for Non-Capitated Medicare	Price Adjusted Reimbursements for Inpatient Hospital Services	Price Adjusted Reimbursements for Professional and Lab. Services	Price Adjusted Reimbursements for Outpatient Services	Price Adjusted Reimbursements for Home Health Services	All Physicians	Physicians in Primary Care	Specialist Physicians
Syracuse	128,300	1,091,054	2.9	13.4	2.7	3,940	2,039	951	324	203	173.2	57.7	114.5
White Plains	120,940	1,063,794	3.3	14.1	3.8	4,551	2,366	1,227	285	207	333.5	105.1	227.0
North Carolina													
Asheville	90,640	522,456	2.6	13.9	3.5	4,051	1,746	869	405	459	181.8	67.6	113.5
Charlotte	194,000	1,689,258	2.8	13.2	3.5	4,466	2,283	881	370	419	158.0	53.2	103.9
Durham	143,580	1,112,805	2.9	15.4	3.5	4,176	2,182	828	397	304	167.0	53.6	112.2
Greensboro	62,220	503,135	2.6	12.0	3.5	3,862	1,956	834	306	260	160.6	55.2	104.4
Greenville	81,940	721,867	3.2	14.3	3.9	4,698	2,498	964	416	336	155.7	52.0	102.9
Hickory	30,060	250,356	3.0	14.2	3.9	4,313	2,290	865	323	305	137.1	47.7	88.6
Raleigh	132,340	1,416,777	2.7	12.8	3.3	4,669	2,431	948	398	394	157.5	53.9	102.7
Wilmington	40,360	315,710	3.1	15.1	3.7	5,290	2,490	1,062	368	637	164.7	54.0	109.9
Winston-Salem	119,000	931,839	2.8	14.0	3.7	4,436	2,367	848	348	342	147.3	49.1	97.3
North Dakota													
Bismarck	31,220	203,420	4.9	20.0	4.5	4,577	2,454	876	515	278	154.5	54.4	98.9
Fargo Moorhead -Mn	69,360	481,267	3.0	12.3	3.1	3,713	1,929	728	421	205	138.7	60.4	76.5
Grand Forks	24,980	178,360	3.9	17.4	4.0	4,404	2,174	725	584	327	147.2	65.8	79.0
Minot	19,260	124,656	5.0	17.6	4.3	4,384	2,360	814	627	181	170.8	69.1	100.7
Ohio													
Akron	86,120	682,339	2.9	17.8	3.4	5,003	2,643	973	400	363	182.0	65.3	115.8
Canton	84,480	621,016	3.0	12.2	2.9	4,261	2,116	960	376	286	148.6	54.2	93.5
Cincinnati	183,500	1,576,226	2.9	14.3	3.6	4,453	2,168	870	458	277	192.8	64.8	127.1
Cleveland	274,040	2,115,071	3.4	16.5	3.8	5,084	2,508	1,028	430	389	210.2	71.0	138.1
Columbus	294,480	2,661,834	3.0	14.5	3.7	4,451	2,269	869	396	294	158.2	57.9	99.3
Dayton	137,400	1,118,493	3.1	16.1	4.3	4,479	2,259	951	402	277	147.7	55.3	91.4
Elyria	29,360	246,230	3.2	13.7	3.4	4,682	2,245	1,050	327	314	162.1	56.6	104.7
Kettering	46,600	376,920	2.6	13.1	3.3	4,302	2,082	967	382	327	210.5	76.7	133.0
Toledo	126,200	993,905	3.1	16.6	4.4	5,099	2,625	1,009	474	308	179.6	63.6	115.1
Youngstown	118,500	696,849	3.5	16.7	4.6	5,218	2,656	1,090	477	392	175.6	66.1	108.6
Oklahoma													
Lawton	23,380	199,870	3.9	14.7	2.4	5,558	2,528	864	539	894	154.1	62.6	90.0
Oklahoma City	198,700	1,624,681	3.5	15.0	3.1	5,488	2,308	910	416	1,168	160.9	58.0	101.8
Tulsa	141,720	1,198,154	3.2	13.8	3.0	5,406	2,246	887	481	1,148	161.9	62.8	98.0
Oregon													
Bend	20,360	139,460	2.5	10.8	3.9	4,014	1,734	746	336	710	171.1	60.2	110.0
Eugene	83,260	643,098	1.9	10.1	3.0	3,533	1,735	680	294	309	179.1	70.1	107.9
Medford	59,100	380,925	2.1	10.4	2.7	3,815	1,802	726	370	400	166.7	62.5	103.0
Portland	149,800	2,117,067	1.9	10.2	3.3	3,680	1,802	680	409	265	190.4	68.0	121.4
Salem	26,840	254,854	1.7	8.9	2.7	3,410	1,641	632	373	238	169.3	57.4	111.0
Pennsylvania													
Allentown	149,240	1,046,197	2.7	13.0	3.4	4,802	2,241	1,150	394	369	180.7	64.0	115.8
Altoona	45,500	302,509	3.1	13.3	3.1	5,073	2,434	865	464	532	148.4	53.2	94.3
Danville	74,020	548,307	3.0	13.3	3.0	4,566	2,220	936	558	312	170.3	60.9	108.6
Erie	113,240	739,828	3.3	14.5	3.7	4,870	2,412	971	420	375	159.8	54.2	104.7
Harrisburg	124,380	923,527	2.2	10.8	2.3	4,517	2,256	975	417	215	172.5	65.6	106.1
Johnstown	42,540	238,917	3.8	18.5	4.8	5,704	3,028	912	635	528	178.2	66.1	111.3
Lancaster	69,460	563,618	2.2	11.1	2.5	4,254	2,090	1,006	406	207	157.8	59.3	97.5

Hospital Referral Region	Medicare Enrollees (1995)	Total Population (1995)	Acute Care Beds	Hospital Employees	Hospital-based Registered Nurses	Price Adjusted Reimbursements for Non-Capitated Medicare	Price Adjusted Reimbursements for Inpatient Hospital Services	Price Adjusted Reimbursements for Professional and Lab. Services	Price Adjusted Reimbursements for Outpatient Services	Price Adjusted Reimbursements for Home Health Services	All Physicians	Physicians in Primary Care	Specialist Physicians
Philadelphia	458,740	3,913,956	3.3	16.6	4.3	5,402	2,782	1,291	372	304	263.5	89.4	173.1
Pittsburgh	509,880	3,057,775	3.6	16.4	4.1	5,545	2,785	1,104	426	495	191.9	64.5	126.4
Reading	81,060	525,543	2.6	12.0	2.8	4,510	2,074	1,008	408	241	166.0	62.4	102.8
Sayre	27,540	196,822	3.3	12.4	3.4	4,053	2,181	776	377	247	158.3	58.1	99.1
Scranton	55,400	299,324	2.9	12.5	3.3	4,779	1,986	1,128	378	528	190.2	69.6	119.7
Wilkes-Barre	44,620	255,080	3.1	13.3	3.0	5,495	2,274	1,131	437	719	200.1	78.6	120.9
York	49,380	359,300	2.1	11.8	3.0	3,683	1,763	812	344	186	161.7	64.3	96.4
Rhode Island													
Providence	145,220	1,151,437	2.4	13.2	2.8	4,511	2,181	956	367	481	209.6	72.4	136.3
South Carolina													
Charleston	81,400	767,555	3.4	16.0	4.8	4,707	2,155	967	464	469	180.0	57.9	121.2
Columbia	111,640	1,036,171	3.0	13.6	3.4	4,000	1,882	846	386	316	163.4	55.1	107.4
Florence	39,820	355,153	4.0	16.2	4.0	4,966	2,412	967	388	574	132.7	50.9	80.4
Greenville	85,700	724,640	2.8	12.1	3.3	4,192	2,108	878	341	316	164.9	58.8	105.2
Spartanburg	43,160	321,110	3.2	14.6	3.3	4,297	2,256	856	357	374	146.2	51.4	93.9
South Dakota													
Rapid City	21,920	194,449	3.7	14.1	3.3	4,335	2,082	775	394	597	172.0	71.6	98.9
Sioux Falls	113,760	715,918	3.9	14.3	4.1	4,081	2,124	783	505	159	149.6	63.6	84.5
Tennessee													
Chattanooga	74,520	587,633	3.3	14.0	3.9	6,012	2,405	937	484	1,522	161.2	55.8	104.6
Jackson	45,660	296,452	3.5	13.6	3.0	5,408	2,289	991	534	1,019	135.0	55.0	79.0
Johnson City	30,680	228,757	3.5	13.7	3.7	5,222	2,503	838	419	808	189.9	72.0	117.3
Kingsport	66,780	475,243	3.9	15.0	3.4	5,343	2,529	781	465	868	160.8	62.5	97.5
Knoxville	148,520	1,147,521	3.3	14.5	3.2	5,431	2,406	911	414	1,181	164.7	60.1	103.7
Memphis	179,440	1,656,593	3.8	15.7	3.5	5,176	2,399	998	361	776	149.9	49.5	99.6
Nashville	240,580	2,132,830	3.4	13.5	3.6	6,000	2,579	936	470	1,258	168.4	57.7	109.8
Texas													
Abilene	43,860	279,801	3.4	15.2	3.4	5,735	2,339	862	490	1,289	154.0	55.8	97.2
Amarillo	51,560	396,166	4.0	17.0	3.7	5,465	2,308	855	422	977	152.0	54.0	97.0
Austin	77,080	1,014,387	1.8	8.4	1.9	4,476	1,711	945	388	625	179.3	62.6	115.7
Beaumont	58,680	444,993	4.6	16.9	3.9	7,444	3,123	1,122	502	1,632	162.8	55.7	106.2
Bryan	17,760	198,132	2.3	10.9	2.2	4,703	1,770	803	468	797	145.3	58.7	85.7
Corpus Christi	48,020	527,470	3.4	15.3	3.1	6,875	2,694	1,107	458	1,591	156.8	55.1	100.8
Dallas	280,940	3,350,616	2.9	13.3	3.6	5,546	2,321	1,004	434	879	168.3	54.0	113.4
El Paso	79,140	927,960	2.6	10.3	2.5	5,215	2,395	832	364	847	141.7	41.6	99.8
Fort Worth	126,140	1,543,710	2.5	12.3	3.2	5,783	2,197	950	437	1,029	152.8	53.0	99.0
Harlingen	42,320	433,491	2.6	11.1	2.6	7,264	3,324	1,052	447	1,877	100.4	34.0	65.8
Houston	325,460	4,654,165	3.4	15.6	3.5	6,216	2,894	1,074	497	827	171.3	53.4	117.1
Longview	23,360	178,258	2.8	13.4	3.7	5,319	2,333	968	469	755	138.0	48.9	88.1
Lubbock	76,480	654,516	4.5	15.3	3.5	6,039	2,761	987	481	1,013	153.0	54.5	97.3
Mcallen	32,800	419,177	2.3	8.3	2.3	8,384	3,723	1,141	434	2,380	88.2	33.8	53.3
Odessa	31,000	318,045	3.5	14.2	3.0	5,791	2,516	1,079	346	889	124.3	36.4	87.6
San Angelo	21,680	154,120	3.8	13.6	3.3	5,445	2,464	916	562	904	156.5	50.7	104.9
San Antonio	163,060	2,005,038	2.7	11.9	2.8	6,434	2,490	1,058	496	1,445	182.7	55.9	126.0
Temple	30,360	369,253	2.2	11.9	2.4	4,345	2,170	650	431	561	124.1	44.9	78.1
Tyler	70,720	452,122	3.3	15.9	3.5	6,294	2,532	1,083	673	1,050	164.1	57.9	105.1

Hospital Referral Region	Medicare Enrollees (1995)	Total Population (1995)	Acute Care Beds	Hospital Employees	Hospital-based Registered Nurses	Price Adjusted Reimbursements for Non-Capitated Medicare	Price Adjusted Reimbursements for Inpatient Hospital Services	Price Adjusted Reimbursements for Professional and Lab. Services	Price Adjusted Reimbursements for Outpatient Services	Price Adjusted Reimbursements for Home Health Services	All Physicians	Physicians in Primary Care	Specialist Physicians
Victoria	18,340	140,251	4.0	15.2	3.6	5,818	2,479	919	466	1,114	156.7	54.9	101.0
Waco	41,020	292,850	2.6	11.4	2.3	3,761	1,609	708	408	515	151.4	54.9	95.7
Wichita Falls	28,560	196,171	3.4	12.8	2.5	5,415	2,117	919	435	888	172.2	60.1	111.1
Utah													
Ogden	27,380	343,189	2.3	11.2	2.9	3,980	1,582	637	330	943	137.1	41.7	95.3
Provo	25,700	352,423	2.3	11.0	2.8	4,474	1,852	669	368	1,002	131.5	43.5	87.6
Salt Lake City	134,000	1,553,931	2.6	13.3	3.5	4,165	1,747	658	370	737	155.6	48.3	107.1
Vermont													
Burlington	68,420	617,328	2.7	14.4	3.2	4,035	2,108	773	450	389	192.7	74.0	117.7
Virginia													
Arlington	100,640	1,653,868	1.9	8.2	2.2	3,871	1,820	1,015	317	241	208.3	70.2	137.1
Charlottesville	58,780	462,687	2.6	13.8	3.8	4,185	2,171	784	466	254	188.2	63.1	124.0
Lynchburg	30,060	220,257	2.8	10.5	3.7	2,929	1,483	675	322	144	145.6	53.6	91.1
Newport News	50,760	511,940	2.7	11.0	2.5	3,961	1,791	969	340	380	181.0	62.3	117.7
Norfolk	108,020	1,194,664	2.9	12.6	3.5	4,539	2,222	1,049	405	335	192.7	63.1	128.8
Richmond	152,100	1,356,790	3.0	13.2	3.9	4,072	2,102	957	316	282	174.7	63.7	110.1
Roanoke	94,860	669,247	3.5	14.0	3.6	4,234	2,193	786	334	412	177.1	63.0	113.2
Winchester	38,040	323,755	2.9	11.7	3.2	4,133	2,264	772	302	356	159.1	51.2	107.0
Washington													
Everett	40,520	506,893	1.6	9.3	2.4	4,072	1,808	800	483	276	173.3	65.1	106.9
Olympia	35,020	313,358	2.2	9.6	2.2	4,021	1,800	819	361	358	170.7	63.0	106.6
Seattle	198,460	2,323,430	1.8	10.7	2.6	4,060	1,862	831	373	296	219.3	80.9	137.6
Spokane	144,880	1,222,904	2.6	10.2	2.7	4,018	1,845	840	373	297	172.2	65.8	105.2
Tacoma	56,160	654,628	1.8	10.4	2.2	4,256	1,989	856	425	300	179.7	59.8	119.0
Yakima	27,800	254,946	2.3	10.4	2.7	4,298	2,025	891	331	334	161.4	63.7	96.0
West Virginia													
Charleston	125,280	868,182	3.8	15.7	3.7	5,085	2,685	819	433	483	167.0	65.5	100.5
Huntington	49,920	355,646	3.8	15.4	4.3	4,701	2,469	978	325	218	167.3	61.5	104.9
Morgantown	57,720	386,430	3.0	14.0	3.2	5,156	2,660	811	480	380	174.1	64.9	108.5
Wisconsin													
Appleton	37,000	282,642	2.4	10.0	2.5	3,323	1,550	690	432	83	142.4	58.4	82.7
Green Bay	66,920	471,256	2.6	11.7	3.0	3,671	1,746	723	460	207	143.0	51.9	90.2
La Crosse	47,560	332,104	2.8	11.7	3.0	3,215	1,743	624	292	165	159.2	60.8	97.4
Madison	110,940	935,588	2.6	12.3	3.0	3,812	1,980	669	351	272	168.7	69.1	98.7
Marshfield	53,320	356,526	3.1	10.7	2.9	3,768	1,934	805	341	227	174.5	68.2	105.2
Milwaukee	280,300	2,405,169	2.8	12.9	3.2	4,231	2,108	877	434	175	190.3	64.4	124.9
Neenah	28,400	212,358	2.7	11.6	3.0	4,339	2,172	831	465	197	163.7	57.0	105.9
Wausau	27,340	179,319	2.5	11.7	2.9	3,988	1,816	872	434	249	168.4	65.0	102.5
Wyoming													
Casper	21,060	170,887	4.2	17.0	4.5	4,889	2,475	730	502	640	177.3	69.6	106.6
United States													
United States	28,341,260	262,306,124	3.0	13.7	3.4	4,878	2,315	1,004	408	495	188.9	65.0	122.9

Variation, Practice Style and Hospital Capacity

Variation, Practice Style and Hospital Capacity

Medical science and medical opinion narrowly constrain clinical decisions about some conditions. For example, the severity of the illness dictates that patients with hip fracture are almost always hospitalized. But in treating other conditions, physicians have a good deal of discretion; for example, not all patients who break their arms are hospitalized. In these cases, physicians differ in their propensity to treat patients either in or outside the hospital and in their inclination to use surgery or to treat the fracture with a cast. Differences in clinical decision making such as these are the immediate source of a good deal of the variation in rates of service among hospital referral regions. Although the patterns of practice vary across regions, they are to a remarkable degree constant within a region from year to year. These patterns of practice create practice profiles. Health service researchers have dubbed these patterns the region's surgical and medical signatures.

This chapter asks several questions:

■ How much variability is there in the rates of hospitalization?

■ Do most conditions have the low variation pattern of hospitalization exhibited by hip fracture? Or are most conditions highly variable, suggesting the influence of practice style on rates of hospitalization?

■ How much of the variation in the rates of hospitalization is associated with hospital capacity?

Most hospitalizations are for conditions that have high or very high patterns of variation in their discharge rates. Medical discharges are more variable than surgical discharges. For medical conditions, the majority of variation is associated with hospital capacity (as measured by the per capita supply of hospital beds).

Practice Style and Hospitalization for Hip, Ankle and Forearm Fractures

Medical decision making about treatment for patients with hip fractures is narrowly constrained by the dictates of medical science and patient needs.

■ It is virtually certain that patients will seek care. Hip fractures are very painful, and patients whose hips are fractured cannot walk. The need for immediate medical help is easily recognized.

■ Correct diagnosis of hip fracture, by physical examination or X-ray, is virtually certain.

■ The likelihood that the attending physician will recommend hospitalization for a patient with hip fracture is a virtual certainty, both because hip fracture is a life-threatening injury, and because the medical profession agrees unanimously on the need for hospitalization for treatment.

As a result, the probability that physicians will accurately diagnose and prescribe hospitalization for patients with fractured hips approaches 100%.

Similarly, all patients with ankle or forearm fractures will seek care, and the correct diagnosis will be made. But the conditions themselves are not so severe that all patients suffering with them need to be hospitalized. Moreover, physicians differ in their opinions about the benefits of available treatments, some preferring to treat with surgery, which requires hospitalization, others preferring to use a cast, which can be applied in an outpatient setting. Consequently, the probability that a given physician will prescribe hospitalization for a patient with ankle or forearm fracture is less than 100%.

In a study of hip fractures among the Medicare population, 99% of cases were hospitalized, and the hospitalization rate and the incidence rate were closely correlated ($R^2 = .99$). But among patients with ankle fractures, only 41% were hospitalized, and only about one-third of the variation in hospitalization rates among regions was explained by variation in incidence ($R^2 = .33$). Only 35% of patients with forearm fractures were hospitalized, and a little more than 25% of the variation in hospitalization was associated with incidence ($R^2 = .27$).

The Pattern of Variation In Hospitalizations for Hip, Ankle, and Forearm Fractures

Figure 3.1 demonstrates the variability in hospitalization rates of ankle and forearm fractures, compared to hip fractures. Hospitalizations for ankle fractures are more variable than hospitalization for hip fractures; and hospitalizations for forearm fracture are more variable than hospitalizations for ankle fractures.

Epidemiologists sometimes use the interquartile ratio as a measure of variation. This statistic is the ratio of the rate in the region ranked at the 75th percentile to

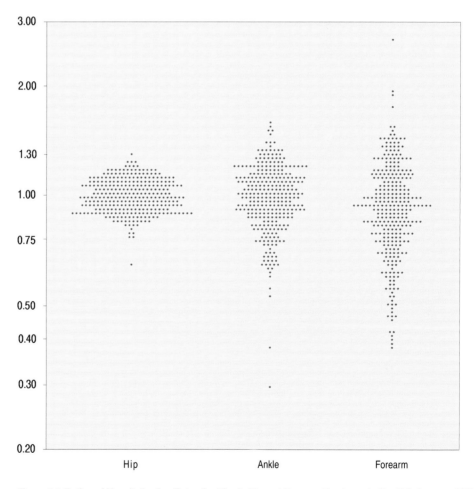

Figure 3.1. Ratios of Hospitalization Rates for Hip, Ankle and Forearm Fractures to the U.S. Average (1994-95)
A log scale, centered about the national average (1.0), was used for clarity. Hospitalizations for hip fractures have a low-variation pattern; the rate closely reflects the incidence of the condition. The variability in the rates of hospitalizations for ankle and forearm fractures reflects the importance of practice style as a determinant of hospitalization rates. Each point represents one of the 306 hospital referral regions in the United States.

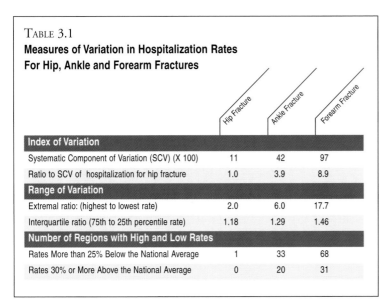

TABLE 3.1
**Measures of Variation in Hospitalization Rates
For Hip, Ankle and Forearm Fractures**

	Hip Fracture	Ankle Fracture	Forearm Fracture
Index of Variation			
Systematic Component of Variation (SCV) (X 100)	11	42	97
Ratio to SCV of hospitalization for hip fracture	1.0	3.9	8.9
Range of Variation			
Extremal ratio: (highest to lowest rate)	2.0	6.0	17.7
Interquartile ratio (75th to 25th percentile rate)	1.18	1.29	1.46
Number of Regions with High and Low Rates			
Rates More than 25% Below the National Average	1	33	68
Rates 30% or More Above the National Average	0	20	31

Table 3.1. Measures of Variation in Hospitalization Rates For Hip, Ankle and Forearm Fractures (1994-95)
Hospitalization rates for hip, ankle and forearm fractures are ranked from low to high according to the systematic component of variation (SCV). The SCV of hospitalizations for ankle fractures is almost 4 times greater than the SCV of hospitalizations for hip fractures; and the SCV of hospitalizations for forearm fractures is almost 9 times greater than the SCV of ankle fractures. The differences in variability are statistically and clinically significant. The extremal ratio (calculated by dividing the rate of the highest region by the rate of the lowest region) of hip fracture is 2.0; of ankle fracture 6.0; and of forearm fracture, 17.7. (See the Appendix on Methods for a description of the Systematic Component of Variation.)

the rate in the region ranked at the 25th percentile. For hospitalization for hip fracture, the interquartile ratio is 1.18; for ankle fracture it is 1.29; and for forearm fracture it is 1.46.

Table 3.1 gives the number of regions with rates that are 30% or more above the national average, as well as the number with rates that are more than 25% below the national average. By definition, when variability increases, more regions have rates that are substantially different from the average. In the case of hospitalization for hip fracture, there is only one region with a rate more than 25% below the national average, and no region is 30% or more above the average. In contrast, thirty-three regions have rates of hospitalization for ankle fracture more than 25% below the national average, and 20 regions are 30% or more above the national average. Sixty-eight regions have rates of hospitalization for forearm fracture that are more than 25% below the national average, and 31 regions are 30% or more above the national average.

Variation in Rates of Hospitalization for Hip, Ankle, and Forearm Fractures

There is relatively little variation in the rates of hospitalization for hip fracture. No regions are 30% or more above the national average; only one is more than 25% below the average. Hospitalization rates are closely correlated with the incidence rate of hip fracture. Rates are higher than average in parts of the South and in Texas, and lower than average in parts of New York, the Midwest, Utah, Southern Idaho and Western Oregon (Map 3.1). The rates of hospitalization for ankle fracture are more variable than for hip fracture. Twenty regions are 30% or more above the national average; 33 are more than 25% below the national average (Map 3.2). Rates of hospitalizations for forearm fractures are the most variable: 31 regions are 30% or more above the national average, and 68 are more than 25% below it. Unlike rates of hospitalization for hip fracture, hospitalization rates for ankle and forearm fractures do not closely follow the incidence of the injury (Maps 3.2 and 3.3). Rates in neighboring regions are sometimes at the extremes, as indicated by the contrasting blue (high rate) and green (low rate) regions on the maps.

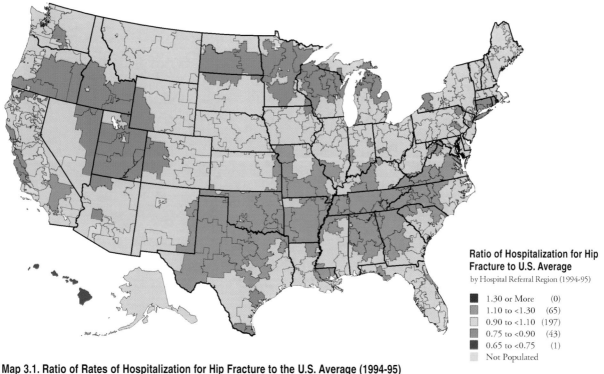

Ratio of Hospitalization for Hip Fracture to U.S. Average
by Hospital Referral Region (1994-95)

- ■ 1.30 or More (0)
- ▨ 1.10 to <1.30 (65)
- ▢ 0.90 to <1.10 (197)
- ▨ 0.75 to <0.90 (43)
- ■ 0.65 to <0.75 (1)
- □ Not Populated

Map 3.1. Ratio of Rates of Hospitalization for Hip Fracture to the U.S. Average (1994-95)
Hospitalization rates for hip fracture are closely correlated with incidence rates; there is relatively little variation among hospital referral regions.

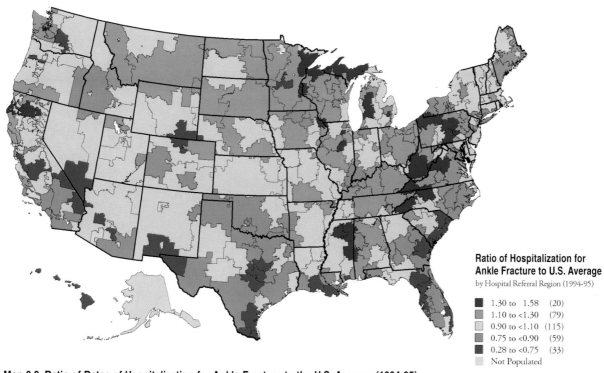

Ratio of Hospitalization for Ankle Fracture to U.S. Average
by Hospital Referral Region (1994-95)

- 1.30 to   1.58   (20)
- 1.10 to <1.30   (79)
- 0.90 to <1.10   (115)
- 0.75 to <0.90   (59)
- 0.28 to <0.75   (33)
- Not Populated

Map 3.2. Ratio of Rates of Hospitalization for Ankle Fracture to the U.S. Average (1994-95)

Hospitalization rates for ankle fracture are more variable than rates of hospitalization for hip fracture but less variable than rates of hospitalization for forearm fractures.

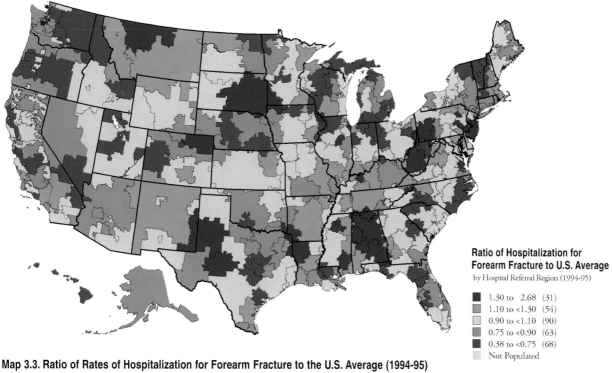

Ratio of Hospitalization for Forearm Fracture to U.S. Average
by Hospital Referral Region (1994-95)

- 1.30 to   2.68   (31)
- 1.10 to <1.30   (54)
- 0.90 to <1.10   (90)
- 0.75 to <0.90   (63)
- 0.38 to <0.75   (68)
- Not Populated

Map 3.3. Ratio of Rates of Hospitalization for Forearm Fracture to the U.S. Average (1994-95)

Hospitalization rates for forearm fracture are not closely related to incidence rates, and vary widely among regions.

Variation in Rates of Hospitalization

Is the low variation in rates of hospitalization for hip fracture the exception, or the rule? If hospitalizations for most conditions had low variation, then professional discretion — practice style— would not have an influence on the health care economy. On the other hand, if the rates of hospitalizations for most conditions were as variable — or even more variable — than the rates of hospitalizations for ankle or forearm fractures, the implications would be quite different.

Research conducted in conjunction with the Atlas examined the pattern of variation in hospitalizations among the national Medicare population by "modified diagnosis-related groups" (M-DRGs). Variations in rates were calculated for 103 M-DRGs, 60 for medical and 43 for surgical hospitalizations. (See Appendix on Methods for definition of M-DRGs). The amount of variation was estimated using the systematic coefficient of variation (SCV). The M-DRGs were then put into four groups, according to their SCVs:

- SCV less than hip fracture   Low Variation Conditions
- SCV between hip and ankle fractures   Moderate Variation Conditions
- SCV between ankle and forearm   High Variation Conditions
- SCV greater than forearm fractures   Very High Variation Conditions

Most hospitalizations were for high or very high variation conditions (Figure 3.2).

- **Medical hospitalizations** constituted 70.3% of all Medicare hospitalizations in 1995. None of the 60 M-DRGs had hospitalization rates that were less variable than the hospitalization rate for hip fracture. Only 6 M-DRGs, representing 13.8% of medical hospitalizations, were "moderately variable" conditions. Twenty-five M-DRGs (49.2% of all medical hospitalizations) were "high variation," and 29 (37.0% of medical hospitalizations) were "very high variation" — that is, they exhibited greater variation than hospitalizations for fractures of the forearm.

■ **Surgical hospitalizations** constituted 29.7% of Medicare hospitalizations in 1995. Two of the 43 surgical M-DRGs, representing 11.3% of hospitalizations for surgical M-DRGs, were less variable than hospitalizations for hip fracture; 15 (34.2% of surgical M-DRGs) were moderately variable. The rates of 54.5% of hospitalizations for surgical M-DRGs were more variable than the rates of hospitalization for ankle fractures; the rates of 15 M-DRGs (35.7% of surgical M-DRGs) and 11 M-DRGs (18.8% of surgical M-DRGs) were classified as "high" or "very high" variation procedures.

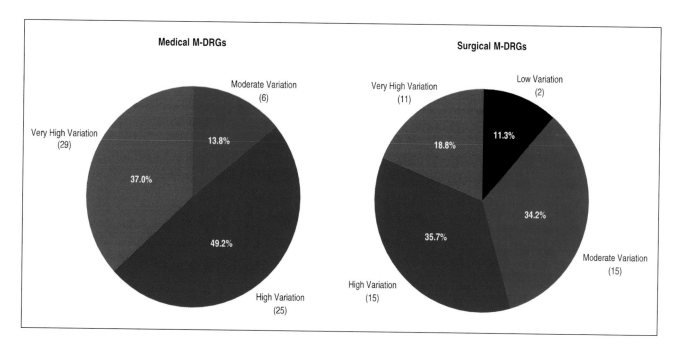

Figure 3.2. Percent of Hospitalizations for Medical and Surgical Major Diagnosis-Related Groups According to Degree of Variation (1994-95)
The figure shows the proportion of medical and surgical M-DRGs according to the degree of variation in their discharge rates. Most causes of hospitalization have high or very high patterns of variation. The number of M-DRGs in each group is given in parentheses.

Discharges for Surgical and Medical Conditions

Discharges for surgical conditions were less variable than discharges for medical conditions. In 1994-95, the rate of surgical discharges per thousand Medicare enrollees varied by a factor of almost two among hospital referral regions (Map 3.4). The rate in the lowest region was 64.5 discharges per thousand enrollees; in the highest region it was 119.8 per thousand enrollees.

Surgical discharges were higher in parts of Michigan, the Middle Atlantic states, Alabama, Louisiana, Texas and California. Rates were lower in Alaska and Hawaii and in parts of the Northeast, Northwest and Southwest.

The rate of medical discharges per thousand Medicare enrollees varied by a factor of almost three (Map 3.5). The rate in the lowest region was 122.3 discharges per thousand enrollees; in the highest region it was 353.5 per thousand enrollees.

Medical discharges were highest in the South, the Dakotas, Montana, the Chicago area, parts of Michigan, New York and New Jersey. Rates of medical discharges were low throughout most of West, particularly in Utah, Idaho, Oregon and Washington.

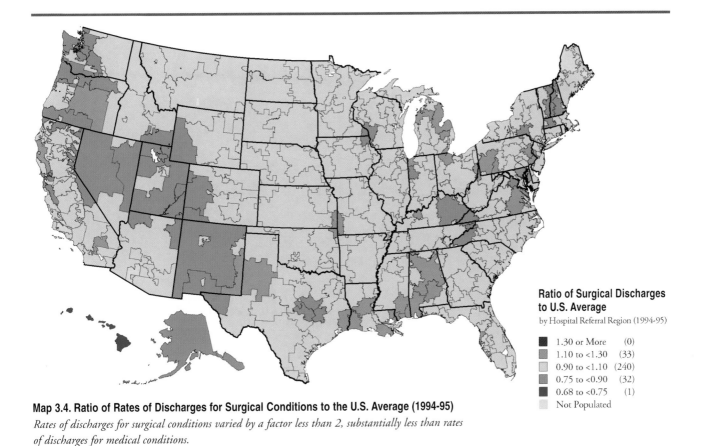

Map 3.4. Ratio of Rates of Discharges for Surgical Conditions to the U.S. Average (1994-95)

Rates of discharges for surgical conditions varied by a factor less than 2, substantially less than rates of discharges for medical conditions.

Ratio of Surgical Discharges
to U.S. Average
by Hospital Referral Region (1994-95)

	1.30 or More	(0)
1.10 to <1.30	(33)
0.90 to <1.10	(240)
0.75 to <0.90	(32)
0.68 to <0.75	(1)
Not Populated	

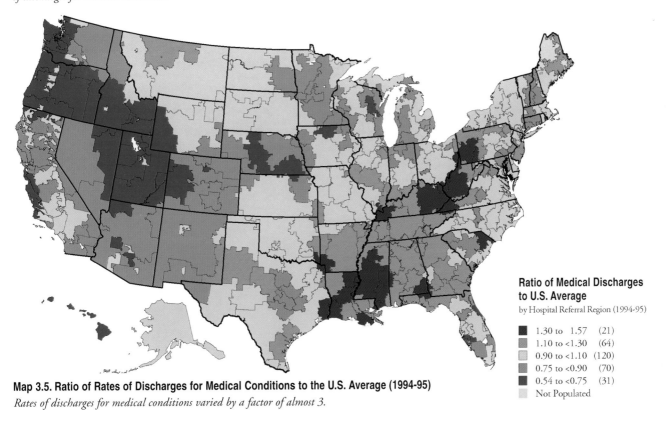

Map 3.5. Ratio of Rates of Discharges for Medical Conditions to the U.S. Average (1994-95)

Rates of discharges for medical conditions varied by a factor of almost 3.

Ratio of Medical Discharges
to U.S. Average
by Hospital Referral Region (1994-95)

1.30 to 1.57	(21)
1.10 to <1.30	(64)
0.90 to <1.10	(120)
0.75 to <0.90	(70)
0.54 to <0.75	(31)
Not Populated	

The Surgical Signature

There are striking differences in the likelihood of undergoing particular surgical procedures such as prostate operations, back surgery and coronary artery bypass grafting, even among neighboring regions with very similar populations. Because the differences in rates tend to persist from year to year, communities become recognizable by their "surgical signatures."

Surgical signatures reflect the practice patterns of individual physicians and local medical culture, rather than differences in need — or even differences in the local supply of surgeons. For example, neighboring regions with about the same per capita numbers of urologists can have very different surgical signatures for prostate surgery. The seven southwest Florida hospital referral regions bounded on the north by the Hudson region and, on the south, the Fort Myers region, provide a good example of this phenomenon (Map 3.6).

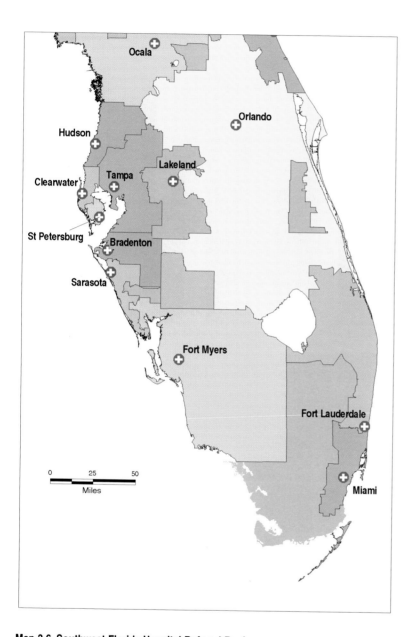

Map 3.6. Southwest Florida Hospital Referral Regions

Surgical signatures often vary substantially from one community to another, even in areas which are demographically similar. The retirement communities of southwest Florida (Hudson, Clearwater, St. Petersburg, Tampa, Bradenton, Sarasota and Fort Myers) provide a good example of the idiosyncratic way in which surgical signatures vary in contiguous communities. The following pages illustrate the sometimes striking contrasts in the risks of surgical intervention among Medicare enrollees, depending on where they live.

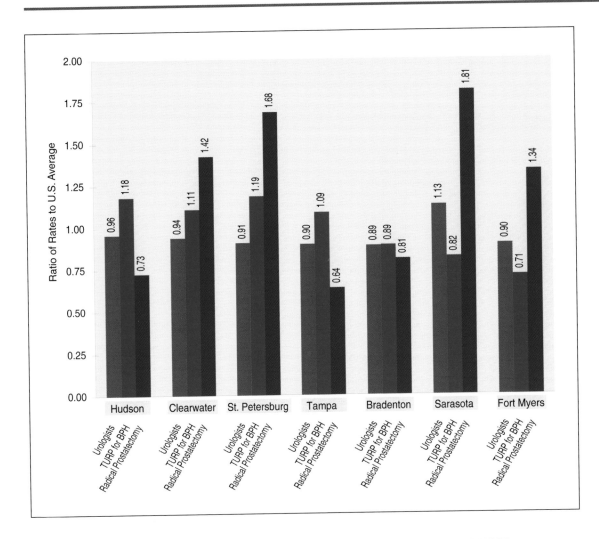

Figure 3.3. The Urological Surgical Signature Of Seven Southwest Florida Hospital Referral Regions (1994-95)

The figure gives the ratio of rates of urologists and of prostate surgery relative to the national average. Although the number of urologists per 100,000 residents is nearly the same in each of the seven hospital referral regions, the amount and kind of prostate surgery varies substantially. The urologists treating patients who live in the Hudson hospital referral region perform surgery for benign prostatic hyperplasia ("TURP for BPH") at a rate 18% higher than the national average, but perform relatively little surgery (27% below the national average) for prostate cancer (radical prostatectomy). Urologists treating Medicare residents of the St. Petersburg hospital referral region perform 2.6 times more radical prostate procedures per 1,000 male Medicare enrollees than the urologists treating residents of the neighboring Tampa hospital referral region, who perform the surgery at a rate that is 36% below the national average. In the Bradenton hospital referral region, rates for both procedures are below the national average; in Sarasota, surgery for benign prostate disease is below the national average but rates of surgery for prostate cancer are 1.8 times the national average. The urologists serving Medicare residents of the Fort Myers hospital referral region perform more surgery for prostate cancer than the national average, but less surgery than the national average for benign prostate disease.

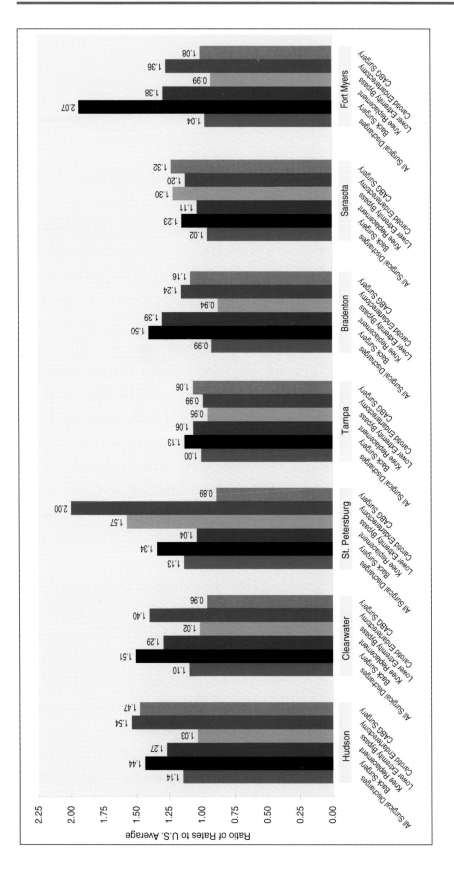

Figure 3.4. The Surgical Signatures of Seven Southwestern Florida Hospital Referral Regions for Five Common Procedures (1994-95)

The overall rate of surgery in each of these communities is close to the national average. However, as in the case of prostate surgery, the likelihood of undergoing specific procedures differs markedly from one community to another. Medicare residents of the St. Petersburg hospital referral region underwent carotid endarterectomy at a rate that was twice the national average. By contrast, Medicare residents of the St. Petersburg hospital referral region had the lowest rate of coronary artery bypass grafting among the seven regions. Surgeons treating Medicare residents of the Fort Myers hospital referral region perform back surgery at twice the national average. For each of the five procedures, rates among Medicare residents of the Tampa hospital referral region are close to the national average. See Chapter Five for a discussion of the clinical reasons for variation in the use of these procedures.

The Medical Signature

The patterns of variation in the discharge rates for medical conditions have their own recognizable "medical signatures." The medical signature, however, is strikingly unlike the surgical signature. The typical surgical signature reflects the idiosyncratic way in which surgery varies — high rates of one procedure and low rates of another. Moreover, the overall likelihood of having surgery (the total surgical discharge rate) does not correlate closely with the likelihood of having any specific procedure.

By contrast, the risk of hospitalization for a specific high variation medical condition tends to be closely associated with the total discharge rate for all medical conditions in the hospital referral region. Indeed, the practice profiles captured by the medical signature suggest that the rules governing decisions about whether to hospitalize patients (rather than treat them elsewhere) are subject to a kind of "thermostat" of supply, set for the hospital referral region, that establishes the level of risk of hospitalization for high variation medical conditions. The level at which the thermostat is set is independent of morbidity levels in the community or the specific condition for which the patient is being treated.

The populations living in the Boston and New Haven hospital service areas, which are remarkably similar in demographic features and other factors that predict the need for care, provide a good example of the thermostat effect. Most Bostonians and New Havenites, when they are hospitalized, are admitted to hospitals associated with some of the nation's most prestigious medical schools. Such an advantage would seem to assure that the residents of these communities are treated in the best, most scientific, high-quality way. Yet studies dating back to the mid 1970s show, year in and year out, that the per capita amount of hospital care provided to Boston residents has been much greater than the amount provided to residents of New Haven. The most consistent differences in hospital care between the two hospital markets are in the capacity of hospitals and the associated discharge rates for high variation medical conditions.

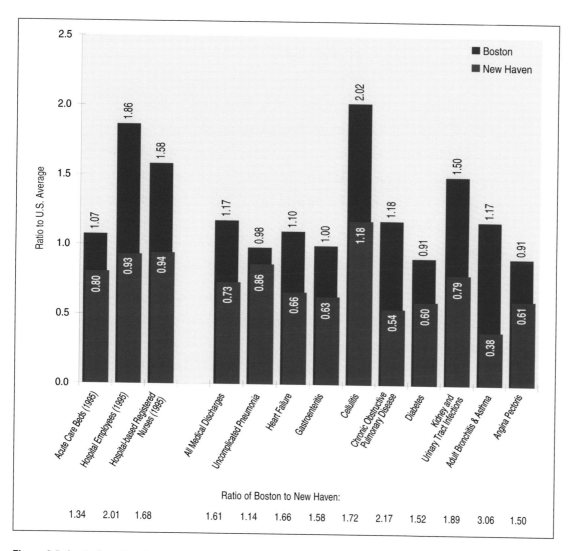

Figure 3.5. Acute Care Hospital Resources and the Medical Signatures of the Boston and New Haven Hospital Service Areas (1994-95)

The figure gives the ratio of hospital resources and discharge rates for all medical discharges and selected high and very high variation medical M-DRGs, relative to the national average. In numbers of hospital beds, personnel, and hospital-employed registered nurses allocated to care of the local population, Boston is well above the national average, but New Haven is below it. There is an increased likelihood of hospitalization among Bostonians, compared to residents of New Haven. The increase in rates among Bostonians range from 1.14 for uncomplicated pneumonia to 3.06 for bronchitis and asthma. The rate of hospitalization for all medical discharges is 1.61 times greater.

The Association Between Hospital Beds and Hospitalizations for Hip Fracture and Medical and Surgical Conditions

The influence of the supply of hospital beds on clinical decision making does not uniformly apply to all conditions. Because the incidence of hip fracture determines the rate of hospitalization for hip fracture victims, one would expect that the local supply of hospital beds would have little influence on the rate at which patients with broken hips are hospitalized. The data bear this out; there is almost no correlation (R^2 = .08) between the supply of beds and the rates of discharges for hip fracture (Figure 3.6).

The local supply of hospital beds has a modest relationship with the discharge rates for surgical conditions (R^2 = .22). The supply of hospital beds has virtually no relationship with discharge rates for low variation procedures (R^2 = .05) or with moderate variation surgical procedures (R^2 = .04) (plot not shown).

In the case of common medical conditions, however, the local supply of staffed hospital beds has a critical influence on the relative risk of hospitalization. The association between hospital beds per thousand residents and hospitalization rates for medical conditions is strong (R^2 = .56), indicating that beds account for the majority of variation in hospitalization rates. Even the hospitalization rates for moderate variation medical conditions are strongly associated with bed capacity (R^2 = .45) (plot not shown).

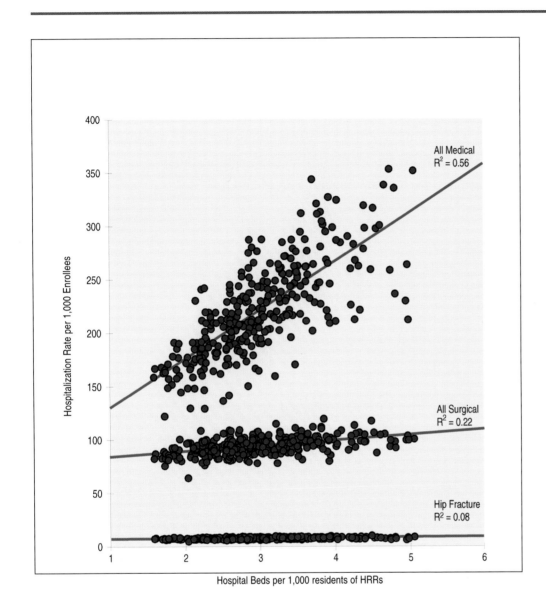

Figure 3.6. The Association Between Allocated Hospital Beds and Medicare Hospitalizations for Medical and Surgical Care and for Hip Fracture (1994-95)

The hospitalization rate for medical conditions is strongly correlated with bed supply (R^2 = .56); surgical hospitalizations are less strongly correlated (R^2 = .22); and hip fracture hospitalizations have little correlation (R^2 = .08).

Chapter Three Table   Rates are adjusted for differences in age, sex, and race composition of areas' populations. The rates represent the health care utilization of persons living in the specified area, regardless of where services were obtained. Hospitalization rates are per thousand enrollees and are for the years 1994-95. Data exclude Medicare enrollees who were members of risk bearing health maintenance organizations. Specific codes used to define the numerator for rates, and methods of age, sex, and race adjustment are given in the Appendix on Methods.

CHAPTER THREE TABLE

Hospitalizations for Total, All Surgical, All Medical, and Selected Medical Conditions Among Non-HMO Medicare Enrollees by Hospital Referral Regions (1994-95)

Hospital Referral Region	Hip Fracture	Ankle Fracture	Radius/Ulna/Wrist Fracture	C.O.P.D.	Adult Bronchitis and Asthma	CHF	Angina Pectoris	Adult Gastroenteritis	Cellulitis	Diabetes Age 35+	Kidney and Urinary Tract Infections	Adult Simple Pneumonia	All Medical Discharges	All Surgical Discharges
Alabama														
Birmingham	9.2	0.80	0.61	14.4	3.6	22.5	3.9	13.4	3.4	3.0	9.2	16.1	283.3	113.8
Dothan	8.7	0.67	0.67	19.5	5.9	29.4	7.2	19.1	5.1	3.6	8.9	21.2	321.3	103.4
Huntsville	8.7	0.72	0.59	11.7	3.9	27.6	4.1	12.6	2.5	3.3	7.9	13.3	256.0	100.0
Mobile	8.5	0.74	0.56	15.0	3.6	24.8	4.8	13.6	3.6	2.9	7.7	16.8	280.9	112.2
Montgomery	8.7	0.72	0.60	15.8	3.4	24.6	4.4	13.0	3.4	2.9	6.5	12.5	262.6	104.6
Tuscaloosa	8.9	0.54	0.66	15.3	4.0	21.7	4.4	19.9	4.5	3.9	11.4	19.3	287.9	101.6
Alaska														
Anchorage	7.3	0.72	0.36	11.9	2.3	19.1	5.2	8.9	3.0	1.8	5.8	17.9	220.6	78.3
Arizona														
Mesa	7.7	0.44	0.33	8.3	1.4	14.7	3.9	5.4	1.7	1.3	4.0	13.3	162.9	89.4
Phoenix	8.4	0.60	0.37	8.6	1.6	15.3	4.2	6.8	2.2	1.6	5.1	13.2	181.7	92.8
Sun City	7.0	0.49	0.35	5.6	1.0	9.7	2.7	4.4	1.1	0.8	2.8	7.8	129.8	97.3
Tucson	8.0	0.56	0.40	8.3	1.6	14.4	4.1	6.6	2.1	1.7	4.5	11.6	172.9	86.3
Arkansas														
Fort Smith	9.4	0.59	0.33	13.4	2.8	30.0	7.7	10.4	2.6	2.8	6.9	18.9	279.4	91.6
Jonesboro	8.7	0.80	0.52	15.5	4.2	24.7	6.0	12.8	2.7	4.2	9.4	20.0	272.5	102.5
Little Rock	8.9	0.68	0.54	12.4	3.8	23.6	4.7	13.2	2.7	3.2	7.6	17.6	264.5	100.5
Springdale	8.5	0.63	0.39	8.2	2.8	22.5	4.4	11.5	2.0	2.1	5.7	16.2	219.5	89.2
Texarkana	8.9	0.85	0.62	17.0	4.2	28.7	6.4	11.6	3.3	3.8	9.3	21.7	298.4	98.3
California														
Orange Co.	7.8	0.56	0.37	8.8	1.6	19.2	4.5	6.6	2.4	1.8	6.0	12.1	201.5	90.2
Bakersfield	8.4	0.65	0.36	9.3	1.9	21.0	7.3	6.7	2.6	2.5	7.5	20.4	219.9	100.4
Chico	8.5	0.68	0.41	8.5	1.1	16.6	5.7	6.5	1.9	1.5	6.0	13.9	191.0	99.7
Contra Costa Co.	7.3	0.71	0.49	6.2	1.1	14.6	3.0	5.3	1.7	1.2	3.9	11.6	168.4	83.2
Fresno	7.2	0.48	0.24	6.4	1.3	17.7	5.1	4.8	1.5	1.5	5.5	14.1	168.3	86.3
Los Angeles	7.6	0.57	0.52	10.8	2.0	22.4	5.9	7.4	3.3	2.5	7.5	13.6	232.6	98.1
Modesto	8.1	0.61	0.34	11.0	1.3	19.0	6.1	6.2	2.0	1.7	6.1	18.6	212.7	92.2
Napa	7.8	0.79	0.29	7.5	0.7	15.7	3.7	5.5	2.0	1.1	4.0	15.1	189.2	109.3
Alameda Co.	7.1	0.66	0.40	6.9	1.1	19.5	3.0	5.1	2.0	1.4	3.3	10.8	185.5	87.4
Palm Spr/Rancho Mir	8.4	0.63	0.43	7.2	1.1	14.6	4.2	6.3	2.0	1.4	5.3	12.1	180.8	108.9
Redding	7.2	0.89	0.37	7.9	1.0	14.8	2.7	5.6	1.7	1.1	5.5	13.6	178.2	102.7
Sacramento	7.9	0.66	0.41	7.9	1.2	16.6	3.8	6.3	2.1	1.3	4.3	14.3	185.8	86.2
Salinas	6.9	0.61	0.47	6.5	1.3	13.7	3.9	6.8	1.7	1.3	3.7	10.3	160.5	100.9
San Bernardino	8.9	0.58	0.50	12.5	2.1	21.4	9.9	8.0	2.9	2.7	7.2	17.0	241.2	98.9
San Diego	7.7	0.58	0.41	8.7	1.2	16.7	3.8	5.7	2.1	1.7	5.1	11.5	177.3	90.8
San Francisco	6.8	0.67	0.46	5.7	1.3	16.6	3.2	4.5	2.4	1.3	3.4	10.6	174.3	76.5
San Jose	6.6	0.49	0.30	6.0	1.1	15.7	3.1	4.6	1.9	1.5	3.5	11.1	166.0	83.3
San Luis Obispo	7.0	0.76	0.49	4.8	1.5	12.8	5.3	6.9	1.6	1.5	3.3	11.2	158.8	91.3
San Mateo Co.	7.2	0.52	0.34	4.4	1.2	13.6	2.0	4.1	1.9	1.3	2.6	9.2	145.0	80.5
Santa Barbara	7.9	0.50	0.33	5.4	1.1	13.4	3.3	5.4	1.7	1.1	4.5	10.4	152.0	92.8

Hospital Referral Region	Hip Fracture	Ankle Fracture	Radius/Ulna/Wrist Fracture	C.O.P.D.	Adult Bronchitis and Asthma	CHF	Angina Pectoris	Adult Gastroenteritis	Cellulitis	Diabetes Age 35+	Kidney and Urinary Tract Infections	Adult Simple Pneumonia	All Medical Discharges	All Surgical Discharges
Santa Cruz	6.7	0.60	0.22	5.9	1.0	16.1	6.3	5.1	1.6	1.0	3.7	11.1	163.7	87.7
Santa Rosa	6.9	0.77	0.47	7.0	1.1	16.3	1.9	5.4	2.0	1.0	2.5	10.4	171.1	86.3
Stockton	8.1	0.55	0.45	9.2	1.7	19.4	4.4	5.8	1.9	1.7	5.2	12.6	194.0	98.1
Ventura	7.7	0.59	0.23	6.8	1.7	14.0	5.1	6.9	1.8	1.4	5.1	11.2	177.5	97.5
Colorado														
Boulder	8.1	0.20	0.18	12.6	2.0	12.7	5.1	6.8	2.0	1.2	3.3	10.4	167.2	87.4
Colorado Springs	8.3	0.67	0.39	7.6	1.5	12.5	4.2	8.4	1.7	1.6	3.9	15.7	180.5	85.4
Denver	8.4	0.60	0.37	8.1	1.9	14.4	3.7	8.0	2.6	1.7	4.1	13.6	182.1	85.3
Fort Collins	8.0	0.49	0.36	7.1	2.5	10.5	2.8	9.2	2.0	1.3	3.8	13.1	172.3	96.9
Grand Junction	7.0	0.55	0.30	7.2	1.8	13.5	5.0	8.1	1.6	1.4	3.5	10.8	166.4	84.2
Greeley	8.1	0.75	0.59	10.3	2.3	15.4	5.4	11.0	2.1	1.6	4.0	14.5	193.9	95.1
Pueblo	8.5	0.53	0.55	6.2	1.9	13.9	2.8	7.7	2.0	1.9	3.5	14.1	179.5	93.0
Connecticut														
Bridgeport	7.4	0.54	0.32	6.1	2.0	17.3	5.4	5.6	2.9	1.8	3.2	10.6	177.3	88.0
Hartford	7.0	0.65	0.37	7.0	1.3	16.5	7.2	5.8	2.7	1.7	3.6	12.3	176.1	90.6
New Haven	7.0	0.59	0.38	6.9	1.4	16.7	5.2	6.1	3.3	1.6	4.3	13.2	185.6	91.9
Delaware														
Wilmington	8.0	0.62	0.54	10.6	2.4	21.6	5.7	7.8	2.6	2.4	5.2	13.7	215.3	94.0
District of Columbia														
Washington	7.7	0.73	0.39	10.2	2.4	21.9	7.5	7.4	3.1	2.5	6.2	13.9	229.1	95.9
Florida														
Bradenton	7.4	0.43	0.17	7.1	1.3	15.0	3.8	7.5	1.3	1.1	3.3	7.7	162.1	94.0
Clearwater	8.4	0.45	0.36	9.4	1.7	18.1	4.5	8.4	1.8	1.7	4.6	7.4	204.2	104.0
Fort Lauderdale	8.0	0.49	0.35	7.6	1.5	18.7	5.6	5.7	2.6	1.5	3.4	6.6	190.2	95.7
Fort Myers	7.6	0.55	0.40	8.4	1.2	17.5	3.2	6.5	1.7	1.7	3.8	7.6	176.1	98.9
Gainesville	8.3	0.45	0.28	13.0	2.2	22.5	7.3	10.8	2.6	2.1	7.1	15.7	229.9	88.5
Hudson	7.6	0.44	0.32	12.5	2.3	24.0	7.8	9.6	2.1	2.2	5.1	8.1	237.7	108.6
Jacksonville	8.5	0.53	0.37	13.1	2.3	25.0	4.3	9.1	2.9	2.2	8.2	13.0	248.6	99.2
Lakeland	7.7	0.52	0.26	9.7	1.9	17.5	4.5	6.1	1.9	1.3	6.2	10.3	205.0	94.1
Miami	8.0	0.46	0.44	13.1	2.5	22.6	8.6	6.4	3.9	3.4	5.7	9.0	241.1	92.6
Ocala	7.4	0.37	0.30	10.1	1.7	17.2	4.3	7.0	1.6	1.7	4.2	7.4	176.6	92.3
Orlando	7.8	0.51	0.34	9.5	1.3	19.1	5.9	7.5	2.0	1.6	5.0	10.1	207.8	95.7
Ormond Beach	8.7	0.55	0.47	6.6	0.8	15.2	3.1	5.0	1.6	1.3	3.6	6.8	167.2	91.3
Panama City	9.0	0.65	0.27	16.0	3.4	26.3	2.6	10.7	3.3	2.9	8.9	16.1	261.6	103.2
Pensacola	8.6	0.58	0.41	13.5	2.1	22.1	4.4	10.0	2.9	2.6	6.9	12.6	254.8	100.8
Sarasota	8.1	0.54	0.31	7.2	1.2	14.6	4.3	5.4	1.7	1.1	3.2	7.3	166.8	97.1
St Petersburg	8.9	0.49	0.46	10.1	1.2	20.2	3.7	7.0	1.8	1.7	5.2	7.9	205.3	107.6
Tallahassee	8.7	0.60	0.43	12.5	4.6	20.9	6.2	13.1	3.2	3.1	6.6	17.0	248.3	95.7
Tampa	8.5	0.46	0.34	10.3	1.9	18.4	3.7	7.0	2.3	2.0	5.1	8.7	208.3	95.2
Georgia														
Albany	9.8	0.51	0.55	14.5	3.0	22.1	5.8	11.7	3.2	3.0	6.9	18.5	246.4	102.0
Atlanta	9.3	0.69	0.40	13.1	2.7	20.9	5.8	10.0	3.0	2.5	8.9	17.3	252.3	95.5
Augusta	8.7	0.50	0.31	9.6	2.6	19.4	4.3	12.1	3.1	2.8	8.6	20.8	243.0	95.9
Columbus	9.3	0.73	0.54	8.7	2.4	20.4	4.7	9.2	2.7	3.4	5.9	14.2	221.5	99.1
Macon	8.9	0.54	0.45	11.5	3.1	23.0	8.1	11.8	3.2	3.0	10.1	19.3	268.8	102.1
Rome	9.6	0.66	0.44	14.3	3.2	23.5	2.7	9.9	2.2	2.9	10.7	14.7	264.7	102.9

Hospital Referral Region	Hip Fracture	Ankle Fracture	Radius/Ulna/Wrist Fracture	C.O.P.D.	Adult Bronchitis and Asthma	CHF	Angina Pectoris	Adult Gastroenteritis	Cellulitis	Diabetes Age 35+	Kidney and Urinary Tract Infections	Adult Simple Pneumonia	All Medical Discharges	All Surgical Discharges
Savannah	8.3	0.42	0.41	12.7	4.5	23.0	5.6	11.2	3.0	2.7	7.5	19.8	262.2	99.9
Hawaii														
Honolulu	5.2	0.25	0.23	4.4	1.7	12.0	2.5	3.9	1.9	1.6	2.9	8.5	148.6	64.5
Idaho														
Boise	7.1	0.58	0.42	6.8	2.2	12.5	4.8	6.8	1.7	1.3	3.8	12.7	164.0	92.8
Idaho Falls	6.9	0.63	0.24	4.5	1.9	9.4	2.1	6.3	2.3	1.4	3.9	13.9	150.5	88.1
Illinois														
Aurora	7.9	0.91	0.49	8.0	1.7	18.5	3.3	7.0	2.9	2.0	6.0	16.6	206.1	95.9
Blue Island	7.5	0.69	0.59	9.9	2.3	25.6	4.9	8.9	4.0	2.7	7.8	16.4	266.0	101.3
Chicago	7.3	0.67	0.57	10.8	2.6	27.4	6.6	9.4	4.8	3.3	8.3	15.9	279.0	98.3
Elgin	7.6	0.59	0.36	10.2	2.6	21.9	4.5	9.4	3.1	2.8	6.2	15.7	230.7	92.1
Evanston	7.2	0.75	0.50	5.9	1.8	19.1	4.0	9.1	3.8	1.9	5.7	13.2	219.6	93.5
Hinsdale	7.7	0.68	0.42	6.9	2.0	17.0	2.8	6.7	3.1	2.0	6.5	14.6	191.3	93.1
Joliet	7.3	0.85	0.39	14.6	3.9	25.9	5.5	12.0	4.7	4.3	8.3	19.9	276.5	103.8
Melrose Park	7.4	0.68	0.41	8.1	2.0	21.7	4.4	7.8	3.4	2.4	6.5	13.2	219.8	94.8
Peoria	7.9	0.82	0.46	9.8	2.6	19.8	5.3	7.8	2.3	2.2	4.8	13.8	204.1	94.2
Rockford	7.7	0.61	0.32	9.2	2.7	20.0	5.7	9.4	2.8	2.3	5.1	15.1	210.8	90.8
Springfield	8.4	0.74	0.41	12.5	4.4	22.2	6.0	11.8	3.0	3.1	6.4	19.5	248.8	100.2
Urbana	8.0	0.64	0.38	11.3	3.4	21.8	8.0	10.5	2.7	2.6	6.2	18.3	223.1	92.5
Bloomington	7.9	0.89	0.63	7.8	2.0	18.9	4.2	8.6	2.0	2.0	3.4	12.2	203.8	95.2
Indiana														
Evansville	8.7	0.58	0.51	14.5	4.7	24.3	6.5	12.4	2.8	3.3	9.1	17.9	263.0	90.6
Fort Wayne	8.2	0.67	0.22	7.1	2.5	18.8	5.8	7.2	2.2	1.8	5.0	12.4	186.1	86.2
Gary	7.2	0.74	0.51	12.4	3.9	26.5	5.3	10.5	3.6	4.3	7.0	16.0	262.7	106.8
Indianapolis	8.6	0.69	0.40	12.0	2.9	23.2	6.3	9.9	2.6	2.9	7.5	17.5	237.8	91.0
Lafayette	8.5	0.61	0.16	8.6	2.4	16.0	4.4	7.8	1.8	1.9	4.0	13.3	187.0	84.3
Muncie	9.2	0.81	0.31	11.6	3.9	22.3	5.9	11.3	2.7	4.1	8.5	16.6	234.6	91.1
Munster	7.3	0.62	0.50	10.8	3.1	29.7	5.8	9.9	3.9	3.7	6.8	14.8	268.2	105.9
South Bend	7.9	0.55	0.28	7.8	2.5	19.2	5.2	7.1	2.3	2.4	4.5	12.4	183.9	88.0
Terre Haute	9.1	0.85	0.42	11.6	2.3	22.9	4.2	9.1	2.6	3.5	6.8	15.6	231.9	100.5
Iowa														
Cedar Rapids	7.3	0.66	0.39	8.0	1.6	13.8	3.2	6.7	2.4	1.5	3.8	15.2	170.8	97.9
Davenport	8.1	0.80	0.29	10.1	2.0	19.9	6.5	9.0	2.2	2.4	4.5	17.4	217.9	90.3
Des Moines	7.9	0.77	0.41	8.9	2.8	19.1	5.1	10.8	2.7	2.1	5.4	18.1	222.1	98.0
Dubuque	7.9	1.05	0.59	8.3	1.6	19.5	6.0	10.6	2.4	2.1	3.2	12.7	215.2	97.5
Iowa City	7.6	0.72	0.55	8.6	2.9	17.3	10.3	11.3	2.7	2.7	5.1	18.4	229.3	87.2
Mason City	7.9	0.58	0.25	6.0	1.9	14.8	3.6	7.0	2.5	1.5	3.2	12.6	165.1	93.0
Sioux City	7.8	0.71	0.34	7.0	2.0	16.6	3.8	9.6	2.0	1.9	3.9	18.7	191.7	97.5
Waterloo	8.3	0.57	0.41	9.8	2.6	18.4	5.4	9.2	2.8	2.0	4.7	15.2	202.8	92.4
Kansas														
Topeka	8.5	0.60	0.48	7.6	1.9	16.4	4.8	9.2	2.0	2.2	4.6	15.6	179.5	91.7
Wichita	8.7	0.69	0.39	8.6	2.9	18.9	5.8	11.3	2.6	3.7	4.9	19.9	229.0	103.3
Kentucky														
Covington	8.8	0.55	0.30	12.9	2.1	27.0	2.5	12.3	2.4	2.7	8.2	23.0	275.2	90.8
Lexington	8.7	0.73	0.33	24.1	4.2	27.2	8.2	13.8	2.9	4.1	11.1	23.7	312.3	81.8
Louisville	9.2	0.75	0.48	16.3	3.5	25.8	5.4	12.0	2.8	3.5	8.8	21.4	272.2	95.7

Hospital Referral Region	Hip Fracture	Ankle Fracture	Radius/Ulna/Wrist Fracture	C.O.P.D.	Adult Bronchitis and Asthma	CHF	Angina Pectoris	Adult Gastroenteritis	Cellulitis	Diabetes Age 35+	Kidney and Urinary Tract Infections	Adult Simple Pneumonia	All Medical Discharges	All Surgical Discharges
Owensboro	8.5	0.81	0.64	13.0	3.4	28.7	11.2	14.1	2.2	3.0	7.9	23.9	280.6	105.2
Paducah	8.3	0.83	0.41	16.3	4.4	24.0	6.7	15.1	2.7	3.4	7.3	20.6	295.2	103.3
Louisiana														
Alexandria	7.6	0.71	0.54	13.7	6.0	31.3	7.8	15.9	5.4	4.0	12.9	23.1	319.5	104.9
Baton Rouge	9.0	0.59	0.30	11.9	3.8	23.8	4.8	10.0	4.0	2.3	10.5	20.1	262.9	95.4
Houma	7.3	0.42	0.43	17.6	7.5	32.9	7.9	13.0	5.5	3.3	8.5	18.5	301.9	119.8
Lafayette	7.5	0.40	0.33	12.3	3.5	26.3	5.1	10.9	3.0	3.5	9.4	17.6	260.3	103.8
Lake Charles	8.2	0.51	0.56	10.6	3.4	33.6	5.5	12.1	4.1	3.6	14.2	24.5	317.0	106.7
Metairie	9.1	0.64	0.34	13.2	3.9	32.6	6.9	9.4	5.0	3.6	10.2	18.5	285.0	108.9
Monroe	9.1	0.69	0.43	19.3	7.8	29.2	8.8	19.9	5.5	4.7	12.6	23.8	352.0	100.8
New Orleans	8.4	0.50	0.49	12.2	2.3	31.3	5.3	8.1	4.8	2.6	8.9	14.5	263.9	103.8
Shreveport	8.2	0.61	0.63	11.6	4.1	22.4	5.3	12.5	4.1	2.7	8.6	23.2	265.4	99.4
Slidell	8.2	0.84	0.55	18.1	4.0	37.7	8.9	18.1	6.6	3.4	12.1	22.6	343.9	112.2
Maine														
Bangor	7.4	0.80	0.37	13.5	2.8	21.3	13.0	11.5	2.7	3.0	5.0	16.8	256.9	94.3
Portland	7.7	0.75	0.39	9.9	2.1	19.0	7.9	9.0	2.2	2.1	3.9	12.5	213.0	90.4
Maryland														
Baltimore	7.9	0.65	0.49	11.4	2.0	24.8	9.6	8.9	3.7	2.2	7.8	15.4	276.9	108.2
Salisbury	7.2	0.66	0.43	11.6	1.8	25.2	7.3	9.3	2.8	2.7	4.6	14.9	244.3	97.5
Takoma Park	7.4	0.73	0.40	6.1	1.3	18.4	5.5	6.5	2.5	1.8	5.7	11.2	207.4	94.7
Massachusetts														
Boston	7.4	0.65	0.50	11.6	2.2	23.1	5.9	8.3	4.2	2.1	6.0	14.0	241.5	91.6
Springfield	7.5	0.61	0.28	8.0	2.4	20.7	8.8	8.1	3.0	2.5	5.0	15.7	196.9	81.5
Worcester	8.1	0.80	0.55	11.7	1.9	24.6	6.7	8.5	4.5	2.2	6.6	18.2	242.3	95.3
Michigan														
Ann Arbor	7.2	0.60	0.32	10.6	2.5	21.9	6.9	8.2	3.3	2.2	6.2	13.6	229.5	96.1
Dearborn	6.8	0.78	0.32	11.2	1.6	29.3	9.2	6.9	4.5	2.3	7.9	13.8	244.1	100.1
Detroit	7.2	0.62	0.31	11.8	2.2	27.5	10.4	7.2	3.7	2.3	7.4	14.8	246.7	100.5
Flint	7.5	0.50	0.32	12.2	2.4	26.9	9.2	8.6	2.7	2.7	6.0	15.0	247.1	111.4
Grand Rapids	7.9	0.86	0.42	6.7	1.8	18.0	4.5	6.4	2.4	1.6	4.1	13.9	173.7	87.5
Kalamazoo	7.6	0.66	0.24	7.5	1.9	17.8	4.2	6.5	2.3	1.6	4.7	14.8	181.9	102.4
Lansing	7.3	0.68	0.34	9.5	2.2	21.9	7.2	8.2	3.0	2.0	4.3	14.5	213.1	102.2
Marquette	7.2	0.89	0.17	6.8	2.8	19.8	8.0	9.3	3.0	1.8	4.0	16.1	211.4	92.8
Muskegon	7.8	0.67	0.26	5.5	1.5	17.2	3.8	6.3	2.1	1.4	4.5	12.3	170.3	93.3
Petoskey	6.2	0.70	0.22	6.8	1.8	18.0	7.3	7.7	1.9	1.9	3.9	12.2	193.0	95.7
Pontiac	7.7	0.87	0.26	12.6	1.9	26.0	9.1	9.1	3.5	2.1	6.4	14.1	253.1	100.9
Royal Oak	7.3	0.59	0.47	8.1	1.6	21.4	6.3	6.0	3.2	1.8	5.9	10.7	212.5	100.4
Saginaw	7.0	0.72	0.33	10.3	2.7	24.5	6.6	8.2	2.5	2.6	5.1	14.0	232.8	108.1
St Joseph	6.4	0.77	0.26	7.1	1.5	19.0	4.2	7.3	2.3	2.0	4.4	13.5	190.8	96.6
Traverse City	6.6	0.77	0.37	8.0	1.9	19.9	4.8	8.6	1.8	1.9	4.1	12.9	207.1	106.3
Minnesota														
Duluth	7.0	0.87	0.51	7.0	2.0	17.0	6.5	8.8	2.2	2.0	4.3	13.0	203.3	93.6
Minneapolis	7.1	0.75	0.44	6.8	2.0	16.6	5.4	8.5	2.3	1.7	3.6	15.1	194.7	90.1
Rochester	7.2	0.74	0.53	6.7	2.1	16.5	5.6	6.9	3.2	1.9	4.0	15.4	187.9	86.6
St Cloud	7.1	0.43	0.20	7.0	2.8	15.6	4.5	10.8	2.6	2.0	3.3	16.6	192.3	87.7
St Paul	7.8	1.03	0.41	7.6	1.8	17.4	7.6	8.9	2.4	2.0	4.9	14.3	209.8	92.2

Hospital Referral Region	Hip Fracture	Ankle Fracture	Radius/Ulna/Wrist Fracture	C.O.P.D.	Adult Bronchitis and Asthma	CHF	Angina Pectoris	Adult Gastroenteritis	Cellulitis	Diabetes Age 35+	Kidney and Urinary Tract Infections	Adult Simple Pneumonia	All Medical Discharges	All Surgical Discharges
Mississippi														
Gulfport	8.4	0.43	0.35	15.1	2.4	39.3	3.3	17.9	3.4	3.1	10.6	15.2	324.5	106.0
Hattiesburg	7.5	0.69	0.76	18.0	6.1	28.0	10.1	22.5	4.0	4.3	11.0	22.4	338.7	105.7
Jackson	8.3	0.62	0.46	14.9	5.6	25.4	8.6	17.0	3.8	3.4	8.9	19.3	297.8	88.0
Meridian	7.9	0.93	0.49	15.8	5.2	28.3	5.8	20.4	4.6	4.0	11.0	32.3	353.5	94.0
Oxford	8.8	1.01	1.16	18.5	5.2	30.1	7.4	19.4	4.1	4.0	7.4	23.4	335.7	98.5
Tupelo	8.6	0.99	0.50	17.7	5.6	24.7	8.5	17.4	3.6	3.8	8.3	21.5	290.6	90.7
Missouri														
Cape Girardeau	8.0	0.64	0.32	11.1	1.4	24.1	4.2	9.6	2.2	2.8	5.5	19.3	218.0	86.1
Columbia	8.5	0.70	0.42	11.6	2.6	19.4	3.3	10.1	2.3	2.7	5.8	18.0	222.5	100.7
Joplin	9.5	0.61	0.41	14.5	4.7	24.0	4.6	14.9	3.0	3.5	9.5	21.0	277.3	106.0
Kansas City	9.1	0.71	0.44	12.0	2.7	20.9	3.9	10.1	3.0	2.3	6.3	19.0	229.0	97.8
Springfield	9.0	0.80	0.35	9.6	2.1	20.1	3.0	9.2	1.6	2.3	5.0	12.9	205.3	95.3
St Louis	8.9	0.72	0.50	10.1	2.3	22.8	5.1	8.9	3.1	2.6	6.1	17.3	236.4	99.2
Montana														
Billings	7.4	0.81	0.48	9.4	2.6	17.0	4.7	10.5	2.5	2.2	4.1	16.3	211.4	91.0
Great Falls	8.0	0.72	0.62	13.5	4.3	19.4	3.3	15.4	2.9	2.7	5.4	19.1	259.6	93.9
Missoula	7.9	0.79	0.56	10.5	3.2	14.8	3.5	13.1	2.0	1.9	4.3	16.5	210.3	94.5
Nebraska														
Lincoln	7.6	0.73	0.30	4.9	2.4	13.7	4.4	8.1	2.0	1.5	3.0	15.1	159.8	88.4
Omaha	8.0	0.72	0.37	8.7	3.1	17.5	4.5	8.5	2.7	1.6	4.3	18.1	196.3	94.3
Nevada														
Las Vegas	8.5	0.47	0.30	12.3	0.9	19.9	3.0	5.7	2.2	1.8	5.4	13.6	191.2	95.1
Reno	8.1	0.68	0.36	8.5	1.1	15.4	3.5	6.0	2.2	1.7	4.2	14.6	173.8	80.6
New Hampshire														
Lebanon	7.6	0.60	0.30	8.3	1.7	16.5	8.5	8.2	2.6	2.3	4.1	15.7	195.5	78.2
Manchester	7.5	0.62	0.35	8.7	1.7	17.1	4.6	7.3	2.2	1.8	3.4	12.0	181.4	82.5
New Jersey														
Camden	7.5	0.65	0.63	10.5	2.2	25.9	9.8	9.7	3.1	3.0	5.5	12.7	247.9	98.6
Hackensack	7.2	0.65	0.46	8.4	2.0	21.7	8.8	8.5	3.1	2.6	4.8	10.3	216.9	98.5
Morristown	7.5	0.69	0.41	8.0	1.9	19.1	7.1	8.2	2.9	2.2	4.4	12.4	210.4	93.4
New Brunswick	7.1	0.75	0.63	8.2	1.9	23.9	9.9	8.7	3.4	2.9	5.3	13.2	237.6	96.6
Newark	6.7	0.68	0.67	11.1	2.0	27.0	11.9	10.1	4.0	4.0	5.4	12.5	258.9	100.0
Paterson	7.5	0.70	0.44	9.1	2.1	24.4	9.4	9.1	3.2	3.0	5.3	15.0	232.8	99.1
Ridgewood	7.5	0.68	0.51	7.3	2.4	20.6	5.9	8.8	3.3	2.1	5.0	14.9	215.8	93.0
New Mexico														
Albuquerque	8.7	0.63	0.55	7.3	2.8	13.6	3.3	8.4	2.6	2.1	6.3	18.9	188.1	83.0
New York														
Albany	7.1	0.65	0.36	11.0	2.2	20.9	8.1	9.0	3.5	2.3	4.7	16.2	217.8	87.2
Binghamton	7.2	0.71	0.52	10.4	2.1	23.4	9.3	10.1	2.7	2.8	4.6	18.2	220.1	82.5
Bronx	7.6	0.62	0.57	9.2	3.0	24.2	8.6	7.6	4.1	3.3	5.6	15.2	236.6	92.7
Buffalo	7.0	0.58	0.38	9.3	2.2	22.8	7.9	8.5	3.2	2.7	5.2	13.2	218.0	89.5
Elmira	7.2	0.56	0.44	13.8	3.5	21.5	6.4	10.9	3.6	2.9	4.6	14.2	232.7	88.3
East Long Island	7.1	0.59	0.51	7.7	1.8	20.0	7.0	7.2	3.5	2.5	5.2	12.8	212.3	92.1
New York	7.2	0.58	0.60	8.5	2.1	20.1	6.7	6.6	4.1	3.1	5.5	12.3	212.7	93.2
Rochester	7.4	0.76	0.45	8.8	2.6	20.1	7.8	9.1	3.6	2.2	5.1	13.7	207.3	95.4

Hospital Referral Region	Hip Fracture	Ankle Fracture	Radius/Ulna/Wrist Fracture	C.O.P.D.	Adult Bronchitis and Asthma	CHF	Angina Pectoris	Adult Gastroenteritis	Cellulitis	Diabetes Age 35+	Kidney and Urinary Tract Infections	Adult Simple Pneumonia	All Medical Discharges	All Surgical Discharges
Syracuse	7.2	0.67	0.40	11.3	2.4	20.7	8.3	9.6	3.0	2.4	4.8	15.0	210.5	89.2
White Plains	7.4	0.74	0.50	8.7	2.5	21.5	8.3	8.8	3.1	2.8	4.7	13.3	230.5	93.3
North Carolina														
Asheville	9.0	0.99	0.43	11.2	2.8	16.2	7.0	9.0	1.8	1.9	5.0	14.9	203.0	80.8
Charlotte	9.3	0.64	0.27	8.9	2.2	19.5	4.6	7.8	2.1	1.7	5.3	13.7	206.3	89.8
Durham	9.0	0.75	0.40	9.3	2.2	18.0	4.7	7.4	2.0	1.7	5.3	12.7	201.5	86.7
Greensboro	9.4	0.64	0.45	8.9	1.9	18.7	5.2	7.9	1.9	1.8	5.3	12.9	197.1	91.9
Greenville	8.6	0.51	0.23	11.1	3.5	22.3	9.3	9.9	2.6	2.1	6.2	15.7	237.0	91.0
Hickory	9.4	0.65	0.20	9.1	1.6	16.4	2.9	8.5	1.8	1.7	4.8	15.5	205.2	90.7
Raleigh	8.6	0.59	0.41	11.0	1.9	20.5	7.0	8.9	2.4	2.0	6.2	14.3	225.5	93.2
Wilmington	8.6	0.50	0.27	10.9	3.2	21.8	8.6	11.4	2.8	2.1	6.7	13.4	235.2	95.8
Winston-Salem	9.4	0.93	0.51	11.3	2.7	19.5	5.8	10.1	2.2	2.1	6.0	14.8	230.2	93.2
North Dakota														
Bismarck	6.3	0.63	0.42	9.1	4.7	21.6	6.6	12.6	3.3	3.4	5.0	20.9	230.2	99.9
Fargo Moorhead -Mn	7.1	0.79	0.32	7.3	2.9	16.6	5.8	8.6	2.5	2.1	4.3	18.0	190.5	89.8
Grand Forks	7.4	0.82	0.26	7.3	3.2	18.8	5.9	10.6	2.5	1.8	5.3	20.5	209.3	86.0
Minot	7.7	0.76	0.47	10.7	4.9	20.2	3.6	10.8	3.7	3.1	4.2	20.7	212.3	100.1
Ohio														
Akron	8.1	0.83	0.36	11.0	2.4	27.2	6.6	8.9	4.0	2.3	11.0	18.8	261.1	96.4
Canton	7.6	0.74	0.29	11.4	2.1	20.7	4.8	7.9	2.9	2.0	5.4	14.2	212.3	89.4
Cincinnati	8.7	0.71	0.39	10.0	1.9	21.9	4.8	7.8	2.6	2.2	6.4	18.8	220.2	92.2
Cleveland	8.0	0.74	0.45	12.7	2.3	26.8	8.2	8.7	3.9	2.3	7.1	14.9	244.4	100.2
Columbus	8.2	0.80	0.43	12.6	2.8	24.0	8.9	9.9	3.1	2.7	6.9	17.9	243.1	99.6
Dayton	8.4	0.58	0.28	10.6	3.2	22.2	8.5	8.6	2.5	2.2	5.9	14.3	215.4	99.2
Elyria	6.7	0.56	0.50	13.6	2.2	26.8	7.0	8.9	3.5	3.0	7.3	16.5	249.4	115.3
Kettering	8.9	0.65	0.35	8.3	2.0	17.6	4.4	7.3	2.2	2.1	5.1	12.5	188.4	93.3
Toledo	8.0	0.81	0.42	12.2	2.3	25.8	8.9	9.8	3.3	2.6	6.6	15.5	241.5	104.8
Youngstown	7.8	0.86	0.51	12.3	3.3	29.1	8.0	10.4	3.2	3.4	6.7	16.4	262.7	100.9
Oklahoma														
Lawton	8.9	0.53	0.22	7.4	1.8	18.9	5.9	8.8	2.3	2.1	8.3	16.3	221.3	89.2
Oklahoma City	8.9	0.54	0.36	10.3	2.4	21.2	6.3	10.3	2.3	2.3	6.7	17.5	233.4	100.9
Tulsa	9.2	0.67	0.39	9.2	2.2	19.8	4.5	8.4	2.0	2.0	5.4	15.5	215.7	90.9
Oregon														
Bend	6.8	0.63	0.21	5.2	1.0	9.6	2.6	5.8	1.2	0.9	3.3	11.4	136.9	106.1
Eugene	7.2	0.68	0.30	6.4	1.4	15.7	4.7	7.0	1.4	1.2	3.4	11.0	157.9	85.1
Medford	6.9	0.76	0.36	5.9	1.4	11.5	3.5	5.7	1.5	1.2	3.3	13.2	148.5	82.2
Portland	7.6	0.67	0.34	5.8	1.4	15.0	3.8	6.3	1.8	1.3	3.8	11.5	166.2	81.9
Salem	7.1	0.35	0.20	4.2	1.1	12.1	2.1	4.8	1.2	1.1	2.5	9.3	122.3	76.1
Pennsylvania														
Allentown	7.3	0.80	0.44	9.5	3.3	25.4	7.3	10.2	4.2	2.7	5.8	12.5	244.3	109.6
Altoona	7.8	0.63	0.37	13.5	3.7	28.6	15.2	12.5	3.4	2.7	5.5	12.5	265.3	96.2
Danville	7.8	0.94	0.45	10.7	3.3	24.1	11.3	9.4	3.2	3.4	6.0	16.8	243.4	94.4
Erie	8.0	0.88	0.43	12.8	3.9	24.8	9.6	11.3	3.8	3.4	5.8	16.9	255.6	94.3
Harrisburg	7.8	0.88	0.45	8.3	2.0	23.4	5.7	8.2	2.7	2.4	4.4	12.4	212.0	94.8
Johnstown	7.2	0.71	0.81	15.8	3.8	32.6	10.9	14.3	3.3	3.4	7.7	15.8	313.5	110.7
Lancaster	7.7	0.61	0.51	8.3	2.1	17.4	2.9	7.8	2.5	2.1	4.0	11.0	186.3	98.0

Hospital Referral Region	Hip Fracture	Ankle Fracture	Radius/Ulna/Wrist Fracture	C.O.P.D.	Adult Bronchitis and Asthma	CHF	Angina Pectoris	Adult Gastroenteritis	Cellulitis	Diabetes Age 35+	Kidney and Urinary Tract Infections	Adult Simple Pneumonia	All Medical Discharges	All Surgical Discharges
Philadelphia	8.1	0.74	0.83	11.0	2.3	26.5	8.8	8.9	3.9	2.4	6.7	13.3	260.0	106.6
Pittsburgh	7.4	0.79	0.58	15.5	3.7	30.8	9.0	11.7	4.3	3.3	8.0	17.2	295.0	108.5
Reading	7.0	0.80	0.61	8.8	3.1	23.9	6.6	9.2	3.4	2.6	4.4	12.7	218.6	98.9
Sayre	7.5	0.74	0.55	13.0	3.8	24.9	10.6	13.0	3.1	3.1	6.0	18.4	261.1	96.5
Scranton	7.0	0.80	0.55	9.5	3.3	27.2	7.8	8.9	3.6	2.8	6.2	15.0	246.1	95.0
Wilkes-Barre	7.5	0.79	0.59	12.6	3.2	28.8	6.5	9.7	3.7	3.6	4.9	11.5	256.1	98.7
York	7.3	0.85	0.39	6.8	2.3	20.8	7.6	8.0	3.1	1.9	4.0	10.7	191.3	93.1
Rhode Island														
Providence	7.0	0.62	0.38	9.5	1.7	21.3	8.2	6.7	3.2	2.1	4.6	11.4	209.7	88.1
South Carolina														
Charleston	8.3	0.44	0.40	9.5	2.4	20.4	3.8	10.3	2.3	2.4	5.8	11.7	217.0	97.9
Columbia	8.2	0.61	0.39	7.4	2.6	17.0	3.9	8.6	2.2	2.1	5.6	14.1	194.9	87.9
Florence	8.8	0.46	0.44	13.2	5.8	28.0	5.9	14.2	4.0	3.9	8.3	18.5	299.0	100.2
Greenville	9.7	0.73	0.26	8.6	2.2	18.5	5.8	8.0	2.0	1.9	5.7	11.9	192.7	90.7
Spartanburg	9.9	0.62	0.30	10.4	3.1	20.9	5.1	10.4	2.7	2.5	6.5	14.4	214.6	85.9
South Dakota														
Rapid City	8.2	0.81	0.43	9.8	2.5	17.5	5.8	10.8	2.9	2.2	4.5	21.5	202.0	94.5
Sioux Falls	7.2	0.76	0.60	8.4	3.2	16.6	6.4	11.0	3.1	2.3	4.0	22.1	215.1	100.3
Tennessee														
Chattanooga	9.0	0.67	0.34	12.5	3.3	24.4	5.1	11.6	2.4	3.2	10.1	15.7	264.6	94.0
Jackson	9.5	0.66	0.52	16.4	3.3	20.5	5.2	10.8	2.5	3.0	8.0	19.1	254.5	91.7
Johnson City	9.0	0.86	0.58	12.6	2.7	20.1	2.8	10.6	2.2	2.0	6.8	16.0	252.0	84.8
Kingsport	9.3	0.86	0.48	23.9	4.7	28.4	10.8	14.5	3.1	3.9	11.2	22.1	327.1	80.0
Knoxville	9.4	0.73	0.45	16.7	3.9	25.4	7.0	12.7	2.5	3.0	9.5	19.7	285.2	90.1
Memphis	9.0	0.64	0.43	13.3	3.2	23.2	5.4	11.1	2.7	2.9	7.3	15.3	247.6	94.9
Nashville	9.0	0.79	0.50	14.9	3.3	26.5	4.5	11.0	2.8	2.7	8.8	16.9	287.7	93.8
Texas														
Abilene	9.4	0.64	0.40	12.5	3.0	22.0	3.9	12.1	2.9	3.2	7.2	17.0	255.8	97.2
Amarillo	9.4	0.53	0.43	9.9	2.3	16.8	4.4	8.7	2.7	2.7	6.8	17.0	211.3	94.1
Austin	9.1	0.46	0.28	7.9	2.2	15.1	3.8	6.7	2.2	1.9	6.6	12.7	178.4	85.8
Beaumont	8.2	0.60	0.40	15.6	3.2	26.6	6.0	11.4	3.6	4.2	12.0	21.2	301.0	104.8
Bryan	9.0	0.55	0.36	8.7	2.1	17.9	4.5	8.4	2.8	2.8	8.5	18.0	195.8	81.4
Corpus Christi	8.3	0.49	0.49	13.0	3.0	31.1	6.9	10.5	4.7	3.7	10.7	13.8	270.0	102.5
Dallas	9.1	0.53	0.37	9.7	2.0	20.1	4.2	6.9	2.2	2.0	7.3	14.9	204.8	92.9
El Paso	7.2	0.48	0.41	7.2	2.1	16.5	2.2	7.0	2.1	3.2	7.6	12.0	184.6	81.7
Fort Worth	9.7	0.55	0.37	9.7	1.8	18.9	4.5	6.4	2.0	1.9	6.2	13.7	195.2	86.1
Harlingen	6.6	0.44	0.35	8.2	1.7	22.7	5.1	8.0	2.6	4.4	10.3	12.2	209.3	95.6
Houston	8.6	0.57	0.46	10.9	2.3	22.5	4.1	8.5	3.4	2.7	8.8	14.4	236.2	99.0
Longview	8.8	0.59	0.54	12.5	1.8	21.5	3.2	7.2	2.1	1.6	6.6	16.7	233.4	94.8
Lubbock	10.2	0.73	0.64	12.0	2.6	23.7	4.1	11.5	2.5	3.1	7.3	22.0	259.4	117.8
Mcallen	7.0	0.43	0.34	9.4	1.8	22.2	5.3	9.0	3.6	4.7	9.0	13.0	209.6	99.5
Odessa	9.7	0.59	0.34	14.0	2.4	19.7	3.2	7.6	1.9	2.9	8.3	15.8	218.2	103.0
San Angelo	9.1	0.69	0.62	12.2	2.7	20.0	5.7	10.1	3.0	3.6	8.7	20.8	227.3	96.7
San Antonio	7.8	0.54	0.41	7.4	2.3	21.8	3.6	7.5	3.2	2.9	8.0	13.3	202.4	91.9
Temple	7.8	0.40	0.18	7.3	2.4	19.1	5.1	6.8	2.5	2.1	7.8	17.2	191.9	79.0
Tyler	8.5	0.61	0.39	10.7	2.2	23.1	4.0	8.3	2.8	2.4	9.1	20.8	238.7	96.7

Hospital Referral Region	Hip Fracture	Ankle Fracture	Radius/Ulna/Wrist Fracture	C.O.P.D.	Adult Bronchitis and Asthma	CHF	Angina Pectoris	Adult Gastroenteritis	Cellulitis	Diabetes Age 35+	Kidney and Urinary Tract Infections	Adult Simple Pneumonia	All Medical Discharges	All Surgical Discharges
Victoria	6.8	0.65	0.21	11.9	3.3	26.8	5.4	13.6	4.4	5.7	9.5	21.2	287.0	96.3
Waco	8.8	0.42	0.31	7.0	1.7	18.2	4.8	6.5	2.0	1.7	6.0	15.6	176.3	82.3
Wichita Falls	9.0	0.58	0.38	8.7	3.0	22.3	6.8	9.9	2.9	2.6	6.8	22.7	243.9	88.2
Utah														
Ogden	7.2	0.81	0.25	3.4	1.0	10.0	1.5	4.3	1.7	1.3	2.4	8.5	129.5	84.7
Provo	7.0	0.62	0.20	2.9	1.8	12.3	2.9	5.6	2.0	1.3	3.6	13.7	146.9	99.0
Salt Lake City	6.8	0.63	0.40	3.7	1.4	10.4	2.7	5.6	1.9	1.3	3.8	11.7	141.9	84.7
Vermont														
Burlington	7.6	0.62	0.28	10.7	2.5	21.0	8.3	11.0	2.8	2.5	4.8	17.6	230.8	91.6
Virginia														
Arlington	8.6	0.74	0.43	7.8	1.7	15.9	5.1	7.3	2.4	1.4	4.7	10.3	190.6	83.9
Charlottesville	8.5	0.88	0.49	11.3	3.3	22.5	5.7	11.6	2.6	2.4	5.1	16.8	245.3	86.0
Lynchburg	9.2	0.75	0.40	8.1	3.6	17.0	3.5	9.9	2.3	2.5	4.8	13.5	195.0	86.5
Newport News	8.5	0.62	0.24	8.2	1.9	19.0	3.4	8.6	2.3	1.6	4.3	11.8	208.6	100.3
Norfolk	8.6	0.66	0.37	11.5	2.4	20.3	5.2	9.9	2.7	2.2	6.0	13.6	223.7	100.1
Richmond	9.0	0.82	0.43	10.9	2.3	20.3	4.9	10.2	2.5	2.2	5.8	11.7	230.0	104.2
Roanoke	9.0	0.79	0.44	15.0	2.2	22.6	6.1	11.9	2.2	2.6	5.8	17.0	257.4	94.3
Winchester	9.3	0.70	0.52	16.0	4.4	30.2	9.3	14.1	3.6	2.7	7.6	19.1	287.6	94.7
Washington														
Everett	7.5	0.72	0.24	5.0	1.0	13.4	3.2	5.3	1.4	1.1	2.7	10.5	159.0	82.9
Olympia	7.6	0.73	0.34	6.9	1.3	15.3	5.7	5.7	1.4	1.0	3.4	14.0	160.5	88.3
Seattle	7.6	0.75	0.36	5.8	1.2	13.4	3.4	6.1	1.9	1.2	3.4	10.3	157.7	84.1
Spokane	7.5	0.60	0.27	7.6	1.4	13.8	4.7	7.0	1.6	1.5	3.3	13.0	171.1	88.5
Tacoma	7.8	0.59	0.34	6.9	0.7	14.3	2.0	5.2	1.3	1.0	3.0	10.3	149.1	81.6
Yakima	6.7	0.42	0.27	6.9	1.3	15.7	3.4	7.9	1.8	1.2	3.4	12.9	172.3	79.5
West Virginia														
Charleston	8.4	0.89	0.56	20.7	3.3	26.7	13.5	14.5	3.1	3.9	9.0	20.8	311.5	97.7
Huntington	8.4	0.68	0.49	17.1	5.1	28.1	10.4	14.8	3.0	4.0	10.4	20.6	304.8	91.4
Morgantown	8.5	0.80	0.31	16.7	3.8	30.0	11.1	11.7	3.4	4.0	8.5	19.8	288.0	93.5
Wisconsin														
Appleton	6.8	0.85	0.37	5.8	1.9	16.6	3.0	7.3	2.0	1.7	2.7	11.2	164.7	90.4
Green Bay	6.7	0.81	0.39	6.5	2.3	18.4	4.5	7.9	2.0	1.8	3.7	10.5	186.1	91.4
La Crosse	6.9	0.79	0.29	6.1	2.1	15.7	7.0	9.5	2.5	1.9	3.6	15.6	200.2	79.4
Madison	7.2	0.75	0.56	7.7	2.0	17.2	5.5	9.5	2.7	1.9	4.4	12.8	201.3	89.2
Marshfield	6.3	0.75	0.25	7.2	2.0	18.1	6.6	9.0	2.3	1.9	4.0	13.3	201.2	88.5
Milwaukee	7.2	0.71	0.46	7.5	1.6	19.8	4.5	7.4	3.0	2.1	4.3	11.6	197.6	97.6
Neenah	7.1	0.54	0.37	7.0	2.1	16.4	2.9	8.3	2.5	1.9	3.2	13.1	182.9	100.9
Wausau	6.1	0.76	0.18	5.4	1.9	16.5	3.9	8.0	2.7	1.5	3.7	12.6	170.1	90.3
Wyoming														
Casper	8.5	0.67	0.39	10.3	2.8	18.1	4.1	12.6	2.7	2.9	5.0	20.3	226.4	97.9
United States														
United States	8.0	0.66	0.43	10.3	2.4	21.2	6.0	8.9	2.9	2.4	6.1	14.6	224.7	94.9

The American Experience of Death

The American Experience of Death

Modern technology has vastly extended the ability to intervene in the lives of patients, most dramatically so when life itself is at stake. But the capability to intervene is not uniformly deployed, and health care providers do not share a uniform propensity to hospitalize dying patients or to use technology at the end of life. The American experience of death varies remarkably from one community to another. For example, in 1994-95:

■ The chance that when death occurred, it occurred in a hospital, varied more than twofold among hospital referral regions, from as few as 20% of deaths to more than 50%.

■ The chance of being in an intensive care unit one or more times during the last six months of life varied by a factor of more than 5, from 9% of deaths in one region to about 48% in another.

■ The number of days Medicare enrollees spent in hospitals during the last six months of life varied by a factor of more than 5 in 1995, from an average of 4.4 days in one hospital referral region to 22.9 days in another.

■ The number of days Medicare enrollees spent in intensive care units during the last six months of life varied by a factor of more than 9 in 1995, from an average of 0.5 days in one hospital referral region to 4.9 days in another.

■ The price-adjusted reimbursements by the Medicare program for hospital (inpatient) care during the last six months of life varied by a factor of 2.8 in 1995, from $5,831 per decedent in the least costly hospital referral region to $16,571 in the most costly region.

Like other medical decisions, end of life decisions about the use of resources are usually influenced by the available supply. The amount of acute care hospital resources allocated to residents of hospital referral regions has a strong influence on the American experience of death.

The Likelihood That Death Will Occur in a Hospital, Rather Than Elsewhere

What are the chances that, when a Medicare enrollee dies, he or she will do so as an inpatient in a hospital? In 1994-95, the chances varied according to where the enrollee lived. In some hospital referral regions, as few as 20% of Medicare deaths occurred in the hospital; in one region, the proportion was more than 50%.

In 48 of the nation's hospital referral regions, the chance of dying in the hospital was 40% or greater. (Areas in dark blue on the map.) Among these regions were Camden, New Jersey (46.0%); Hackensack, New Jersey (45.6%); Memphis, Tennessee (42.2%); and Little Rock, Arkansas (40.3%).

In 84 regions, fewer than 30% of deaths occurred in the hospital. (Light blue areas on the map.) Among these regions were Salt Lake City (22.9%); San Francisco (28.7%); and Cincinnati (29.3%).

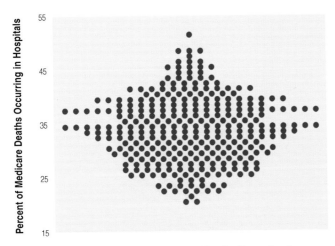

Figure 4.1. Percent of Medicare Deaths Occurring in Hospitals (1994-95)

The percent of Medicare deaths that occurred while the decedent was an inpatient in a hospital ranged from 20% to 51% of all deaths. Rates are age, sex, and race adjusted. Each point represents one of the 306 hospital referral regions in the United States.

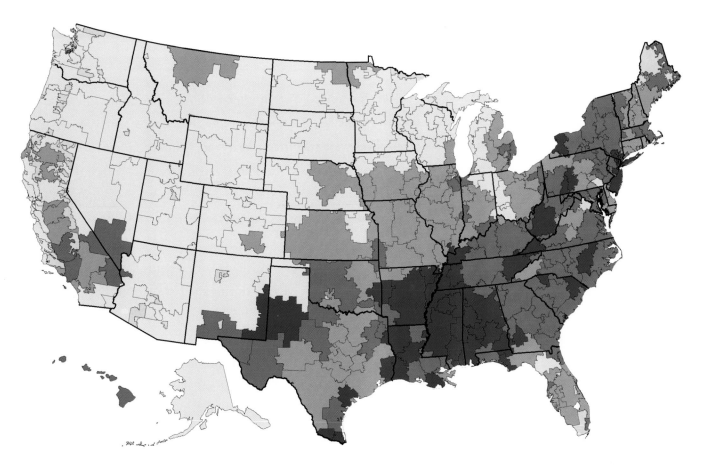

Map 4.1. Percent of Medicare Deaths Occurring in Hospitals (1994-95)

Regions where residents had an above average likelihood of a hospitalized death were primarily in the Middle and South Atlantic states. Medicare enrollees living in Boston, Detroit, Chicago, Los Angeles and parts of Texas also had higher than average likelihoods of dying as inpatients. Lower than average regions were primarily on the West Coast, Alaska, Mountain States and upper Midwest, including Minnesota and parts of Michigan.

Percent of Medicare Deaths Occurring in Hospitals

by Hospital Referral Region (1994-95)

- 40 to   51 (48)
- 35 to < 40 (84)
- 30 to < 35 (90)
- 20 to < 30 (84)
- Not Populated

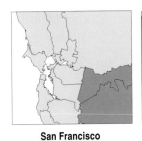
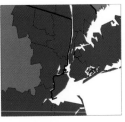
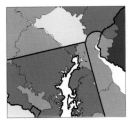
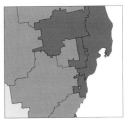

San Francisco   Chicago   New York   Washington-Baltimore   Detroit

The Likelihood of Intensive Care Treatment During the Last Six Months of Life

What are the chances that a Medicare enrollee will be treated in an intensive care unit at some time during the last six months of life? In one region in 1994-95, only 9% of Medicare enrollees were admitted one or more times to intensive care units (either a coronary care or an intensive care unit) during the last six months of their lives; in other regions, more than five times as many enrollees — about 48% — were admitted at least once to intensive care.

Several of the hospital referral regions in which Medicare enrollees had the highest chances for spending time in intensive care during the last six months of their lives were in Florida; they included Miami (47.5% chance of admission to an intensive care unit); St. Petersburg (46.8%); Fort Lauderdale (40.5%); and Jacksonville (40.4%). Hospital referral regions in other parts of the country also had high rates, including Munster, Indiana (47.9%); Gulfport, Mississippi (40.3%); Harlingen, Texas (40.0%); El Paso, Texas (40.0%); Dearborn, Michigan (39.9%); Youngstown, Ohio (39.4%); Texarkana, Arkansas (39.2%); Orange County, California (39.2%); and Elgin, Illinois (39.0%).

The hospital referral regions where Medicare enrollees had the lowest chances of one or more intensive care admissions during the last six months of life included Sun City, Arizona (less than 9%); Bloomington, Illinois (15.6%); Wausau, Wisconsin (17.6%); Topeka, Kansas (18.1%); Bend, Oregon (16.3%); Salt Lake City (21.1%); Portland, Oregon (21.5%); and Providence, Rhode Island (22.0%).

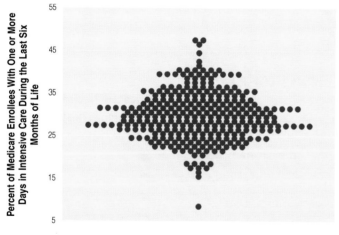

Figure 4.2. Percent of Medicare Enrollees With One or More Admissions to Intensive Care During the Last Six Months of Life (1994-95)

The percent of Medicare enrollees spending one or more days in a coronary care or intensive care unit during the last six months of their lives, after adjusting for differences in age, sex, and race, ranged from less than 9% to more than 45%. Each point represents one of the 306 hospital referral regions in the United States.

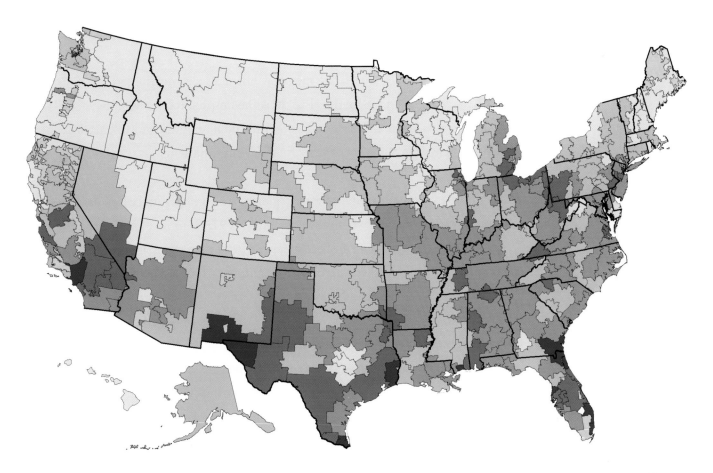

Map 4.2. Percent of Medicare Enrollees Experiencing Intensive Care During the Last Six Months of Life (1994-95)

Medicare residents of southern California, parts of Texas, New Mexico, Florida and the Midwest, Pennsylvania and New Jersey were more likely to spend part of their last six months of life in an intensive care or coronary care unit than Medicare residents of the Northwest, northern New England, central Texas or northern California.

Percent of Medicare Enrollees Experiencing Intensive Care During the Last Six Months of Life

by Hospital Referral Region (1994-95)

■ 40 to 48	(12)
■ 35 to < 40	(44)
■ 30 to < 35	(86)
■ 25 to < 30	(102)
□ 9 to < 25	(62)
Not Populated	

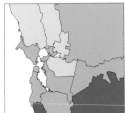

San Francisco

Chicago

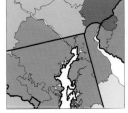

New York

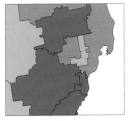

Washington-Baltimore

Detroit

Days in Hospitals During the Last Six Months of Life

The amount of time Americans spend in hospitals during the last six months of their lives depends on where they live. In some hospital referral regions in 1994-95, the average was a low as 4.4 days. In other hospital referral regions, enrollees spent, on average, as many as 22.9 of their final days as inpatients.

In 75 of the nation's hospital referral regions, the average number of days spent in hospitals during the last six months of life was 12 or more. The hospital referral regions in which Medicare enrollees spent the most time as inpatients during the last six months of their lives were in New York and New Jersey. The four highest regions in the nation were Newark, New Jersey (22.9 days); Manhattan (22.0); the Bronx, New York (20.9); and Paterson, New Jersey (20.7). All of New Jersey's seven hospital referral regions, and six of New York's 10 regions, ranked in the top 13 hospital referral regions in the nation for days spent in hospitals during the last six months of life. Other regions with high use of hospitals during the last six months of life included Philadelphia (14.4 days); Miami (14.3); Pittsburgh (13.8); Chicago (13.8); Detroit (13.6); Baltimore (12.9); Boston (12.5); and Birmingham, Alabama (12.2).

In 72 hospital referral regions, the number of days spent in hospitals during the last six months of life was fewer than eight. Among the lowest were Salt Lake City (5.3 days); Denver (7.1); Phoenix, Arizona (7.4); Albuquerque, New Mexico (7.4); and San Francisco (7.5).

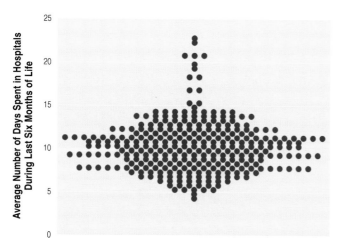

Figure 4.3. Average Number of Days Spent in Hospitals During the Last Six Months of Life (1994-95)

The average number of days of hospital care during the last six months of life, after adjusting for age, sex and race, ranged from 4.4 to 22.9. Each point represents one of the 306 hospital referral regions in the United States.

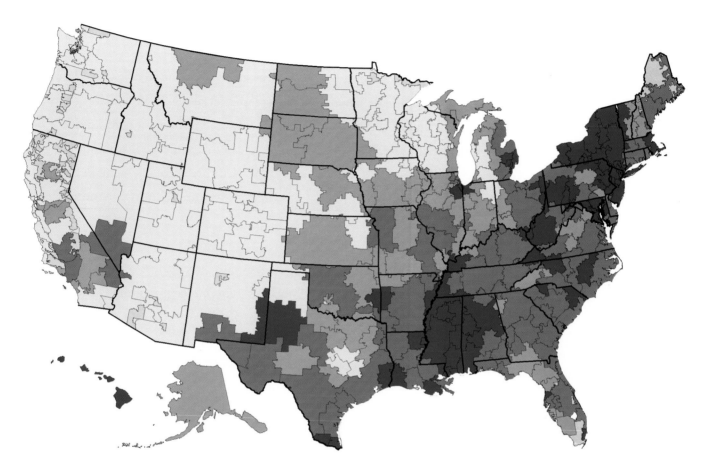

Map 4.3. Average Number of Days Spent in Hospitals During the Last Six Months of Life (1994-95)

Regions with high use of hospitals for Medicare enrollees in the last six months of life included New York, New Jersey, the South, Hawaii, the Chicago area and parts of Texas, New England and Michigan. Regions with low use included Minnesota, the Mountain States, the Desert Southwest and much of the West Coast.

Average Number of Days Spent in Hospitals During the Last Six Months of Life

by Hospital Referral Region (1994-95)

- 12.0 to 22.9 (75)
- 10.0 to < 12.0 (87)
- 8.0 to < 10.0 (72)
- 4.4 to < 8.0 (72)
- Not Populated

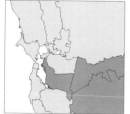

San Francisco

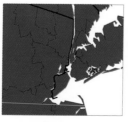

Chicago

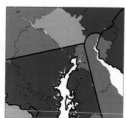

New York

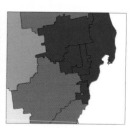

Washington-Baltimore

Detroit

Days in Intensive Care During the Last Six Months of Life

The number of days that Medicare enrollees spend in intensive care units during the last six months of life depends on the hospital referral region in which they live. In 1994-95, the region with the lowest use rate was the retirement community of Sun City, Arizona; the region with the highest was another retirement community — St. Petersburg, Florida. On average in 1994-95, Medicare enrollees living in St. Petersburg spent nine times more days (4.9) in intensive care than their counterparts in Sun City (0.5).

There were 47 regions that had average stays in intensive care of three or more days; 47 regions had stays of between 2.5 and less than 3.0 days. Among the hospital referral regions with high rates of days spent in intensive care during the last six months of life were St. Petersburg, Florida (4.9 days); Munster, Indiana (4.9); Miami (4.8); Beaumont, Texas (4.2); Los Angeles (4.1); Jacksonville, Florida (3.7); New Brunswick, New Jersey (3.6); and Palm Springs, California (3.5).

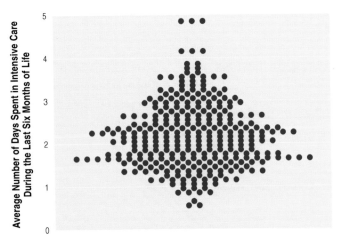

Figure 4.4. Average Number of Days Spent in Intensive Care During the Last Six Months of Life (1994-95)

The average number of days of stay in intensive care (ICU and CCU) during the last six months of life, after adjusting for age, sex and race, ranged from 0.5 days to 4.9. Each point represents one of the 306 hospital referral regions in the United States.

There were 55 hospital referral regions in which enrollees in the last six months of life had average stays in intensive care of fewer than 1.5 days. Seventy-eight regions had between 1.5 and 2.0 days in intensive care during the last six months of life. The average number of days were low in Portland, Oregon (1.0); Salt Lake City (1.1); Austin, Texas (1.4); Denver (1.5); Cincinnati (1.7); and Tallahassee, Florida (1.7). The number of days that Medicare residents of Los Angeles spent in intensive care during their last six months of life was 2.4 times higher than the number of days in intensive care among Medicare residents of San Francisco (1.7).

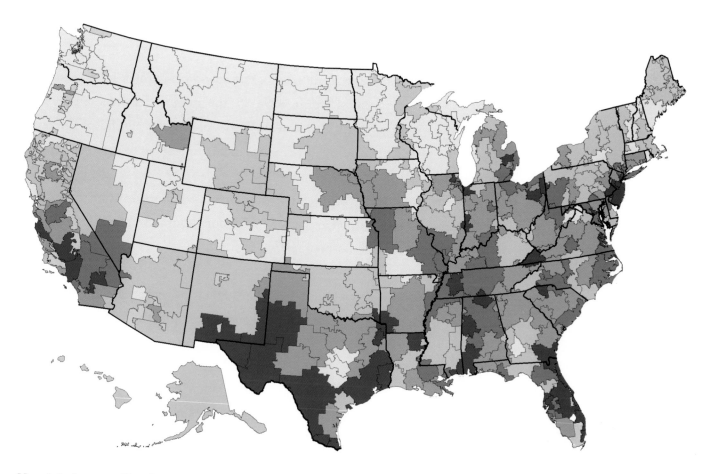

Map 4.4. Average Number of Days Spent in Intensive Care During the Last Six Months of Life (1994-95)

There were high rates of use of intensive care beds in Florida, southern California, south Texas, parts of New York, New Jersey, Alabama, Louisiana, Michigan and Illinois. Regions with low use included northern California, the Northwest, Mountain States, Minnesota, and much of New England.

**Average Number of Days
Spent in Intensive Care
During the Last Six Months of Life**

by Hospital Referral Region (1994-95)

- 3.0 to   4.9 (47)
- 2.5 to < 3.0 (47)
- 2.0 to < 2.5 (79)
- 1.5 to < 2.0 (78)
- .5 to < 1.5 (55)
- Not Populated

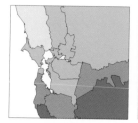

San Francisco

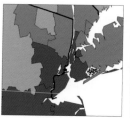

Chicago

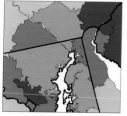

New York

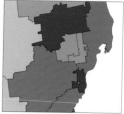

Washington-Baltimore

Detroit

Reimbursements for Inpatient Care During the Last Six Months of Life

How much money does the Medicare program spend per enrollee for hospital care during the last six months of life? In 1994-95, the amount depended on the hospital referral region in which the enrollee lived. Among the 306 hospital referral regions, the lowest price adjusted reimbursements for inpatient care per enrollee during the last six months of life in 1994-95 were $5,831 for residents of Bend, Oregon. The highest price adjusted reimbursements were for Medicare residents of Manhattan, who received, on average, $16,571, or about 2.8 times more than enrollees living in the Bend hospital referral region.

Among the hospital referral regions with the highest per enrollee reimbursements during the last six months of life were the Bronx, New York ($15,950); Harlingen, Texas ($15,399); McAllen, Texas ($14,359); Miami ($14,212); and Chicago ($12,543).

Among the hospital referral regions with the lowest per enrollee reimbursements during the last six months of life were Salem, Oregon ($6,174); Ogden, Utah ($6,193); Appleton, Wisconsin ($6,492); and Grand Junction, Colorado ($6,534).

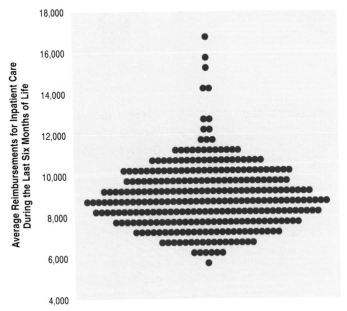

Figure 4.5. Average Reimbursements per Enrollee for Inpatient Care During the Last Six Months of Life (1994-95)

The average reimbursement for inpatient care during the last six months of life, after adjusting for price, age, sex, and race, ranged from $5,831 to $16,571. Each point represents one of the 306 hospital referral regions in the United States.

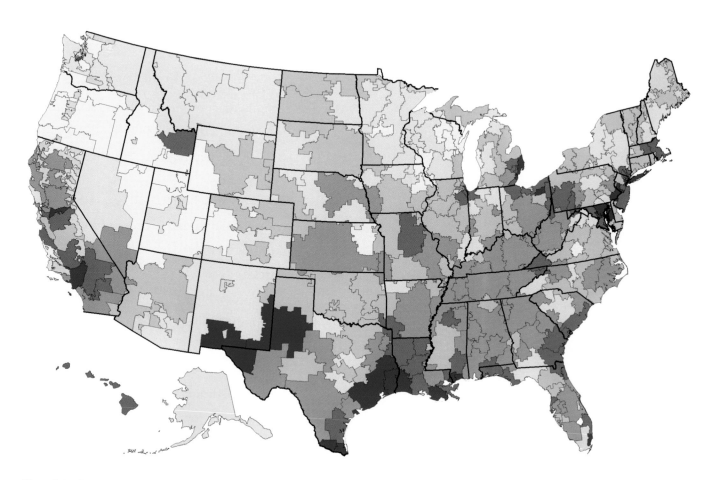

Map 4.5. Average Price Adjusted Reimbursements for Inpatient Care During the Last Six Months of Life (1994-95)

Reimbursements per person during the last six months of life were high in southern New York, New Jersey, Pennsylvania, the Detroit and Chicago areas, southern California, parts of Texas and the east coast of Florida. They were low in northern New England, the upper Midwest, the Mountain states, and the Northwest.

Average Reimbursements for Inpatient Care During the Last Six Months of Life ($)

by Hospital Referral Region (1994-95)

- 11,000 to 16,571 (24)
- 10,000 to 11,000 (50)
- 9,000 to 10,000 (66)
- 8,000 to 9,000 (83)
- 7,000 to 8,000 (59)
- 5,831 to 7,000 (24)
- Not Populated

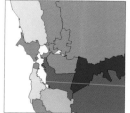

San Francisco

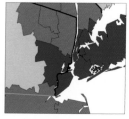

Chicago

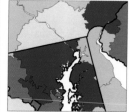

New York

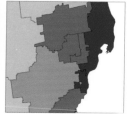

Washington-Baltimore

Detroit

Report Card on The American Experience of Death

Medicare claims data make it possible to "profile" care in the last six months of life for hospital referral regions, as well as for individual hospitals. This section profiles care in 23 hospital referral regions, each with more than 180,000 Medicare enrollees, to display the variability of strategies for managing the care of Medicare patients who are dying.

The experiences of Medicare enrollees with hospital care and with stays in intensive care units during the last six months of their lives are recorded in Table 4.1. The table gives for each selected region the chance that an enrollee was treated in an intensive care unit during the last six months of life, and the chance that when death occurred, it was in a hospital.

The percent of Medicare deaths that occurred in a hospital ranged from a low of 22.2% in Portland, Oregon, to a high of 51.3% in Newark, New Jersey. Among the regions with the highest percents of deaths in hospitals were Birmingham, Alabama (42.5%); Philadelphia (39.6%); Detroit (38.0%); Pittsburgh (39.1%); Atlanta (38.4%); Miami (39.5%); and Chicago (37.1%). Among the regions with low percentages of deaths in hospitals were Seattle (25.0%); Minneapolis (25.5%); and San Diego (27.2%). The chances of dying in a hospital were more than twice as high for Medicare residents of the Manhattan hospital referral region, 1.9 times higher for Medicare residents of the Birmingham, Alabama hospital referral region, and 1.8 times higher for residents of the Miami hospital referral region, than they were for Medicare residents of the Portland, Oregon hospital referral region.

TABLE 4.1
Report Card on the Hospital Experiences of Medicare Enrollees During the Last Six Months of Life
According to the Hospital Referral Region of Residence, 1994-95.
(Ratio to Portland, OR in parentheses)

Hospital Referral Region	The Percent of Enrollees Who Experienced: death as an inpatient	intensive care during last six months
Newark	51.3 (2.3)	41.5 (1.9)
Manhattan	48.8 (2.2)	29.4 (1.4)
Birmingham	42.5 (1.9)	34.9 (1.6)
Philadelphia	39.6 (1.8)	36.9 (1.7)
Miami	39.5 (1.8)	47.5 (2.2)
Pittsburgh	39.1 (1.8)	35.5 (1.7)
Atlanta	38.4 (1.7)	31.1 (1.5)
Detroit	38.0 (1.7)	33.4 (1.6)
Chicago	37.1 (1.7)	39.8 (1.9)
Baltimore	35.9 (1.6)	30.2 (1.4)
Boston	35.9 (1.6)	28.5 (1.3)
Los Angeles	35.1 (1.6)	44.6 (2.1)
St Louis	34.3 (1.6)	33.6 (1.6)
Cleveland	34.2 (1.5)	35.9 (1.7)
Houston	33.9 (1.5)	38.2 (1.8)
Indianapolis	33.4 (1.5)	29.9 (1.4)
Dallas	33.2 (1.5)	30.3 (1.4)
Kansas City	32.0 (1.4)	33.7 (1.6)
Milwaukee	31.5 (1.4)	26.8 (1.3)
San Diego	27.2 (1.2)	31.2 (1.5)
Minneapolis	25.5 (1.2)	23.1 (1.1)
Seattle	24.5 (1.1)	25.0 (1.2)
Portland	22.2 (1.0)	21.5 (1.0)

47.5% of the Miami Medicare enrollees who died experienced at least one episode of care in an intensive care unit during the last six months of their lives. In the Portland, Oregon hospital referral region, only 21.5% of Medicare residents spent time in intensive care. Among the regions where Medicare residents had the highest chance of being admitted to an intensive care unit during the last six months of life were Los Angeles (44.6% of enrollees); Chicago (39.8%); and Houston (38.2%). Among the regions where Medicare residents had the lowest chance of being admitted to an intensive care unit at the end of life were Milwaukee (26.8%); Seattle (21.5%); and Minneapolis (23.1%)

The per-enrollee amounts of inpatient resources used during the last six months of life (Part A Medicare payments) varied substantially in 1994-95 (Table 4.2). Resources expended on residents of the Manhattan and Miami hospital referral regions (among others) were far higher than reimbursements for enrollees in the hospital referral regions in Minneapolis, Seattle, and Portland, Oregon. Medicare residents of the Manhattan hospital referral region spent, on average, 22 days, or more than 12% of their last six months of life, in hospitals. In Portland, Oregon, Medicare enrollees spent an average of about 3% of their last six months as inpatients.

The average price adjusted reimbursement for inpatient care during the last six months of life for Medicare enrollees living in Manhattan was $16,571, or 2.4 times more than was reimbursed for residents of the Portland, Oregon hospital referral region ($6,793). Federal spending on inpatient care in the last six months of life was high in Miami ($14,212); Chicago ($12,543); Philadelphia ($12,093); and Los Angeles ($11,800). Medicare spending was low, by comparison, in Minneapolis ($7,246); Seattle ($7,255); and Milwaukee ($8,007).

The report card (Table 4.2) illustrates the commitment of Miami's health care systems to intensive care in 1994-95. On average, Medicare enrollees living in this region spent more time in intensive care during the last six months of their lives than residents of anywhere else in the country — on average, 4.8 days. Miami's rate

TABLE 4.2

Report Card on Hospital Resources Allocated to Medicare Enrollees During the Last Six Months of Life

According to the Hospital Referral Region of Residence, 1994-95.
(Ratio to Portland, OR in parentheses)

Hospital Referral Region	Price-adjusted Medicare reimbursements for hospital care during last 6 mo.	Days in hospital during last 6 months	Days in ICU during last 6 months	ICU days as % of total
Manhattan	$16,571 (2.44)	22.00 (4.04)	3.12 (3.17)	14.20
Miami	$14,212 (2.09)	14.34 (2.63)	4.83 (4.90)	33.68
Chicago	$12,543 (1.85)	13.79 (2.53)	3.23 (3.28)	23.46
Philadelphia	$12,093 (1.78)	14.45 (2.65)	3.23 (3.28)	22.34
Los Angeles	$11,800 (1.74)	11.25 (2.06)	4.14 (4.20)	36.83
Newark	$11,557 (1.70)	22.90 (4.20)	4.17 (4.24)	18.23
Baltimore	$11,549 (1.70)	12.87 (2.36)	2.31 (2.34)	17.92
Detroit	$11,309 (1.66)	13.58 (2.49)	2.90 (2.95)	21.38
Houston	$11,023 (1.62)	10.77 (1.98)	3.5 (3.20)	29.52
Pittsburgh	$10,924 (1.61)	13.81 (2.53)	2.61 (2.65)	18.92
Boston	$10,047 (1.48)	12.46 (2.29)	1.96 (1.99)	15.75
Cleveland	$10,001 (1.47)	11.30 (2.07)	2.83 (2.87)	25.06
San Diego	$9,817 (1.45)	7.95 (1.46)	2.42 (2.46)	30.45
Birmingham	$9,807 (1.44)	12.24 (2.25)	2.91 (2.96)	23.80
Atlanta	$9,707 (1.43)	10.97 (2.01)	2.23 (2.27)	20.37
St Louis	$9,639 (1.42)	10.68 (1.96)	2.64 (2.67)	24.67
Kansas City	$8,893 (1.31)	10.14 (1.86)	2.64 (2.68)	26.08
Dallas	$8,675 (1.28)	9.27 (1.70)	2.07 (2.11)	22.38
Indianapolis	$8,623 (1.27)	9.27 (1.70)	2.27 (2.30)	24.48
Milwaukee	$8,007 (1.18)	9.49 (1.74)	1.90 (1.93)	20.06
Seattle	$7,255 (1.07)	6.25 (1.15)	1.37 (1.39)	21.97
Minneapolis	$7,246 (1.07)	6.78 (1.24)	1.29 (1.31)	19.08
Portland	$6,793 (1.00)	5.45 (1.00)	0.99 (1.00)	18.08

of days spent in intensive care during the last six months of life was almost 5 times higher than the rate among Medicare residents of the Portland, Oregon, hospital referral region. The Miami hospital referral region ranked fourth, behind Newark, Manhattan, and Philadelphia, in the number of days enrollees spent in hospitals during the last six months of life. A full 34% of those hospital days were spent in intensive care, compared to 14.2% among Medicare residents of Manhattan, and 22.3% for those in the Philadelphia hospital referral region.

The health care system in Los Angeles is also heavily committed to intensive care: almost 36.8% of Medicare patient days in hospitals during the last six months of life in 1994-95 were spent in intensive care. Residents of the Los Angeles hospital referral region ranked third in the amount of intensive care they received at the end of life, receiving more than 4 times as much care as residents of Portland, Oregon, and 1.7 times as much as residents of the San Diego hospital referral region.

Level of Acute Hospital Care Resources and the Likelihood of a Hospitalized Death

The level of resource allocation in the acute care hospital sector in hospital referral regions in 1994-95 was correlated with the chance that when a Medicare enrollee's death occurred, it was in a hospital. Figure 4.6 shows the relationship between the percent of Medicare deaths occurring in hospitals and the numbers of acute care hospital beds per thousand residents of hospital referral regions. The chance of dying in a hospital ranged from 20% of all deaths of Medicare enrollees in the region to more than 50%. The R^2 statistic indicates that 38% of the variation in the likelihood of dying as an inpatient was attributable to the intensity of investment in acute hospital capacity in the region.

Although there was substantial variation in spending among hospital referral regions for home health, hospice and hospital care, there is little evidence that greater spending for hospice or home health care led to less investment in acute hospital care for terminal care or inpatient care during the last six months of life. There was little association between Medicare spending for inpatient care and home health care spending (R^2 = .05) or inpatient spending and hospice care (R^2 = .01).

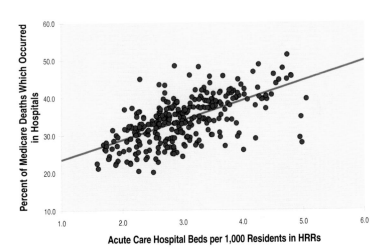

Figure 4.6. The Association Between Percent of Deaths Occurring in Hospitals and the Supply of Hospital Beds (1994-95)

There was a relationship between the percent of all deaths that occurred while the enrollees were in hospitals and the numbers of hospital beds per 1,000 Medicare enrollees (R^2 = .38). Each point represents one of the 306 hospital referral regions in the United States.

Chapter Four Table   All hospitalization and utilization rates are based on Medicare deaths occurring during the period July 1, 1994 — December 31, 1995, and are expressed as rates per person (per decedent). Rates are age, sex and race adjusted and reimbursements are also adjusted for regional differences in prices. Data exclude Medicare enrollees who were members of risk bearing health maintenance organizations.

CHAPTER FOUR TABLE

Hospitalization Rates and Medicare Reimbursements During the Last Six Months of Life Among Non-HMO Medicare Enrollees by Hospital Referral Region (1994-95)

Hospital Referral Region	Medicare Deaths (1994 plus 1995)	Percent of Medicare Deaths Occurring in Hospitals	Percent of Enrollees Admitted to ICU in Last Six Months of Life	Average Days in Hospitals in Last Six Months of Life	Average Days in ICU in Last Six Months of Life	Average Inpatient Reimbursements per Capita During Last Six Months of Life
Alabama						
Birmingham	22,222	42.5	34.9	12.2	2.9	9,807
Dothan	3,570	41.1	31.6	11.7	2.2	9,199
Huntsville	4,332	40.0	36.8	11.3	3.1	8,861
Mobile	6,505	41.2	38.6	12.6	3.3	9,582
Montgomery	4,094	41.6	31.9	10.8	2.2	9,017
Tuscaloosa	2,323	41.2	36.2	13.2	3.6	9,039
Alaska						
Anchorage	1,797	27.9	27.7	8.2	1.8	7,699
Arizona						
Mesa	3,892	26.3	32.8	7.4	2.3	7,996
Phoenix	14,161	26.1	30.2	7.4	2.0	8,517
Sun City	2,925	28.4	8.9	7.5	0.5	7,766
Tucson	6,211	22.7	28.6	6.3	1.8	7,346
Arkansas						
Fort Smith	3,775	43.9	31.7	12.7	1.7	8,572
Jonesboro	2,649	42.0	27.4	11.1	1.7	8,816
Little Rock	16,179	40.3	31.0	11.4	2.2	9,594
Springdale	3,500	31.9	29.7	8.2	1.5	7,012
Texarkana	3,107	39.6	39.2	11.5	3.3	10,666
California						
Orange Co.	10,636	31.8	39.2	9.0	2.9	9,876
Bakersfield	5,159	36.3	34.4	10.9	3.0	10,180
Chico	2,920	30.5	29.9	8.5	2.2	9,886
Contra Costa Co.	4,900	27.6	24.4	7.4	1.7	9,038
Fresno	6,331	31.5	29.7	7.8	2.1	8,319
Los Angeles	38,559	35.1	44.6	11.2	4.1	11,800
Modesto	4,827	33.8	36.4	10.0	2.9	10,948
Napa	3,004	26.8	24.4	7.2	1.6	9,622
Alameda Co.	8,557	29.1	26.0	8.0	1.7	10,088
Palm Spr/Rancho Mir	2,186	30.3	39.1	9.2	3.5	10,932
Redding	3,272	30.2	28.4	7.3	1.8	9,324
Sacramento	13,980	30.0	26.7	8.0	2.0	9,431
Salinas	2,267	23.3	35.1	7.6	3.2	10,770
San Bernardino	8,570	31.2	37.8	9.1	3.0	10,716
San Diego	13,577	27.2	31.2	7.9	2.4	9,817
San Francisco	9,473	28.7	27.3	7.5	1.7	9,043
San Jose	7,119	28.1	29.5	7.8	2.5	8,771
San Luis Obispo	1,800	26.3	31.8	6.3	2.3	6,580
San Mateo Co.	4,562	25.3	28.3	6.9	2.1	7,950
Santa Barbara	2,633	26.5	27.5	6.8	1.5	7,247

Hospital Referral Region	Medicare Deaths (1994 plus 1995)	Percent of Medicare Deaths Occurring in Hospitals	Percent of Enrollees Admitted to ICU in Last Six Months of Life	Average Days in Hospitals in Last Six Months of Life	Average Days in ICU in Last Six Months of Life	Average Inpatient Reimbursements per Capita During Last Six Months of Life
Santa Cruz	1,869	27.1	35.0	7.7	2.8	9,304
Santa Rosa	3,377	23.9	17.7	6.8	0.9	7,174
Stockton	3,152	32.9	29.8	8.4	2.0	11,142
Ventura	3,225	31.6	29.9	9.7	2.3	9,343
Colorado						
Boulder	1,190	21.2	28.9	6.2	1.9	6,694
Colorado Springs	4,301	28.3	23.2	7.9	1.3	7,648
Denver	12,239	24.2	25.8	7.1	1.5	8,061
Fort Collins	1,698	25.8	23.2	7.4	1.5	7,899
Grand Junction	2,059	23.0	17.8	5.6	0.7	6,534
Greeley	2,157	27.0	23.0	7.8	1.5	8,515
Pueblo	1,460	30.8	26.7	8.0	1.7	8,564
Connecticut						
Bridgeport	6,401	35.9	27.9	12.9	2.4	8,554
Hartford	14,244	32.4	27.5	10.1	2.0	8,406
New Haven	13,294	32.0	28.1	10.9	2.0	8,233
Delaware						
Wilmington	5,799	34.8	32.5	11.9	2.7	8,778
District of Columbia						
Washington	16,766	37.1	31.5	13.4	2.7	10,710
Florida						
Bradenton	3,533	33.0	39.8	8.9	2.9	8,853
Clearwater	7,348	32.3	35.6	10.2	2.9	9,442
Fort Lauderdale	23,068	32.8	40.5	11.7	3.7	10,468
Fort Myers	10,091	32.3	33.1	9.3	2.4	9,009
Gainesville	4,152	29.0	31.5	9.0	2.6	8,589
Hudson	5,741	37.3	40.6	12.6	3.2	10,714
Jacksonville	10,123	36.0	40.4	11.1	3.7	10,209
Lakeland	3,133	34.2	35.4	10.2	3.0	9,554
Miami	17,999	39.5	47.5	14.3	4.8	14,212
Ocala	5,279	30.9	28.1	8.5	1.8	8,196
Orlando	24,840	33.5	38.4	10.3	3.1	9,375
Ormond Beach	3,348	32.8	39.6	10.1	3.1	9,227
Panama City	1,714	40.3	31.8	11.4	2.8	10,442
Pensacola	5,472	38.2	32.7	11.5	2.4	10,064
Sarasota	6,314	30.3	32.9	9.2	2.7	8,624
St Petersburg	5,865	34.6	46.8	11.9	4.9	10,509
Tallahassee	6,136	30.7	26.7	9.8	1.7	7,705
Tampa	7,465	34.7	39.9	11.0	3.5	9,751
Georgia						
Albany	1,886	40.5	24.6	10.9	1.4	9,143
Atlanta	28,081	38.4	31.1	11.0	2.2	9,707
Augusta	5,141	38.5	27.6	11.7	2.2	9,215
Columbus	2,825	39.6	30.3	10.9	1.9	8,264
Macon	6,397	39.9	31.6	10.8	1.9	9,488
Rome	2,558	37.5	31.8	9.0	2.2	9,157

Hospital Referral Region	Medicare Deaths (1994 plus 1995)	Percent of Medicare Deaths Occurring in Hospitals	Percent of Enrollees Admitted to ICU in Last Six Months of Life	Average Days in Hospitals in Last Six Months of Life	Average Days in ICU in Last Six Months of Life	Average Inpatient Reimbursements per Capita During Last Six Months of Life
Savannah	5,595	38.7	32.1	12.0	2.4	10,141
Hawaii						
Honolulu	5,403	36.9	23.9	14.4	1.6	10,507
Idaho						
Boise	5,070	25.1	22.5	5.9	1.1	6,455
Idaho Falls	1,180	26.3	23.8	6.6	2.2	10,070
Illinois						
Aurora	1,388	33.0	28.3	8.6	2.1	7,826
Blue Island	8,056	36.1	36.2	12.7	2.6	10,467
Chicago	21,540	37.1	39.8	13.8	3.2	12,543
Elgin	3,426	32.0	39.0	10.4	3.1	8,874
Evanston	7,782	31.1	35.2	11.0	2.6	9,775
Hinsdale	2,431	28.5	32.6	9.4	2.5	8,802
Joliet	3,986	39.7	34.3	12.7	2.3	10,461
Melrose Park	10,672	31.9	34.6	10.4	2.7	9,705
Peoria	7,567	32.6	24.8	9.2	1.5	8,884
Rockford	6,455	32.3	28.5	9.1	2.1	8,258
Springfield	10,501	34.3	26.0	10.4	2.0	8,972
Urbana	4,664	33.5	25.6	8.8	1.7	8,339
Bloomington	1,509	32.4	15.6	9.1	1.1	8,836
Indiana						
Evansville	8,141	33.7	31.5	9.4	2.0	7,964
Fort Wayne	7,644	28.5	31.0	7.3	2.2	7,142
Gary	4,698	39.5	34.5	13.9	3.1	10,622
Indianapolis	23,729	33.4	29.9	9.3	2.3	8,623
Lafayette	1,897	33.0	26.5	8.4	2.1	7,736
Muncie	1,857	34.9	32.6	9.6	2.5	9,189
Munster	3,148	40.2	47.9	13.6	4.9	10,399
South Bend	6,462	28.3	26.3	8.2	1.8	7,152
Terre Haute	2,395	37.4	38.6	10.2	3.5	9,023
Iowa						
Cedar Rapids	2,559	30.1	22.9	9.2	1.8	6,876
Davenport	5,512	34.5	29.1	9.3	1.8	8,230
Des Moines	10,830	33.1	27.9	9.5	2.0	8,057
Dubuque	1,624	27.1	23.0	8.1	1.2	6,648
Iowa City	3,290	34.4	25.0	9.5	1.3	8,407
Mason City	2,021	24.4	18.3	6.1	0.9	7,346
Sioux City	3,051	29.4	29.9	7.9	2.2	7,376
Waterloo	2,468	28.6	27.8	7.8	1.4	7,495
Kansas						
Topeka	4,453	26.9	18.1	7.3	0.9	6,976
Wichita	13,594	34.1	25.2	9.3	1.4	9,053
Kentucky						
Covington	3,113	33.2	33.4	10.2	2.3	8,251
Lexington	12,827	38.9	27.5	11.5	1.9	9,191
Louisville	15,482	37.5	31.2	11.7	2.6	9,056

Hospital Referral Region	Medicare Deaths (1994 plus 1995)	Percent of Medicare Deaths Occurring in Hospitals	Percent of Enrollees Admitted to ICU in Last Six Months of Life	Average Days in Hospitals in Last Six Months of Life	Average Days in ICU in Last Six Months of Life	Average Inpatient Reimbursements per Capita During Last Six Months of Life
Owensboro	1,592	38.7	31.5	9.8	2.4	8,833
Paducah	4,749	40.0	33.0	12.0	2.3	9,421
Louisiana						
Alexandria	2,868	40.4	26.3	11.0	1.6	10,278
Baton Rouge	5,700	38.8	34.6	10.9	2.9	9,278
Houma	1,805	41.8	29.8	13.0	2.3	11,317
Lafayette	4,659	37.9	30.6	10.4	2.3	10,047
Lake Charles	2,069	46.2	26.1	12.9	1.7	11,425
Metairie	3,464	39.5	32.0	12.4	2.3	10,902
Monroe	2,934	39.6	35.5	12.4	3.2	10,220
New Orleans	7,486	34.8	33.6	11.2	2.5	10,666
Shreveport	7,030	41.2	31.6	11.0	2.2	10,651
Slidell	1,339	36.8	33.8	12.5	2.6	11,476
Maine						
Bangor	4,403	37.2	24.8	11.1	1.7	8,067
Portland	9,904	33.5	22.3	10.6	1.4	7,900
Maryland						
Baltimore	22,258	35.9	30.2	12.9	2.3	11,549
Salisbury	4,154	34.7	24.7	10.6	1.6	8,833
Takoma Park	4,725	34.6	33.3	13.9	3.5	12,407
Massachusetts						
Boston	44,305	35.9	28.5	12.5	2.0	10,047
Springfield	8,063	34.2	23.3	10.5	1.4	8,731
Worcester	6,193	36.2	26.9	11.2	1.6	10,220
Michigan						
Ann Arbor	10,184	34.9	36.6	11.1	2.6	9,600
Dearborn	5,468	38.7	39.9	14.5	3.4	11,106
Detroit	19,480	38.0	33.4	13.6	2.9	11,309
Flint	4,589	39.6	35.6	12.8	3.0	10,283
Grand Rapids	8,566	25.0	27.9	7.6	1.8	7,096
Kalamazoo	6,162	29.2	27.1	7.7	1.6	8,000
Lansing	5,125	31.0	27.6	9.7	1.7	8,406
Marquette	2,557	29.5	24.3	8.6	1.2	8,257
Muskegon	2,602	25.6	24.2	7.7	1.3	6,820
Petoskey	1,804	28.3	27.5	8.7	1.8	7,599
Pontiac	2,907	33.2	31.2	12.4	2.1	10,527
Royal Oak	6,081	36.0	28.7	13.3	2.2	10,456
Saginaw	7,166	33.6	33.0	10.4	2.4	8,096
St Joseph	1,521	30.6	25.3	8.9	1.9	8,201
Traverse City	2,254	27.4	26.7	8.5	2.1	8,183
Minnesota						
Duluth	4,435	28.6	27.1	7.3	1.7	7,195
Minneapolis	21,572	25.5	23.1	6.8	1.3	7,246
Rochester	4,108	25.4	24.8	6.8	1.6	7,896
St Cloud	1,893	25.2	26.0	6.8	1.5	6,858
St Paul	5,902	23.7	29.0	7.2	1.9	7,783

Hospital Referral Region	Medicare Deaths (1994 plus 1995)	Percent of Medicare Deaths Occurring in Hospitals	Percent of Enrollees Admitted to ICU in Last Six Months of Life	Average Days in Hospitals in Last Six Months of Life	Average Days in ICU in Last Six Months of Life	Average Inpatient Reimbursements per Capita During Last Six Months of Life
Mississippi						
Gulfport	1,636	40.8	40.3	13.9	3.8	11,319
Hattiesburg	2,824	47.8	27.4	14.1	1.8	10,205
Jackson	10,360	43.7	26.4	12.3	1.9	8,518
Meridian	2,278	44.8	27.9	13.6	1.7	9,253
Oxford	1,418	45.7	25.9	14.3	2.3	10,339
Tupelo	3,691	46.8	31.0	13.3	2.4	9,010
Missouri						
Cape Girardeau	3,367	34.3	32.9	9.4	2.6	8,388
Columbia	7,334	33.6	31.8	9.4	2.2	10,045
Joplin	4,491	35.4	27.5	9.8	1.5	9,297
Kansas City	20,043	32.0	33.7	10.1	2.6	8,893
Springfield	8,468	31.4	27.0	8.5	1.5	8,005
St Louis	34,798	34.3	33.6	10.7	2.6	9,639
Montana						
Billings	4,545	27.5	21.3	7.9	1.1	7,591
Great Falls	1,568	30.1	24.1	8.5	1.3	7,979
Missoula	3,168	26.9	22.0	6.9	1.2	7,502
Nebraska						
Lincoln	6,136	27.3	20.3	6.2	1.2	7,073
Omaha	11,871	31.4	28.2	8.5	2.1	9,007
Nevada						
Las Vegas	6,418	37.3	35.7	10.8	3.0	9,217
Reno	4,500	29.3	25.0	7.4	1.7	7,857
New Hampshire						
Lebanon	4,158	30.8	22.7	9.2	1.4	8,529
Manchester	6,609	31.3	22.7	9.7	1.5	7,090
New Jersey						
Camden	28,246	46.0	35.0	16.9	3.0	10,548
Hackensack	11,352	45.6	31.9	19.1	2.7	10,319
Morristown	7,882	39.6	31.2	15.4	2.4	8,554
New Brunswick	7,140	48.5	35.7	19.9	3.6	10,782
Newark	14,065	51.3	41.5	22.9	4.2	11,557
Paterson	3,525	45.7	31.9	20.7	2.6	10,377
Ridgewood	3,310	43.3	29.9	18.1	2.4	10,021
New Mexico						
Albuquerque	8,152	28.3	25.7	7.4	1.6	7,469
New York						
Albany	19,239	36.4	26.2	14.3	1.9	7,895
Binghamton	4,188	35.8	26.0	12.6	1.4	7,252
Bronx	9,072	45.6	28.2	20.9	2.6	15,950
Buffalo	16,700	41.2	28.6	16.9	2.3	8,811
Elmira	4,390	39.2	28.8	15.4	1.9	7,948
East Long Island	37,583	48.2	30.8	20.5	3.0	12,507
New York	36,642	48.8	29.4	22.0	3.1	16,571
Rochester	11,624	35.5	25.5	14.0	1.9	8,776

Hospital Referral Region	Medicare Deaths (1994 plus 1995)	Percent of Medicare Deaths Occurring in Hospitals	Percent of Enrollees Admitted to ICU in Last Six Months of Life	Average Days in Hospitals in Last Six Months of Life	Average Days in ICU in Last Six Months of Life	Average Inpatient Reimbursements per Capita During Last Six Months of Life
Syracuse	10,657	35.6	24.9	14.2	1.8	7,527
White Plains	9,757	42.7	30.4	18.5	2.7	10,646
North Carolina						
Asheville	6,614	33.2	27.3	8.8	1.9	7,710
Charlotte	15,349	37.3	33.2	11.1	2.7	8,699
Durham	11,334	36.8	27.2	10.2	1.9	8,743
Greensboro	4,744	36.4	31.0	11.1	3.0	7,989
Greenville	6,749	37.4	33.8	10.9	2.6	9,290
Hickory	2,268	35.8	31.9	9.9	2.8	9,517
Raleigh	10,499	41.3	31.7	12.2	2.2	9,217
Wilmington	3,115	38.5	29.9	10.9	1.9	8,665
Winston-Salem	9,629	39.8	32.3	12.4	2.4	9,616
North Dakota						
Bismarck	2,190	29.3	21.7	9.2	1.1	8,908
Fargo Moorhead -Mn	5,639	27.1	22.9	7.6	1.3	7,889
Grand Forks	1,970	30.4	22.4	7.5	1.0	8,323
Minot	1,543	27.8	24.0	8.6	1.4	8,643
Ohio						
Akron	6,959	37.8	30.9	12.6	2.3	11,043
Canton	6,735	33.9	34.0	10.0	3.0	8,494
Cincinnati	15,391	29.3	26.2	8.7	1.7	8,561
Cleveland	22,862	34.2	36.0	11.3	2.8	10,001
Columbus	25,002	33.2	32.8	10.1	2.5	9,144
Dayton	11,557	29.5	29.3	9.5	2.3	8,689
Elyria	2,357	30.3	39.3	10.3	3.3	8,129
Kettering	3,530	29.3	28.5	9.2	2.1	8,101
Toledo	10,250	33.2	35.5	10.7	2.8	10,162
Youngstown	9,036	37.9	39.4	12.3	3.5	10,609
Oklahoma						
Lawton	2,046	33.1	27.1	9.0	1.7	8,413
Oklahoma City	17,003	38.7	27.7	10.3	1.7	8,730
Tulsa	11,997	34.8	27.3	9.3	1.7	8,406
Oregon						
Bend	1,372	20.1	16.3	4.8	0.6	5,831
Eugene	6,153	22.5	19.0	5.4	0.9	6,442
Medford	4,508	22.4	21.2	5.2	1.1	6,472
Portland	13,374	22.2	21.5	5.5	1.0	6,793
Salem	2,220	26.1	30.7	5.9	2.1	6,174
Pennsylvania						
Allentown	11,882	39.0	30.6	14.2	2.2	9,597
Altoona	3,850	40.2	33.4	12.1	2.4	9,683
Danville	6,025	33.0	27.5	9.8	1.6	7,996
Erie	9,187	34.5	27.0	11.2	2.0	8,326
Harrisburg	9,760	34.9	28.4	10.6	1.9	8,485
Johnstown	3,426	41.7	29.7	14.0	1.8	10,987
Lancaster	5,370	27.0	29.2	8.4	2.1	7,124

Hospital Referral Region	Medicare Deaths (1994 plus 1995)	Percent of Medicare Deaths Occurring in Hospitals	Percent of Enrollees Admitted to ICU in Last Six Months of Life	Average Days in Hospitals in Last Six Months of Life	Average Days in ICU in Last Six Months of Life	Average Inpatient Reimbursements per Capita During Last Six Months of Life
Philadelphia	41,008	39.6	36.9	14.4	3.2	12,093
Pittsburgh	40,932	39.1	35.5	13.8	2.6	10,924
Reading	6,667	36.9	27.3	12.2	1.6	8,197
Sayre	2,253	35.0	27.2	12.5	1.6	8,716
Scranton	4,560	39.0	24.3	14.2	1.6	8,633
Wilkes-Barre	4,037	36.4	29.6	13.4	1.8	7,782
York	3,710	32.4	34.2	10.2	3.0	7,733
Rhode Island						
Providence	11,876	32.9	22.0	11.3	1.4	8,781
South Carolina						
Charleston	5,816	37.3	31.1	11.3	2.9	10,223
Columbia	8,798	37.3	29.8	11.1	2.4	7,962
Florence	3,385	43.4	32.6	12.3	2.1	9,716
Greenville	6,865	38.8	30.4	12.0	2.4	9,120
Spartanburg	3,520	42.1	36.6	12.3	3.0	7,899
South Dakota						
Rapid City	1,586	27.1	22.1	8.2	1.3	7,537
Sioux Falls	8,837	29.6	25.3	8.2	1.7	8,341
Tennessee						
Chattanooga	6,106	37.4	34.4	10.3	2.3	9,298
Jackson	4,027	41.1	36.5	11.1	3.8	9,108
Johnson City	2,544	37.3	28.6	10.1	2.3	10,059
Kingsport	5,348	44.8	36.7	13.6	3.1	10,298
Knoxville	12,226	42.0	32.3	11.8	2.4	9,553
Memphis	16,135	42.2	29.1	12.1	2.6	9,633
Nashville	20,315	37.2	34.2	10.4	2.6	9,836
Texas						
Abilene	3,697	39.2	30.7	11.5	2.1	9,707
Amarillo	4,260	26.0	31.3	7.9	2.2	8,185
Austin	5,817	31.4	23.7	8.3	1.4	7,368
Beaumont	4,762	44.6	42.5	13.5	4.2	11,012
Bryan	1,469	32.3	27.3	7.9	2.0	8,083
Corpus Christi	3,883	39.0	35.0	11.4	2.4	10,164
Dallas	23,396	33.2	30.3	9.3	2.1	8,675
El Paso	5,404	35.1	40.0	10.7	3.5	11,274
Fort Worth	10,958	30.7	33.2	8.1	2.2	8,101
Harlingen	2,831	43.5	40.1	13.3	3.8	15,399
Houston	27,687	33.9	38.2	10.8	3.2	11,023
Longview	1,893	37.6	37.6	10.1	3.3	9,984
Lubbock	6,022	40.7	37.7	12.3	3.6	11,124
Mcallen	2,031	45.0	35.4	13.0	3.2	14,359
Odessa	2,437	37.9	36.2	11.4	3.4	9,246
San Angelo	1,694	34.1	28.7	9.3	2.4	8,086
San Antonio	13,359	34.5	35.8	10.8	3.0	9,611
Temple	2,445	30.0	24.6	7.8	1.2	8,853
Tyler	5,631	37.2	30.8	9.9	2.0	9,516

Hospital Referral Region	Medicare Deaths (1994 plus 1995)	Percent of Medicare Deaths Occurring in Hospitals	Percent of Enrollees Admitted to ICU in Last Six Months of Life	Average Days in Hospitals in Last Six Months of Life	Average Days in ICU in Last Six Months of Life	Average Inpatient Reimbursements per Capita During Last Six Months of Life
Victoria	1,525	42.2	31.1	11.5	1.7	9,601
Waco	3,594	30.3	24.5	6.6	1.3	7,410
Wichita Falls	2,489	37.3	29.6	9.7	2.2	7,746
Utah						
Ogden	1,941	20.5	24.0	4.4	1.3	6,193
Provo	1,867	25.5	24.1	5.6	1.6	7,345
Salt Lake City	9,175	22.9	21.1	5.3	1.1	6,572
Vermont						
Burlington	5,446	35.2	26.8	13.5	1.7	8,065
Virginia						
Arlington	7,520	29.5	27.4	9.9	2.0	7,230
Charlottesville	4,635	33.0	28.8	9.4	2.1	8,646
Lynchburg	2,498	34.2	33.6	9.7	2.6	6,517
Newport News	3,873	37.0	37.1	10.7	3.2	8,026
Norfolk	9,073	38.9	34.0	11.8	2.8	8,589
Richmond	12,457	36.5	30.2	11.5	2.5	8,207
Roanoke	7,837	37.7	30.6	11.7	2.4	8,365
Winchester	3,097	35.5	23.9	10.8	1.4	7,703
Washington						
Everett	3,200	22.5	22.1	5.6	1.1	6,785
Olympia	2,696	23.7	26.5	5.4	1.4	7,344
Seattle	15,288	24.5	25.0	6.2	1.4	7,255
Spokane	10,956	25.4	22.0	6.4	1.3	7,274
Tacoma	4,734	23.8	28.0	5.5	1.5	6,904
Yakima	2,134	27.5	24.3	6.7	1.3	7,747
West Virginia						
Charleston	10,703	42.0	30.4	13.1	2.3	9,857
Huntington	4,359	39.7	25.7	12.2	1.7	9,484
Morgantown	4,700	36.7	35.2	11.4	3.0	9,969
Wisconsin						
Appleton	2,916	25.7	22.1	6.6	1.2	6,492
Green Bay	5,033	29.3	23.9	8.1	1.2	6,603
La Crosse	3,837	25.1	22.1	6.5	1.0	6,755
Madison	8,680	27.9	23.1	8.0	1.3	7,377
Marshfield	3,949	29.6	20.5	7.7	1.0	7,075
Milwaukee	22,581	31.5	26.8	9.5	1.9	8,007
Neenah	2,327	26.8	18.7	7.9	1.0	6,537
Wausau	1,962	23.7	17.6	6.7	0.8	6,832
Wyoming						
Casper	1,649	29.0	25.2	7.9	1.7	9,000
United States						
United States	2,305,068	35.2	31.0	11.3	2.4	9,460

The Surgical Treatment of Common Diseases

The Surgical Treatment of Common Diseases

While geographic variation in the use of surgery has long been recognized, not all surgical procedures are equally variable. For example, colon resection (colectomy) exhibits the low variation pattern seen with hospitalization rates for hip fracture (Chapter Three). Others, such as coronary artery bypass grafting, have a high variation profile.

What distinguishes low variation from high variation surgery? In general, low variation procedures are non-discretionary; they are used to treat clinical conditions for which physicians agree on the most appropriate treatment strategy. In addition, patient and doctor preferences are aligned — both parties have the same goals.

Conversely, high variation procedures involve physician discretion; the variability reflects underlying problems in medical decision making that occur because of inadequate science and failure to take patient preferences into account.

■ Sometimes, medical science is inadequate to provide definitive information on which treatment is likely to provide the best outcome for a given patient. In these cases, procedure rates vary because physicians disagree about the effectiveness of surgery.

■ Sometimes, the scientific evidence regarding outcomes is adequate, but the available treatments have different risks and benefits which only the patient can assess. The fact that patient preferences are unevenly incorporated into treatment decisions results in high variations in procedure rates.

In this chapter, we describe how these two factors are reflected in the variation profiles of nine common surgical procedures. Together these procedures comprised about 25% of the inpatient surgery (major and minor) performed on the Medicare population in 1994-95.

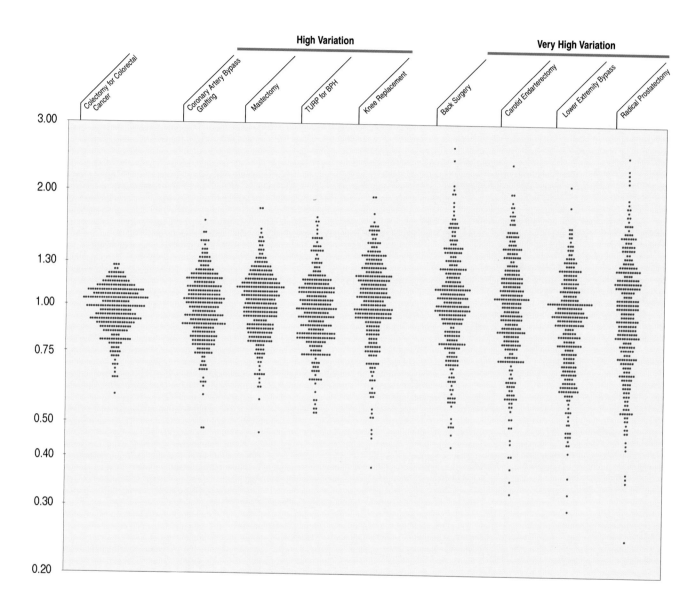

Fig. 5a. Ratios of Rates of Common Surgery to the U.S. Average (1994-95)

A log scale, centered on the national average (1.0) was used for clarity. Colectomy for colorectal cancer was the least variable; radical prostatectomy for cancer of the prostate was the most variable. Each point represents one of the 306 hospital referral regions in the United States.

TABLE 5.1.

Quantitative Measures of Variability of Low, High, and Very High Variation Procedures Among the 306 Hospital Referral Regions (1994-95)

	Colectomy for Colorectal Cancer	Coronary Artery Bypass Grafting	High Variation I				Very High Variation II		
			Mastectomy	TURP for BPH	Knee Replacement	Back Surgery	Carotid Endarterectomy	Lower Extremity Bypass	Radical Prostatectomy
Index of Variation									
Systematic Component of Variation or SCV (X 100)	18.9	40.5	43.9	52.2	64.3	91.2	100.5	109.8	127.6
Ratio to SCV of colectomy for colorectal cancer	1.0	2.1	2.3	2.8	3.4	4.8	5.3	5.8	6.8
Range of Variation									
Extremal ratio: (highest to lowest region)	2.2	3.5	3.8	3.3	5.2	6.0	7.2	7.0	10.0
Interquartile range: (75th to 25th percentile region)	1.21	1.30	1.30	1.34	1.33	1.47	1.50	1.53	1.62
Number of Regions with High and Low Rates									
Rates more than 25% below the national average	15	21	19	30	30	42	56	83	71
Rates 30% or more above the national average	0	23	26	27	55	62	60	30	60

The figure provides a visual impression of variability. Table 5.1 reports the corresponding quantitative measures of variability. The procedures are ranked from low to high, according to the systematic component of variation (SCV). The SCV for coronary artery bypass grafting, a high variation procedure, is more than twice that of colectomy; and back surgery is more than twice as variable as coronary artery bypass surgery. The increases in variability from low to high and from high to very high are statistically and clinically significant. The table also reports the extremal ratio, or the ratio of highest to lowest rates among the 306 hospital referral regions. For colectomy, the extremal ratio is 2.2. For high variation procedures, the extremal ratios are 3.5 to 5.2 times greater in the highest region compared to the lowest. For very high variation procedures, the ratios are between 6 and 10 times greater in the highest, compared to the lowest, region.

Epidemiologists sometimes use the interquartile ratio as a measure of variation. This statistic is the ratio of the rate in the region ranked at the 75th percentile to the region ranked at the 25th percentile. For colectomy, the interquartile ratio is 1.21. For the procedures listed in the table, the interquartile ratio increases from top to bottom and is greatest for radical prostatectomy: the rate in the region ranked at the 75th percentile is 1.62 times higher than the region ranked at the 25th percentile.

Table 5.1 also gives the number of regions with rates that were 30% or more above the national average, as well as the number with rates that were more than 25% below the national average. By definition, when the variability increases, more regions have rates that are substantially different from the average. In the case of colectomy, there were 15 areas where rates were more than 25% below the average, and none were 30% or more above the average. For coronary artery bypass grafting, 21 regions were more than 25% below the average, while 23 were 30% or more above the average. For radical prostatectomy, 71 regions were more than 25% below the average and 60 regions were 30% or more above the average.

Colorectal Cancer

Malignant tumors of the colon or rectum are detected in a number of ways. They can be identified during evaluation of patients presenting with abdominal pain, constipation, or rectal bleeding. Cancers may also be detected by screening asymptomatic patients with fecal occult blood tests (which identify trace amounts of blood in the stool) or endoscopy (examining the rectum and colon with a lighted scope).

The status of science is, by and large, quite good. Once a cancer is identified, there is universal agreement about the need for surgical removal of the tumor (colectomy). In this procedure, the segment of colon containing the tumor is removed and the remaining bowel is reconnected by an anastamosis. In the case of colectomy, physicians and patients share the common goal of extending life expectancy. Even among patients for whom cure is not possible (because of distant cancer spread), surgery is generally recommended for palliative purposes, such as reducing the risks of later bowel obstruction.

The dilemma of choice is virtually a non-issue. Colectomy is the only recognized approach to cancer cure, and the only alternative for attempting to extend patients' life expectancies. Physicians and patients share the same goals and agree on the need for surgery.

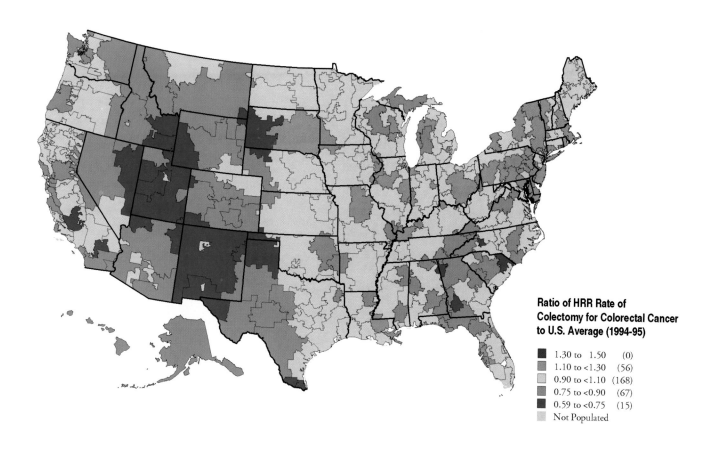

Ratio of HRR Rate of Colectomy for Colorectal Cancer to U.S. Average (1994-95)

■ 1.30 to 1.50   (0)
■ 1.10 to <1.30 (56)
□ 0.90 to <1.10 (168)
■ 0.75 to <0.90 (67)
■ 0.59 to <0.75 (15)
□ Not Populated

Map 5.1. Colectomy for Colorectal Cancer

Rates of colectomy for cancer of the colon and rectum demonstrate relatively little variation. There were no regions with rates 30% or more above the national average (blue); only 15 regions were more than 25% below the national average (green). Rates were lowest in Utah, southeastern Idaho, New Mexico and parts of Texas as well as in isolated regions in the South and California. Rates were higher in the Northeast and Midwest.

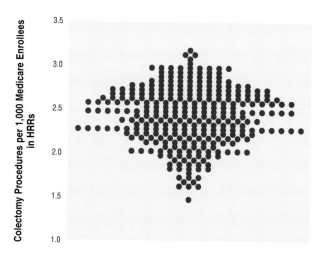

Figure 5.1. Colectomy Among Hospital Referral Regions (1994-95)

The rates varied from 1.5 to 3.2 per thousand Medicare enrollees, after adjustment. Each point represents one of the 306 hospital referral regions in the United States.

Coronary Artery Disease

Patients with coronary artery disease most often present with symptoms of chest pain (angina) or shortness of breath. Occasionally, patients are first diagnosed after a myocardial infarction. There are multiple approaches to treating coronary artery disease: risk factor modification (diet, exercise) and medicines to reduce the frequency and severity of angina; percutaneous transluminal coronary angioplasty (PTCA); and coronary artery bypass grafting (CABG). Decisions to recommend CABG depend on the severity of the patient's symptoms and the severity of the underlying coronary disease. Disease severity is typically determined by diagnostic tests, such as stress tests and coronary angiography.

The status of science in making decisions about whether to perform CABG surgery is imperfect. Several randomized controlled trials initiated in the 1970s have demonstrated that CABG prolongs life in patients who have very severe coronary disease (as determined by specific findings on angiography). However, most patients currently undergoing this procedure do not meet these specific criteria. For the majority of patients, scientific evidence that CABG prolongs life or reduces the long term risks of myocardial infarction is absent.

The dilemma of choice. For many patients, CABG is recommended primarily to improve angina symptoms, a goal shared by patients and physicians. However, the variation in rates of CABG across geographic regions suggests that physicians have different symptom "thresholds" for recommending surgery. Moreover, physicians do not interpret patient preferences in a uniform way. Patients with similar degrees of angina often have different responses to their symptoms; some are bothered more, and some less, by the same degree of discomfort. In addition, individual patients differ in how they feel about the risks of death and complications associated with surgery. Variation in CABG rates will persist until an effective means of incorporating these differences in patient preferences is found and factored explicitly into treatment decisions.

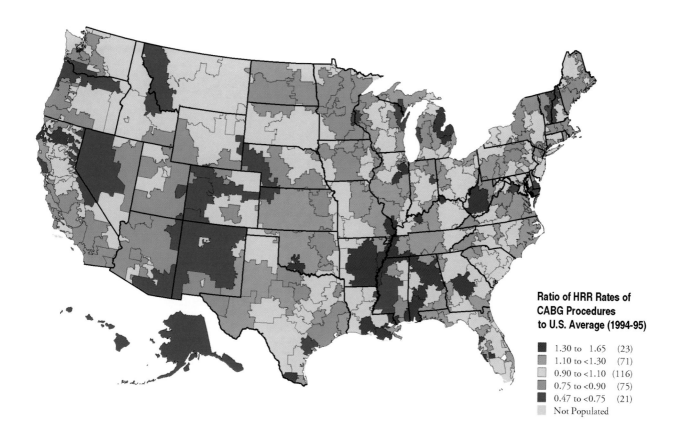

**Ratio of HRR Rates of
CABG Procedures
to U.S. Average (1994-95)**

■ 1.30 to 1.65   (23)
■ 1.10 to <1.30   (71)
□ 0.90 to <1.10 (116)
■ 0.75 to <0.90   (75)
■ 0.47 to <0.75   (21)
  Not Populated

Map 5.2. Coronary Artery Bypass Grafting

Rates of CABG varied more than rates of colectomy for colorectal cancer. Twenty-three regions had rates 30% or more higher than the national average (blue); 21 regions had rates more than 25% below the national average (green). Rates were high in Alabama, Arkansas, parts of Florida, Michigan, and parts of California. Rates were low in the Mountain states, the Northeast, and parts of California, as well as in Hawaii and Alaska.

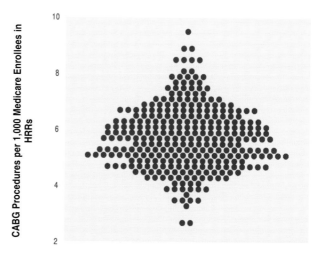

Figure 5.2. CABG Among Hospital Referral Regions (1994-95)

The rates varied from 2.7 to 9.5 per thousand Medicare enrollees, after adjustment. Each point represents one of the 306 hospital referral regions in the United States.

Early Stage Breast Cancer

Breast cancers are usually identified by screening mammography or by the patient herself after the appearance of a breast lump. These findings prompt a biopsy, which establishes the diagnosis of cancer. While occasionally the cancer will have spread to distant organs by the time of first diagnosis, most breast cancers are diagnosed in earlier stages.

The status of science is good. Randomized clinical trials demonstrate the value of early screening in reducing mortality in women who are over 50. Once diagnosed, surgery is universally recommended for treatment of breast cancer. There are two principal surgical approaches: breast sparing surgery (lumpectomy, which is followed by radiation therapy) and mastectomy (complete removal of the breast). Randomized clinical trials have shown that these two approaches have nearly identical rates of cancer cure.

The dilemma of choice concerns preferences, not science. The tradeoffs involve subjective factors that only patients can evaluate for themselves. With breast sparing surgery, a woman accepts the need for radiation and faces the possibility that the tumor will recur locally, requiring a complete mastectomy; but she avoids, at least in the near term, the total loss of her breast. With mastectomy, a woman avoids radiation and reduces the risk of local recurrence, but loses her breast. While reconstructive surgery and prostheses are potential options, the effect of mastectomy on body appearance and self-image is a considerable burden for many women.

Despite the scientific evidence that the survival rate is the same for breast sparing surgery and for mastectomy, and in spite of wide consensus that patient preferences should determine which treatment is chosen (and thus drive the aggregate rates of each procedure), the wide variations in surgical rates suggest that physician, rather than patient, preferences are the deciding factors in most cases.

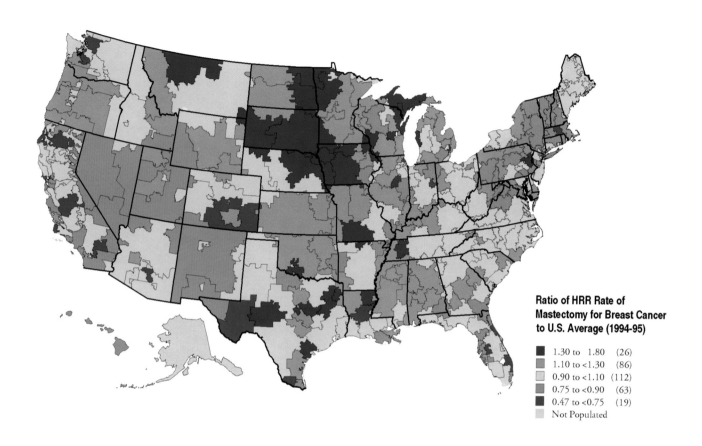

Ratio of HRR Rate of
Mastectomy for Breast Cancer
to U.S. Average (1994-95)

■ 1.30 to 1.80   (26)
■ 1.10 to <1.30   (86)
□ 0.90 to <1.10 (112)
■ 0.75 to <0.90   (63)
■ 0.47 to <0.75   (19)
□ Not Populated

Map 5.3. Mastectomy for Breast Cancer

Mastectomy for breast cancer is a high variation procedure. Twenty-six regions had rates 30% or more higher than the national average (blue); 19 had rates more than 25% below the national average (green). Rates were higher in the Midwest than on the East or West coasts.

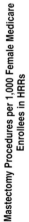
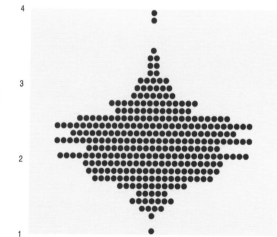

Mastectomy Procedures per 1,000 Female Medicare Enrollees in HRRs

Figure 5.3. Mastectomy Among Hospital Referral Regions (1994-95)

The rates varied from 1.1 to 4.0 per thousand female Medicare enrollees, after adjustment. Each point represents one of the 306 hospital referral regions in the United States.

Benign Prostatic Hyperplasia

Benign prostatic hyperplasia (BPH) is a common condition among older men. The most significant symptom of BPH, which for some men can be very bothersome, is difficulty in urination, caused by an enlargement of the prostate gland. There are multiple ways of treating BPH, including letting nature take its course (symptoms sometimes improve spontaneously); using one of several drugs; and having surgery, usually a transurethral prostatectomy (TURP).

The status of science. Outcomes research conducted over the last few years has done much to clarify the benefits and risks of undergoing treatment for BPH. A number of clinical studies have provided good evidence that surgery improves urinary symptoms. However, surgery carries with it significant risk of side effects, including retrograde ejaculation and a slight risk of incontinence. While not as effective as surgery, pharmaceuticals also improve urinary symptoms, with lower risks.

The dilemma of choice concerns preferences and tradeoffs. There are several possible outcomes associated with the different treatment options. Individual men differ in how they assess the risks and benefits of those outcomes. Men who choose surgery have the best chance of successfully reducing their symptoms, but face a substantial risk of suffering from retrograde ejaculation (or, less commonly, impotence and incontinence) after surgery. Men who choose medications may not realize the same improvement of symptoms as those who undergo surgery, but they avoid the risk of retrograde ejaculation. Men who choose watchful waiting forgo the risks and costs of surgery or drug treatment, but have reduced prospect for substantial improvement in symptoms.

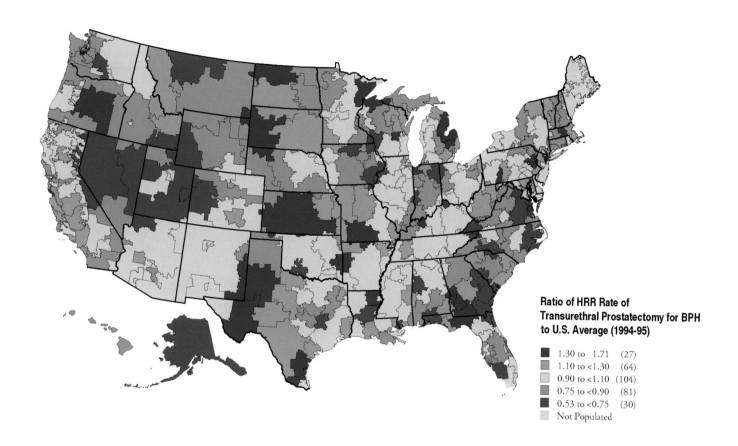

**Ratio of HRR Rate of
Transurethral Prostatectomy for BPH
to U.S. Average (1994-95)**

■	1.30 to 1.71 (27)
■	1.10 to <1.30 (64)
■	0.90 to <1.10 (104)
■	0.75 to <0.90 (81)
■	0.53 to <0.75 (30)
■	Not Populated

Map 5.4. Transurethral Prostatectomy for BPH

Prostatectomy for benign prostate hyperplasia is a high variation procedure. Twenty-seven regions had rates 30% or more higher than the national average (blue); 30 regions had rates more than 25% lower than the national average (green). Rates were high in western Texas, Kansas, parts of North and South Dakota, and central Oregon. Rates were lower in the Mountain states, northern Montana, and many regions on the East Coast.

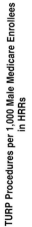

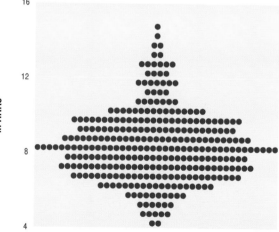

Figure 5.4. TURP for BPH Among Hospital Referral Regions (1994-95)

The rates varied from 4.5 to 14.5 per thousand male Medicare enrollees, after adjustment. Each point represents one of the 306 hospital referral regions in the United States.

Degeneration of the Knee Joint

Joint soreness and stiffness in elderly people are usually related to chronic degeneration of joint surfaces (osteoarthritis). Severe osteoarthritis of the knee causes pain with walking, and can sometimes limit mobility. Because anti-inflammatory medications have limited effectiveness in patients with severe symptoms, total knee replacement — a major surgical procedure involving placement of a prosthesis — is often recommended.

The status of science is fairly good in the case of knee replacement. While joint replacement has not been assessed in randomized clinical trials, most physicians agree that it is effective in improving patients' functional status and quality of life. The well-known risks associated with the procedure include surgical mortality and prosthesis-related complications; and long periods of recovery and rehabilitation after surgery are required.

The dilemma of choice. Orthopedic surgeons and patients share the same goal — to reduce pain and increase mobility. However, only patients are able to determine how much their symptoms affect their lives, and how they feel about the risks and side effects of surgery. The high degree of variation in use rates, even among neighboring regions, suggests that recommendations for joint replacement are driven largely by provider assessments of the tradeoffs between the risks and benefits of surgery.

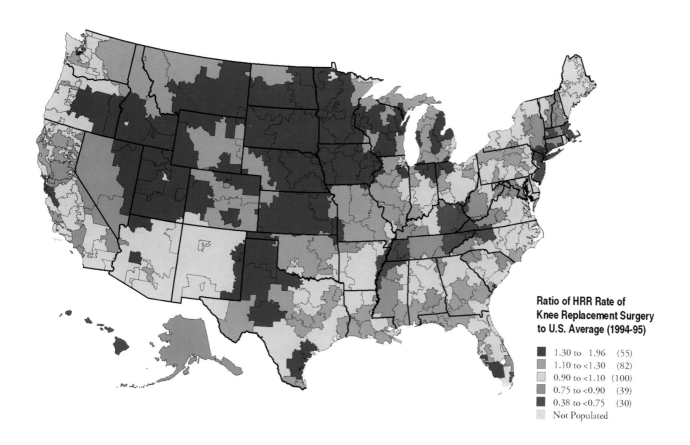

**Ratio of HRR Rate of
Knee Replacement Surgery
to U.S. Average (1994-95)**

■ 1.30 to 1.96   (55)
■ 1.10 to <1.30 (82)
□ 0.90 to <1.10 (100)
■ 0.75 to <0.90 (39)
■ 0.38 to <0.75 (30)
  Not Populated

Map 5.5. Knee Replacement Surgery

Knee replacement surgery is a high variation procedure. Fifty-five regions had rates 30% or more higher than the national average (blue); 30 regions had rates more than 25% below the national average (green). Rates were high in the upper Midwest and the Mountain states, and in parts of Texas and Oklahoma. Rates were low on the East and West coasts.

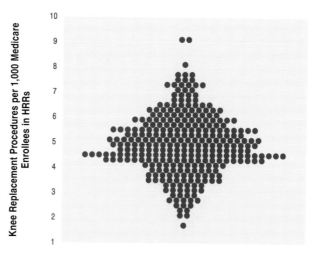

Figure 5.5. Knee Replacement Among Hospital Referral Regions (1994-95)

The rates varied from 1.8 to 9.1 per thousand Medicare enrollees, after adjustment. Each point represents one of the 306 hospital referral regions in the United States.

Back Pain

For most patients with the common problem of back pain, the symptoms are self-limited and the precise cause is never established. In some patients, however, back pain is caused by spinal stenosis (narrowing of the boney spine leading to pressure on the cord) or herniated discs (which "pinch" nerves exiting the spinal cord). These conditions can also cause neurological symptoms, such as leg weakness and numbness. When patient symptoms or findings on physical examination suggest spinal stenosis or a herniated disc, the diagnosis can be supported by imaging procedures such as computed tomography (CT scans) or magnetic resonance imaging (MRI scans).

The status of science concerning back surgery for spinal stenosis and herniated discs is poor. First, the clinical significance of these anatomic abnormalities is unclear — the same X-ray findings are frequently noted in patients without any back pain or neurological symptoms. Second, the effectiveness of back surgery for spinal stenosis or herniated discs has not been established by randomized clinical trials. Although recent studies suggest that symptoms and functional status in selected patients with herniated discs are initially improved after surgery, the long term effectiveness of surgery is still unknown and hotly debated. Moreover, little is known about the natural history of these conditions treated without surgery.

Dilemma of choice. Like any procedure aimed at improving symptoms, patient preferences are central to decision making in back surgery. Only the patient can determine how back-related symptoms affect his or her function or quality of life. In addition, physicians and patients may not always share the same goals in back surgery; for example, a physician may recommend surgery because of leg weakness, while the patient is primarily concerned with back pain.

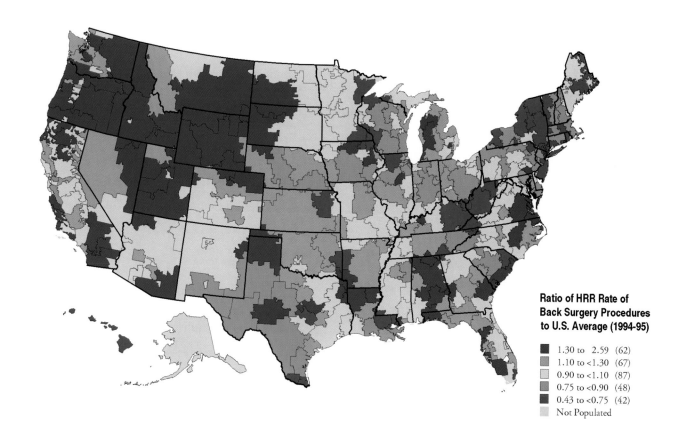

Ratio of HRR Rate of
Back Surgery Procedures
to U.S. Average (1994-95)

■ 1.30 to 2.59 (62)
■ 1.10 to <1.30 (67)
□ 0.90 to <1.10 (87)
■ 0.75 to <0.90 (48)
■ 0.43 to <0.75 (42)
□ Not Populated

Map 5.6. Back Surgery

Back surgery is a very high variation procedure. Sixty-two regions have rates 30% or more higher than the national average (blue); 42 have rates more than 25% below the national average (green). Rates are high in the Northwest and in the Mountain states, parts of Texas, Florida, North and South Carolina, Alabama, and California. Rates are lower in the Northeast and parts of the Midwest.

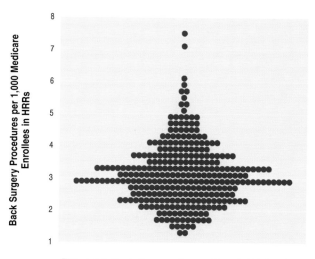

Figure 5.6. Back Surgery Among Hospital Referral Regions (1994-95)

The rates varied from 1.3 to 7.6 per thousand Medicare enrollees, after adjustment. Each point represents one of the 306 hospital referral regions in the United States.

Carotid Artery Disease

Many strokes are caused by narrowing (stenosis) of the carotid arteries, a diagnosis which is made using ultrasound or angiography. While nearly all patients with carotid stenosis are treated with aspirin, carotid endarterectomy is considered a treatment option for patients with severe stenosis (greater than 60% narrowing) and/or symptoms, including transient visual symptoms and numbness or weakness in an extremity. Endarterectomy, which removes plaque from the artery, carries a small risk of death, but has a higher and more variable risk of stroke.

The status of science concerning carotid endarterectomy in patients with symptoms is good, but inadequate for patients who are asymptomatic. Randomized controlled trials have demonstrated that, for patients with severe stenosis and symptoms, surgery is substantially more effective in reducing the risk of stroke than watchful waiting (12% vs. 26% at two years in one well-known trial). Recent clinical trials have demonstrated the effectiveness of surgery in asymptomatic patients, but the benefit is substantially smaller (5% vs. 11% in another trial at five years). Moreover, the studies of asymptomatic patients were based on relatively healthy (and low-risk) patients undergoing surgery at medical centers with proven records of excellent results.

The dilemma of choice is most apparent in treatment decisions for patients with carotid stenosis but no symptoms. Physicians and patients have the same objective — reduction of the risk of debilitating stroke. While physicians often emphasize the *magnitude* of stroke risks with each option, treatment decisions must also account for the *timing* of these risks. While surgery promises slightly lower stroke risks over the long term, strokes occurring as a result of the procedure affect patients immediately. The risk of stroke with watchful waiting rise gradually. For very elderly patients or those who are risk-averse, preferences about risk should play a substantial part in the decision about whether or not to undergo surgery.

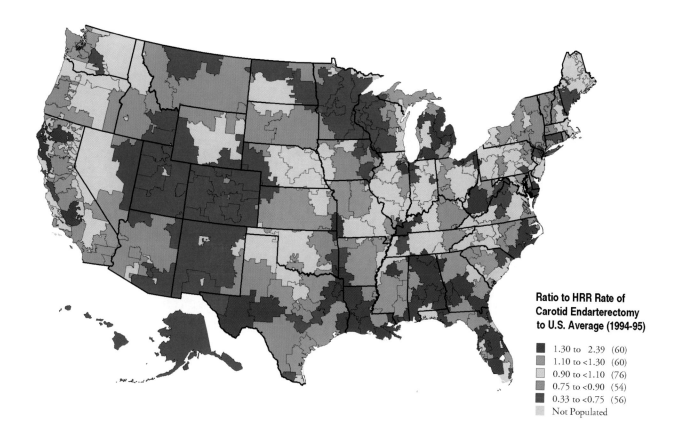

Ratio to HRR Rate of
**Carotid Endarterectomy
to U.S. Average (1994-95)**

■ 1.30 to 2.39 (60)
■ 1.10 to <1.30 (60)
□ 0.90 to <1.10 (76)
■ 0.75 to <0.90 (54)
■ 0.33 to <0.75 (56)
□ Not Populated

Map 5.7. Carotid Endarterectomy

Carotid endarterectomy is a very high variation procedure. Sixty regions have rates that are 30% or more higher than the national average (blue); 56 regions have rates that are more than 25% below the national average (green). Rates are high in parts of California, throughout much of the deep South and Florida, and in parts of Michigan. Rates are lower in the Northwest, in the Plains and Mountain states, and in New England.

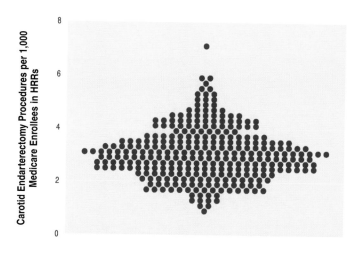

Figure 5.7. Carotid Endarterectomy Among Hospital Referral Regions (1994-95)

The rates varied from 1.0 to 7.1 per thousand Medicare enrollees, after adjustment. Each point represents one of the 306 hospital referral regions in the United States.

Peripheral Vascular Disease

Atherosclerosis ("hardening of the arteries") can affect the arteries supplying blood to the legs, especially in patients with diabetes and those who smoke. Atherosclerosis can cause muscle pain with walking or exercise (claudication). In its most severe forms, patients can experience pain at rest or foot ulcers and infections that will not heal and can ultimately result in the need for amputation of the leg. Other than risk factor modification (such as smoking cessation), there are no effective medications for treating peripheral vascular disease; as a result, many patients undergo lower extremity bypass to improve blood flow to their legs.

The status of science in lower extremity bypass is incomplete. While its effectiveness in different settings has not been established in controlled trials, most physicians agree that bypass surgery can obviate the need for leg amputation in patients with especially severe peripheral vascular disease. For patients with less severe disease (e.g., claudication only), the role of surgery is hotly debated. Conversely, the risks of lower extremity bypass are well known. These include immediate risks of heart attacks and death with the procedure and long term risks of bypass failure and need for subsequent interventions.

Dilemma of choice. Decisions about lower extremity bypass are complicated, and physicians and patients can differ in their assessments of tradeoffs between risks and benefits. In recommending surgery, vascular surgeons might focus on improving patient symptoms and avoiding leg amputations (and the need for limb prostheses). Though many patients no doubt share these primary goals, they might be bothered to different degrees by their symptoms and can differ in their willingness to take risks with surgery. In some cases, even patients with severe, limb-threatening disease can be more concerned about life expectancy than the status of their legs. This fundamental tradeoff can only be assessed by the individual patient.

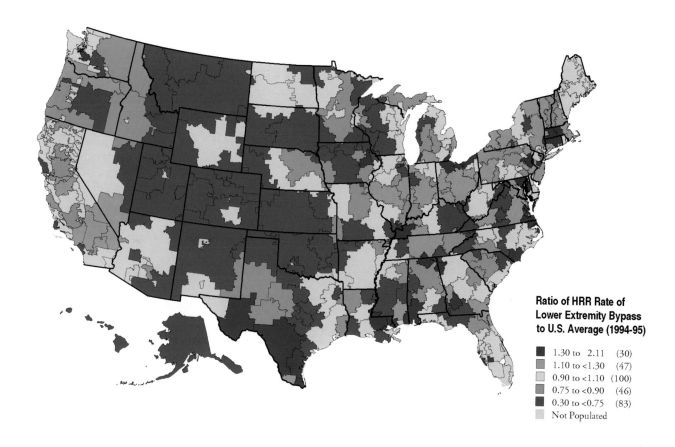

Ratio of HRR Rate of
Lower Extremity Bypass
to U.S. Average (1994-95)

- 1.30 to 2.11   (30)
- 1.10 to <1.30   (47)
- 0.90 to <1.10   (100)
- 0.75 to <0.90   (46)
- 0.30 to <0.75   (83)
- Not Populated

Map 5.8. Lower Extremity Bypass

Lower extremity bypass is a very high variation procedure. Thirty regions have rates that are 30% or more higher than the national average (blue); 83 have rates that are more than 25% lower than the national average (green). Rates are high in parts of Texas, Louisiana, and on the East Coast. Rates are low throughout the Midwest, the Plains and Mountain states, and in parts of Texas.

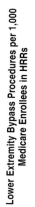
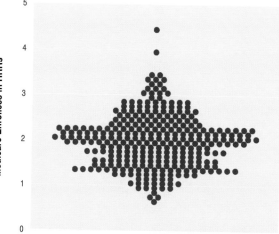

Lower Extremity Bypass Procedures per 1,000 Medicare Enrollees in HRRs

Figure 5.8. Lower Extremity Bypass Procedures Among Hospital Referral Regions (1994-95)

The rates varied from 0.6 to 4.5 per thousand Medicare enrollees, after adjustment. Each point represents one of the 306 hospital referral regions in the United States.

Early Stage Prostate Cancer

Prostate cancer, primarily a disease of older men, can be detected by routine physical examination or during evaluation for difficulties with urination. Prostate cancer can also be identified by screening men with the prostate specific antigen (PSA) blood test; its widespread use has led to the discovery of many more early stage cancers than were previously detected. Treatment of early stage prostate cancer usually involves either radiation therapy or radical prostatectomy, a surgical procedure in which the prostate gland is completely removed.

The status of science is poor. There are no completed clinical trials comparing survival in men who are being treated actively (with radiation or surgery) and those who are employing watchful waiting. Determining a benefit with radiation or surgery is difficult because most forms of early stage prostate cancer are very slow growing; many men, depending on their age, never have symptoms and die from other causes. While the benefits of active treatment are not clearly established, the complications of radiation and surgery are well documented: both carry a substantial risk of incontinence and impotence.

The dilemma of choice concerns preferences in the face of scientific uncertainty. A man who chooses radiation or surgery takes the chance that active treatment will improve his life expectancy, but he gambles on side effects including impotence and incontinence. A man who chooses watchful waiting forgoes the possibility that active treatment works, but avoids the risks associated with surgery. The very high variation profile of radical prostatectomy reflects both physician uncertainty about patient outcomes with each treatment strategy and problems with how patient preferences are incorporated into treatment choices.

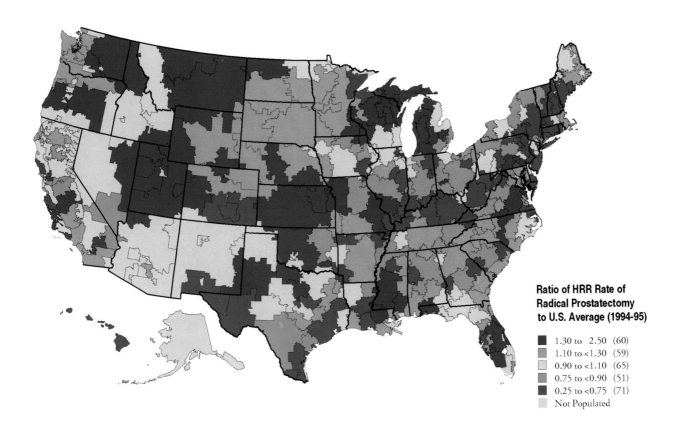

**Ratio of HRR Rate of
Radical Prostatectomy
to U.S. Average (1994-95)**

- 1.30 to 2.50 (60)
- 1.10 to <1.30 (59)
- 0.90 to <1.10 (65)
- 0.75 to <0.90 (51)
- 0.25 to <0.75 (71)
- Not Populated

Map 5.9. Radical Prostatectomy

Radical prostatectomy is a very high variation procedure. Sixty regions have rates that are 30% or more higher than the national average (blue); 71 regions have rates that are more than 25% below the national average (green). Rates are high in the Northwest, the Mountain and Great Plains states, Michigan, and parts of Florida and Mississippi. Rates are low in the Northeast, much of the Midwest, and in parts of Florida and Texas.

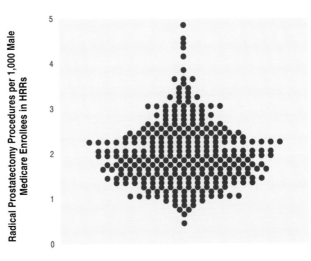

Figure 5.9. Radical Prostatectomy Among Hospital Referral Regions (1994-95)

The rates varied from 0.5 to 4.9 per thousand male Medicare enrollees, after adjustment. Each point represents one of the 306 hospital referral regions in the United States.

Chapter Five Table   All rates are age, sex, and race adjusted, and are expressed as rates per 1,000 Medicare enrollees. Surgical rates are for 1994-95, using a two year "person-year" denominator as given in the column labeled "Medicare Enrollees (1994 plus 1995)." Rates for mastectomy and prostate procedures are sex-specific. Data exclude Medicare enrollees who were members of risk bearing health maintenance organizations.

CABG = coronary artery bypass grafting
TURP for BPH = transurethral resection of the prostate for benign prostatic hyperplasia

Specific codes used to define the numerator for rates, and methods of age, sex, and race adjustment are included in the Appendix on Methods.

CHAPTER FIVE TABLE

Rates of Common Surgical Procedures Among Non-HMO Medicare Enrollees by Hospital Referral Region (1994-95)

Hospital Referral Region	Medicare Enrollees (1994 plus 1995)	Colectomy for Colorectal Cancer	CABG Surgery	Mastectomy for Cancer	TURP for BPH	Knee Replacement	Back Surgery	Carotid Endarterectomy	Lower Extremity Bypass	Radical Prostatectomy
Alabama										
Birmingham	537,479	2.3	8.2	2.4	9.0	4.5	4.2	4.2	1.9	1.6
Dothan	90,492	1.9	7.1	1.9	10.4	5.1	3.7	4.0	1.5	2.0
Huntsville	108,063	2.2	6.6	2.2	8.7	4.2	4.2	4.1	3.3	2.4
Mobile	166,897	2.6	8.4	2.5	6.7	5.1	3.0	4.1	3.9	2.3
Montgomery	98,236	2.2	5.5	2.6	6.8	4.1	5.9	4.0	2.0	2.2
Tuscaloosa	56,503	2.2	6.3	2.8	5.8	4.7	3.8	3.8	1.5	1.4
Alaska										
Anchorage	53,661	2.1	4.1	2.0	4.6	3.8	3.0	1.8	0.9	2.1
Arizona										
Mesa	110,303	2.4	5.1	1.3	7.1	5.6	3.6	2.2	1.8	2.3
Phoenix	378,996	2.1	4.6	2.2	8.4	4.6	3.0	2.5	2.0	2.0
Sun City	95,755	2.3	5.1	2.5	9.5	6.3	3.6	2.4	1.2	2.1
Tucson	158,221	2.1	3.6	2.3	8.1	4.7	4.3	1.4	1.4	2.0
Arkansas										
Fort Smith	88,596	2.2	5.7	1.9	12.8	4.6	2.0	1.9	1.4	1.8
Jonesboro	62,128	2.5	6.6	1.9	9.8	4.9	3.6	3.5	1.7	1.0
Little Rock	388,936	2.4	8.0	2.4	8.3	5.0	3.4	3.5	2.3	2.5
Springdale	93,936	2.4	5.2	2.3	9.4	3.8	2.7	2.4	1.1	1.3
Texarkana	69,870	2.6	6.0	2.4	9.2	4.7	4.2	4.2	2.0	1.2
California										
Orange Co.	277,496	2.2	4.5	1.9	6.4	4.0	3.2	2.4	1.6	2.5
Bakersfield	122,394	1.7	6.4	2.3	9.6	4.4	3.3	4.7	1.6	2.2
Chico	75,738	2.6	6.1	2.1	9.8	5.4	4.0	3.3	1.7	1.7
Contra Costa Co.	135,462	2.0	6.0	1.7	7.6	4.1	2.4	2.9	1.7	2.6
Fresno	167,352	2.2	4.8	1.6	10.0	4.5	3.0	2.6	2.0	2.7
Los Angeles	979,115	2.3	5.1	1.8	9.5	3.5	3.2	2.4	2.6	2.3
Modesto	122,468	2.5	5.3	2.3	9.0	4.7	2.9	3.5	2.4	1.7
Napa	73,922	2.4	6.8	2.2	8.4	5.4	3.5	5.2	2.0	1.8
Alameda Co.	220,774	2.2	4.5	1.8	8.7	3.6	2.9	2.4	2.0	1.7
Palm Spr/Rancho Mir	60,846	1.8	4.8	1.5	9.3	4.8	5.5	3.4	2.6	2.8
Redding	85,526	2.6	9.0	1.6	8.5	5.4	4.4	4.6	2.1	2.5
Sacramento	372,342	2.2	6.2	2.1	7.9	3.9	3.0	2.6	1.6	2.0
Salinas	65,778	2.2	6.3	1.9	9.6	4.6	3.8	3.1	1.7	1.1
San Bernardino	186,067	2.4	4.9	2.0	8.0	4.5	4.0	2.9	2.5	2.0
San Diego	340,069	1.9	4.4	1.8	7.6	4.3	4.1	2.2	2.1	2.3
San Francisco	247,271	2.2	4.3	1.4	6.4	3.2	2.8	1.7	1.7	1.7
San Jose	200,648	2.2	4.7	2.0	7.1	3.0	2.5	2.2	2.3	1.9
San Luis Obispo	45,883	2.6	4.7	2.4	9.4	5.1	5.2	2.9	2.0	2.9
San Mateo Co.	127,808	2.2	4.4	1.9	6.6	3.2	2.8	3.0	2.3	1.9
Santa Barbara	67,633	2.1	4.7	1.4	7.1	4.9	5.8	2.5	1.5	2.6

Hospital Referral Region	Medicare Enrollees (1994 plus 1995)	Colectomy for Colorectal Cancer	CABG Surgery	Mastectomy for Cancer	TURP for BPH	Knee Replacement	Back Surgery	Carotid Endarterectomy	Lower Extremity Bypass	Radical Prostatectomy
Santa Cruz	47,307	2.3	4.6	2.0	11.1	3.3	3.0	2.6	2.0	2.5
Santa Rosa	88,736	2.1	3.7	2.0	6.4	4.4	2.7	3.2	1.5	1.3
Stockton	81,367	2.3	5.9	2.2	6.8	3.6	3.7	3.5	2.6	1.6
Ventura	87,044	2.4	5.3	1.8	9.9	4.2	4.9	2.6	2.1	3.4
Colorado										
Boulder	29,840	2.0	4.4	2.1	9.7	4.1	4.8	2.4	1.0	2.7
Colorado Springs	120,774	2.2	5.4	1.6	8.8	5.3	3.1	2.2	1.5	1.3
Denver	310,515	2.0	3.4	2.2	6.8	5.5	3.6	1.8	1.4	2.3
Fort Collins	48,758	2.6	4.3	2.5	8.8	6.9	7.0	1.8	1.0	2.9
Grand Junction	60,182	1.9	2.7	2.1	5.8	6.5	3.2	1.3	0.8	3.1
Greeley	58,402	2.4	5.5	2.1	7.8	7.4	4.9	1.7	1.1	2.5
Pueblo	38,864	2.1	4.3	2.5	10.9	6.5	3.5	1.8	2.2	1.1
Connecticut										
Bridgeport	177,126	2.5	4.0	1.8	7.7	3.3	3.1	2.2	2.2	1.6
Hartford	379,870	2.5	6.2	1.8	7.0	3.8	2.3	1.9	2.8	1.5
New Haven	355,027	2.9	6.4	2.1	7.2	3.4	2.1	2.4	2.6	1.1
Delaware										
Wilmington	149,894	2.8	4.8	2.2	8.9	4.5	2.7	3.6	2.2	1.8
District of Columbia										
Washington	434,959	2.4	5.2	2.4	9.3	3.9	3.2	3.0	2.4	1.7
Florida										
Bradenton	97,968	3.0	6.7	2.4	7.6	6.5	4.4	3.7	2.0	1.6
Clearwater	190,163	2.8	5.5	1.9	9.4	6.0	4.4	4.1	2.2	2.8
Fort Lauderdale	649,805	2.5	6.8	1.6	8.0	3.8	3.3	3.2	2.2	1.9
Fort Myers	330,485	2.6	6.2	2.1	6.0	6.4	6.1	4.0	2.1	2.6
Gainesville	104,978	2.2	5.6	2.1	8.0	4.6	3.4	3.7	1.7	1.8
Hudson	170,411	3.0	8.5	1.7	10.0	5.9	4.2	4.6	2.2	1.4
Jacksonville	249,798	2.3	6.8	1.7	6.0	4.3	3.0	4.6	2.4	2.3
Lakeland	86,072	2.3	6.3	1.2	6.6	5.6	3.7	4.4	2.3	1.6
Miami	450,631	2.5	5.4	1.7	7.9	3.0	1.7	1.7	2.0	1.7
Ocala	165,669	2.4	6.6	1.7	7.9	5.2	4.1	4.0	2.3	2.2
Orlando	712,980	2.6	5.9	2.0	7.0	4.8	3.1	4.0	2.1	2.9
Ormond Beach	92,611	2.9	5.2	1.0	8.4	4.4	3.0	3.2	2.2	3.8
Panama City	44,279	3.0	6.4	2.0	9.6	5.3	3.3	4.0	2.0	2.1
Pensacola	150,623	2.3	7.0	2.2	5.8	5.4	4.0	3.0	2.1	2.9
Sarasota	192,164	2.8	7.6	1.8	7.0	5.1	3.6	3.6	2.8	3.6
St Petersburg	140,562	2.7	5.1	2.5	10.1	4.8	3.9	5.9	3.3	3.3
Tallahassee	146,298	2.0	5.8	2.2	12.8	5.1	3.4	3.5	1.3	1.9
Tampa	188,237	2.8	6.1	1.8	9.2	4.9	3.3	2.9	2.0	1.2
Georgia										
Albany	44,137	1.8	5.2	2.5	12.2	5.6	3.0	4.9	3.4	2.1
Atlanta	710,713	2.2	5.6	2.0	7.2	4.3	2.7	3.5	2.2	2.3
Augusta	124,772	2.1	6.2	2.8	4.5	4.3	3.5	3.2	1.7	1.5
Columbus	67,659	2.0	6.6	2.1	11.2	4.5	3.9	5.1	2.4	1.4
Macon	145,511	2.3	7.7	2.4	9.9	5.2	3.3	4.3	1.9	1.5
Rome	60,935	1.8	7.1	2.3	9.1	4.0	3.1	5.0	2.9	1.8

Hospital Referral Region	Medicare Enrollees (1994 plus 1995)	Colectomy for Colorectal Cancer	CABG Surgery	Mastectomy for Cancer	TURP for BPH	Knee Replacement	Back Surgery	Carotid Endarterectomy	Lower Extremity Bypass	Radical Prostatectomy
Savannah	141,664	2.5	6.2	2.1	5.5	5.2	4.9	3.6	2.2	2.3
Hawaii										
Honolulu	186,522	1.9	3.5	1.6	6.3	1.8	1.9	1.0	1.1	1.1
Idaho										
Boise	139,886	2.0	5.5	2.1	6.6	7.7	5.3	2.4	1.7	1.8
Idaho Falls	33,432	1.7	5.3	2.5	10.2	6.1	4.2	1.0	1.0	1.9
Illinois										
Aurora	33,523	2.3	6.9	2.1	8.9	7.3	3.7	4.3	1.3	1.9
Blue Island	190,678	3.1	6.9	2.3	8.5	4.5	2.6	3.5	2.4	2.0
Chicago	481,644	2.7	6.1	1.9	10.2	3.3	1.7	2.1	1.9	1.2
Elgin	84,116	2.5	5.8	2.8	7.3	4.9	3.5	2.8	2.1	1.1
Evanston	222,380	2.5	6.4	1.5	8.5	4.3	2.8	2.3	1.4	2.1
Hinsdale	62,711	2.8	7.4	2.3	7.5	4.5	3.1	2.6	1.3	2.0
Joliet	97,925	2.7	8.5	2.3	9.2	6.1	2.4	4.6	1.6	1.9
Melrose Park	266,580	2.7	7.1	2.0	8.7	4.5	2.5	2.6	1.8	1.4
Peoria	189,850	2.8	5.7	2.5	8.2	5.5	2.2	3.2	2.2	2.3
Rockford	172,170	2.7	5.8	2.6	8.1	5.7	2.1	3.0	2.0	1.9
Springfield	258,349	2.7	7.4	2.8	8.8	5.9	3.7	3.1	2.5	1.5
Urbana	113,019	2.8	6.7	1.9	7.8	4.6	2.7	3.3	2.5	1.3
Bloomington	38,340	2.4	8.9	3.5	8.5	5.5	4.2	3.2	1.7	1.4
Indiana										
Evansville	197,344	2.6	6.1	2.4	7.1	5.1	3.0	2.8	1.8	1.4
Fort Wayne	197,467	2.6	5.0	1.8	5.1	6.7	3.5	2.7	2.1	1.3
Gary	115,149	3.1	6.7	2.3	14.1	5.5	3.0	4.2	2.5	2.0
Indianapolis	577,302	2.5	5.5	2.2	7.4	4.8	2.4	3.2	2.4	1.7
Lafayette	46,058	2.5	6.2	2.1	6.4	5.6	3.7	2.1	1.4	1.8
Muncie	46,009	3.0	3.9	1.6	6.9	5.1	3.2	2.2	1.6	1.3
Munster	81,614	3.2	7.6	2.2	9.6	5.2	2.3	4.3	2.4	1.7
South Bend	167,189	2.6	7.1	2.5	6.9	6.1	2.5	3.0	2.2	1.6
Terre Haute	54,462	2.8	6.9	2.6	5.6	4.3	3.3	3.2	2.6	1.5
Iowa										
Cedar Rapids	70,726	2.6	6.1	2.6	6.9	8.1	3.8	2.6	3.0	2.3
Davenport	139,217	3.0	4.6	2.1	5.4	6.4	2.7	3.4	1.9	1.8
Des Moines	281,031	2.7	5.1	2.8	7.2	6.8	2.3	2.3	1.4	2.0
Dubuque	43,412	2.8	4.3	3.0	7.9	6.6	3.3	4.5	1.4	2.1
Iowa City	84,807	2.7	5.9	1.6	4.5	6.1	2.3	2.2	1.6	1.3
Mason City	53,884	2.3	6.7	3.9	5.4	7.3	4.2	2.9	1.3	1.5
Sioux City	80,490	2.7	4.6	3.1	8.1	9.1	2.7	3.2	1.3	1.8
Waterloo	64,000	2.6	4.4	2.4	7.1	7.2	2.9	1.9	1.7	2.5
Kansas										
Topeka	111,252	2.3	4.7	2.7	9.9	7.0	2.1	3.2	1.3	2.8
Wichita	350,947	2.4	6.8	2.7	11.9	7.3	3.4	3.7	1.3	2.6
Kentucky										
Covington	73,891	3.0	8.1	1.7	5.7	3.7	2.7	3.6	2.7	1.2
Lexington	303,869	2.3	6.0	2.2	9.0	2.9	1.8	2.4	1.5	1.3
Louisville	374,076	2.4	6.9	2.6	8.7	4.4	2.8	3.2	2.2	1.4

Hospital Referral Region	Medicare Enrollees (1994 plus 1995)	Colectomy for Colorectal Cancer	CABG Surgery	Mastectomy for Cancer	TURP for BPH	Knee Replacement	Back Surgery	Carotid Endarterectomy	Lower Extremity Bypass	Radical Prostatectomy
Owensboro	36,107	2.0	7.7	2.5	12.7	4.4	4.6	4.3	2.3	1.5
Paducah	113,220	2.9	6.2	2.5	7.2	4.0	3.3	5.6	3.0	1.2
Louisiana										
Alexandria	68,176	2.3	5.9	1.5	4.7	5.3	3.4	4.7	2.1	1.1
Baton Rouge	137,670	2.7	6.1	2.2	8.5	4.6	1.9	3.3	2.8	4.9
Houma	45,986	2.7	9.5	1.8	7.4	5.7	3.7	7.1	1.5	2.3
Lafayette	117,623	2.5	7.4	2.1	9.8	5.7	2.4	5.5	1.9	0.9
Lake Charles	52,492	2.3	6.0	2.3	8.0	6.0	3.0	4.5	1.4	2.4
Metairie	90,099	2.6	7.5	2.0	9.5	5.1	2.1	5.5	3.4	2.4
Monroe	68,195	2.0	5.4	2.9	14.0	5.1	3.9	2.3	1.1	1.5
New Orleans	173,118	2.8	6.5	2.5	8.2	4.5	2.3	4.7	2.2	1.8
Shreveport	169,027	2.3	5.6	2.7	8.6	4.6	3.9	4.2	1.6	2.1
Slidell	31,751	2.6	8.0	2.2	6.2	5.9	3.9	5.9	3.2	1.6
Maine										
Bangor	110,857	2.7	4.7	2.0	9.1	4.6	1.9	2.7	2.2	2.3
Portland	258,754	2.7	4.8	2.1	7.7	4.4	2.6	2.2	2.2	1.1
Maryland										
Baltimore	554,763	2.8	5.9	2.3	10.4	4.8	3.3	3.5	3.4	2.3
Salisbury	105,521	2.8	3.6	2.5	8.2	4.8	2.5	4.5	2.1	0.7
Takoma Park	132,928	2.2	4.6	2.4	7.4	3.5	3.1	2.7	2.3	1.9
Massachusetts										
Boston	1,143,195	2.9	5.1	1.6	10.0	3.3	2.2	2.8	2.7	1.7
Springfield	205,413	2.7	4.3	1.9	7.0	3.3	2.2	2.3	2.9	1.1
Worcester	146,527	2.7	4.7	1.4	11.3	3.6	2.2	3.1	2.8	2.1
Michigan										
Ann Arbor	264,391	2.4	5.4	1.9	9.3	5.4	2.7	3.3	2.0	1.5
Dearborn	146,511	2.6	6.9	2.1	7.7	5.0	2.2	3.9	2.7	1.8
Detroit	464,934	2.7	6.6	2.4	9.4	4.6	2.8	4.0	2.4	1.7
Flint	116,033	2.4	8.4	2.7	11.7	5.8	3.1	4.6	2.2	2.6
Grand Rapids	225,773	2.2	4.9	2.1	8.7	5.9	4.7	2.8	1.7	3.7
Kalamazoo	154,892	2.5	5.3	2.6	7.6	5.7	3.5	4.4	2.6	3.2
Lansing	126,740	2.4	7.1	2.2	7.1	6.1	3.5	4.0	1.9	3.2
Marquette	65,819	2.1	7.0	2.9	6.8	5.7	2.9	3.4	1.8	2.6
Muskegon	69,045	2.0	4.2	3.0	9.3	6.7	3.7	3.7	1.5	3.5
Petoskey	49,979	2.5	5.9	2.5	9.5	5.9	3.4	3.3	2.2	2.7
Pontiac	73,114	2.2	6.3	2.2	7.3	4.8	4.4	3.8	2.0	1.4
Royal Oak	164,071	2.4	5.7	1.4	9.8	4.3	3.2	3.8	1.6	1.7
Saginaw	189,336	2.6	7.9	2.4	11.1	6.2	3.7	4.8	2.2	2.0
St Joseph	39,347	2.4	6.0	2.3	7.5	5.9	3.8	4.2	3.2	3.1
Traverse City	63,020	2.8	6.9	2.6	8.7	5.4	4.2	5.2	1.5	3.0
Minnesota										
Duluth	110,010	2.6	4.8	2.7	13.9	5.7	2.1	1.8	1.0	1.4
Minneapolis	565,246	2.3	5.0	2.7	8.4	6.3	2.9	1.7	1.6	2.5
Rochester	111,140	2.5	4.9	2.7	7.1	6.3	1.9	1.7	1.4	3.0
St Cloud	51,161	2.4	5.0	2.7	7.8	7.1	2.9	2.0	2.0	2.3
St Paul	148,272	2.3	4.3	2.7	7.2	6.4	3.1	1.5	1.9	2.9

Hospital Referral Region	Medicare Enrollees (1994 plus 1995)	Colectomy for Colorectal Cancer	CABG Surgery	Mastectomy for Cancer	TURP for BPH	Knee Replacement	Back Surgery	Carotid Endarterectomy	Lower Extremity Bypass	Radical Prostatectomy
Mississippi										
Gulfport	37,993	2.5	4.7	2.4	9.6	5.2	3.2	5.3	2.3	2.0
Hattiesburg	64,090	2.0	4.9	2.3	8.4	5.7	2.9	3.8	2.4	4.4
Jackson	239,461	2.3	4.3	2.6	8.5	3.9	2.9	3.5	1.6	3.1
Meridian	53,642	2.3	6.0	2.4	10.3	4.4	2.8	3.4	1.3	2.3
Oxford	34,347	2.7	6.8	2.6	8.7	3.6	3.3	4.7	2.2	1.4
Tupelo	89,959	2.0	6.2	2.5	8.4	4.3	2.6	3.3	1.8	2.1
Missouri										
Cape Girardeau	77,117	2.2	7.5	1.8	9.4	4.3	3.1	3.8	1.3	1.3
Columbia	178,064	2.7	7.2	2.5	9.7	5.8	3.5	3.4	1.8	1.5
Joplin	104,872	2.3	5.5	2.8	10.6	7.3	3.2	4.2	1.9	2.5
Kansas City	484,363	2.7	5.3	2.6	9.5	5.9	2.9	3.6	2.2	3.0
Springfield	215,960	2.3	6.2	2.8	11.8	5.2	2.8	2.8	1.2	2.3
St Louis	835,277	2.7	6.8	2.4	8.1	5.5	3.0	2.8	2.3	3.0
Montana										
Billings	124,356	2.2	5.6	2.3	6.7	6.1	4.6	2.5	1.5	4.2
Great Falls	40,385	2.5	5.1	3.3	4.8	5.8	3.1	1.4	1.4	3.3
Missoula	84,737	2.1	3.6	2.5	9.4	5.1	3.3	2.6	1.0	2.0
Nebraska										
Lincoln	158,230	2.6	5.0	2.4	7.1	7.6	2.6	3.1	1.9	2.9
Omaha	304,693	2.7	5.6	2.9	8.3	7.0	3.2	3.0	1.9	2.4
Nevada										
Las Vegas	169,265	2.4	5.4	1.9	7.3	3.5	2.9	3.6	2.7	1.7
Reno	124,388	2.0	3.9	1.9	5.4	4.1	3.3	2.8	1.9	1.8
New Hampshire										
Lebanon	108,521	2.6	3.9	1.9	6.4	4.1	2.4	2.2	1.8	1.3
Manchester	170,161	2.8	5.8	1.9	7.2	3.6	2.4	2.9	2.4	1.1
New Jersey										
Camden	719,405	2.9	5.3	2.3	8.7	3.3	1.9	3.0	2.4	1.3
Hackensack	318,321	2.8	5.1	1.9	12.7	2.5	1.7	1.9	2.5	1.2
Morristown	211,595	2.6	4.6	2.1	10.0	3.1	2.2	2.0	2.0	1.8
New Brunswick	198,391	2.6	5.3	1.9	8.2	2.7	2.1	3.1	2.9	2.0
Newark	354,227	2.8	4.7	2.0	11.9	2.2	1.4	1.7	2.7	1.0
Paterson	83,423	2.9	4.9	1.6	12.9	2.7	1.7	1.8	3.0	1.0
Ridgewood	88,588	2.6	5.1	2.0	8.1	2.4	1.7	1.9	2.1	1.9
New Mexico										
Albuquerque	226,584	1.7	2.7	1.8	7.8	4.5	3.0	1.5	1.2	1.9
New York										
Albany	482,713	2.9	5.6	1.9	8.5	3.5	1.8	2.6	2.7	1.3
Binghamton	111,017	2.5	4.7	1.9	6.3	4.4	2.9	2.5	2.1	0.7
Bronx	209,549	2.6	4.1	2.0	11.0	2.4	1.3	1.1	2.4	1.7
Buffalo	419,829	2.8	5.8	2.1	8.6	4.4	2.1	3.2	2.4	1.7
Elmira	110,385	2.6	5.9	1.7	7.9	3.7	1.7	3.0	1.5	1.8
East Long Island	993,102	2.7	5.7	1.9	9.2	2.2	1.4	1.9	2.2	1.0
New York	921,023	2.6	5.0	2.0	9.6	2.1	1.5	1.6	2.1	0.9
Rochester	297,439	2.6	5.9	2.0	8.6	4.4	2.5	3.3	2.7	2.1

Hospital Referral Region	Medicare Enrollees (1994 plus 1995)	Colectomy for Colorectal Cancer	CABG Surgery	Mastectomy for Cancer	TURP for BPH	Knee Replacement	Back Surgery	Carotid Endarterectomy	Lower Extremity Bypass	Radical Prostatectomy
Syracuse	269,229	2.7	5.1	2.4	6.4	4.4	1.4	3.3	2.3	1.7
White Plains	262,606	2.9	5.1	2.4	10.1	2.8	2.0	2.2	1.9	1.5
North Carolina										
Asheville	182,675	2.1	4.6	2.2	6.8	3.9	2.5	3.1	1.5	2.2
Charlotte	385,571	2.3	5.7	2.1	6.0	4.4	3.1	2.9	1.8	2.3
Durham	289,156	2.3	5.9	2.0	7.5	4.4	2.9	2.4	1.5	2.8
Greensboro	126,534	2.3	6.6	2.2	7.4	4.2	3.8	3.1	2.2	2.2
Greenville	167,054	2.6	7.1	2.1	4.8	4.4	3.3	4.2	1.9	2.1
Hickory	60,987	1.8	7.3	2.5	7.3	3.5	3.0	3.8	2.1	2.2
Raleigh	265,693	2.2	6.0	2.2	8.0	4.4	4.1	3.4	1.9	2.4
Wilmington	81,845	2.0	6.7	2.6	7.5	5.1	2.7	4.3	2.9	2.3
Winston-Salem	246,496	2.4	6.0	2.4	8.4	3.2	3.0	2.7	2.2	2.3
North Dakota										
Bismarck	62,268	2.3	4.8	2.6	9.3	6.9	4.8	3.1	2.3	2.4
Fargo Moorhead -Mn	144,962	2.6	5.1	3.2	6.8	6.1	2.7	1.6	2.0	2.5
Grand Forks	49,542	2.7	5.3	3.0	7.1	6.3	2.8	2.4	1.3	1.8
Minot	39,488	2.5	6.4	2.8	12.1	5.4	2.7	1.9	2.0	4.5
Ohio										
Akron	178,783	2.6	6.4	1.9	7.0	5.6	2.7	3.5	2.1	1.5
Canton	173,295	2.6	6.1	2.3	7.0	5.3	2.8	2.8	2.4	1.2
Cincinnati	368,421	2.7	5.8	2.0	9.2	4.4	3.2	3.3	2.5	1.6
Cleveland	571,022	2.6	6.3	2.2	8.5	4.7	2.9	4.2	2.8	1.6
Columbus	601,479	2.9	5.1	2.2	8.9	5.0	2.6	3.1	2.7	1.6
Dayton	282,726	2.6	7.3	2.6	7.5	5.6	3.2	3.3	2.6	1.5
Elyria	59,128	2.6	6.3	1.7	7.6	5.6	3.3	5.1	4.5	1.1
Kettering	94,569	2.7	6.7	2.3	8.0	4.2	2.9	3.4	2.5	3.6
Toledo	250,645	2.7	5.8	2.1	8.4	6.1	3.3	3.7	2.8	2.0
Youngstown	232,794	2.6	5.7	2.3	10.8	4.9	2.4	3.9	2.1	1.5
Oklahoma										
Lawton	48,734	2.5	7.6	3.2	5.5	5.0	3.0	3.7	1.2	1.8
Oklahoma City	408,313	2.3	6.4	2.6	8.9	5.3	3.3	3.2	1.4	3.1
Tulsa	291,992	2.2	5.0	2.6	7.6	5.7	3.5	2.5	1.3	1.7
Oregon										
Bend	39,516	2.4	5.7	2.4	14.5	6.4	7.6	3.1	1.3	4.4
Eugene	167,889	2.0	4.5	2.6	8.0	4.8	5.0	2.6	1.7	2.8
Medford	122,278	2.3	4.9	2.7	7.0	4.9	4.5	3.4	1.8	2.0
Portland	322,105	2.3	3.9	2.4	6.8	4.4	4.6	2.9	2.5	2.5
Salem	55,675	2.3	4.3	2.7	7.0	5.2	3.8	2.6	1.3	1.6
Pennsylvania										
Allentown	307,875	3.0	5.7	2.9	12.2	4.3	2.3	3.3	2.9	1.3
Altoona	95,524	3.1	7.3	2.5	10.0	4.2	2.4	2.3	1.9	1.3
Danville	154,249	3.0	4.8	1.9	8.3	5.3	3.0	3.1	1.6	1.7
Erie	226,760	2.7	5.5	2.5	8.4	5.3	2.6	2.7	1.9	1.7
Harrisburg	253,802	2.8	6.0	2.2	8.1	4.9	2.8	2.9	2.0	2.7
Johnstown	89,066	2.6	6.9	1.9	11.8	5.3	2.9	2.9	1.7	2.0
Lancaster	140,914	2.5	5.9	1.8	8.4	4.6	4.1	2.2	1.8	2.5

Hospital Referral Region	Medicare Enrollees (1994 plus 1995)	Colectomy for Colorectal Cancer	CABG Surgery	Mastectomy for Cancer	TURP for BPH	Knee Replacement	Back Surgery	Carotid Endarterectomy	Lower Extremity Bypass	Radical Prostatectomy
Philadelphia	989,081	2.8	5.8	1.8	9.7	4.5	2.4	2.7	2.5	1.5
Pittsburgh	1,040,060	2.9	6.7	1.7	9.2	5.0	3.0	3.0	2.6	2.0
Reading	169,509	2.9	6.4	2.0	8.9	5.1	2.7	2.7	2.7	2.1
Sayre	56,304	2.5	4.5	2.5	6.6	5.1	2.3	2.7	1.6	1.1
Scranton	114,614	3.0	5.5	2.5	6.4	4.4	2.1	2.4	2.6	0.7
Wilkes-Barre	96,247	2.8	6.3	2.7	8.0	4.3	2.2	2.6	2.3	1.0
York	97,650	2.9	7.2	1.8	7.8	4.0	2.5	2.7	2.1	0.8
Rhode Island										
Providence	308,154	2.9	4.8	1.8	9.0	4.2	1.7	2.6	2.2	1.0
South Carolina										
Charleston	161,754	2.5	5.2	2.3	9.7	4.5	3.9	2.8	2.2	2.5
Columbia	222,914	2.1	5.3	2.3	6.4	4.6	2.2	3.5	1.7	1.6
Florence	78,959	1.8	5.7	2.7	10.9	4.0	2.2	2.2	1.5	0.9
Greenville	176,406	2.3	6.4	2.3	9.4	3.7	2.9	2.5	1.7	2.2
Spartanburg	85,168	2.0	4.7	2.2	10.2	3.7	2.4	2.6	1.5	2.4
South Dakota										
Rapid City	45,539	1.7	6.2	2.8	13.3	6.3	4.8	2.5	0.9	2.2
Sioux Falls	235,194	2.9	5.8	3.3	10.3	7.6	3.2	2.4	1.2	2.3
Tennessee										
Chattanooga	149,998	2.2	6.6	2.2	9.2	3.7	2.2	2.8	1.4	1.7
Jackson	92,620	2.7	6.8	2.9	9.9	3.1	2.8	2.2	1.0	1.8
Johnson City	61,756	1.9	5.8	1.8	5.8	2.8	1.6	2.8	1.4	1.2
Kingsport	133,235	1.9	4.8	2.3	6.1	2.4	1.8	2.8	1.4	0.9
Knoxville	304,170	2.1	6.1	2.0	8.5	3.2	2.2	3.6	1.7	1.7
Memphis	368,727	2.5	7.8	2.4	8.5	2.7	2.7	3.2	2.0	1.5
Nashville	486,202	2.3	6.6	2.3	8.6	3.7	3.7	3.1	2.5	2.3
Texas										
Abilene	88,885	2.0	7.0	2.3	9.3	5.5	2.6	3.8	1.8	2.0
Amarillo	105,065	1.6	5.7	2.3	7.3	7.5	4.9	3.0	1.5	1.9
Austin	156,434	2.4	5.4	2.5	8.9	5.6	2.9	2.0	1.3	2.2
Beaumont	119,549	2.7	6.7	2.3	9.5	5.6	2.8	4.1	1.8	2.1
Bryan	37,569	2.7	6.5	2.2	4.6	6.0	3.4	2.2	1.0	2.4
Corpus Christi	101,137	2.2	6.2	2.6	12.1	6.1	2.5	3.3	3.2	1.1
Dallas	578,294	2.5	5.3	2.2	8.3	4.7	2.9	3.5	2.1	1.9
El Paso	163,371	1.6	4.8	1.7	9.1	4.9	2.4	1.8	2.0	1.2
Fort Worth	267,069	2.3	4.8	2.5	7.8	4.6	3.2	2.9	1.5	3.1
Harlingen	82,451	1.5	6.4	1.7	8.3	5.5	1.5	2.8	2.9	0.5
Houston	687,852	2.3	5.1	2.2	8.8	4.4	2.9	3.3	2.1	1.4
Longview	46,841	2.1	4.5	3.2	9.3	5.3	4.1	4.4	1.3	2.5
Lubbock	153,660	2.2	6.4	2.2	11.6	9.1	2.4	2.6	1.7	3.2
Mcallen	68,302	1.7	7.5	1.4	11.9	5.4	1.7	2.2	2.7	1.0
Odessa	64,802	1.9	7.2	1.3	13.4	5.9	2.3	4.9	3.1	1.2
San Angelo	42,616	2.0	5.4	3.0	10.2	7.2	4.8	4.3	1.8	1.9
San Antonio	348,366	1.9	5.4	2.2	10.5	4.9	2.4	2.5	2.8	1.7
Temple	64,471	2.3	5.8	1.8	7.0	5.3	1.9	2.3	0.7	2.1
Tyler	138,026	2.4	5.9	2.8	6.4	5.5	2.8	4.9	2.0	2.4

Hospital Referral Region	Medicare Enrollees (1994 plus 1995)	Colectomy for Colorectal Cancer	CABG Surgery	Mastectomy for Cancer	TURP for BPH	Knee Replacement	Back Surgery	Carotid Endarterectomy	Lower Extremity Bypass	Radical Prostatectomy
Victoria	38,961	2.6	4.0	3.3	10.0	6.5	3.2	3.6	1.2	1.7
Waco	85,259	2.4	5.2	2.9	7.2	4.5	4.3	2.5	1.3	1.1
Wichita Falls	57,741	2.3	5.0	1.8	10.8	6.2	3.3	3.2	1.3	3.6
Utah										
Ogden	57,185	1.9	5.2	2.7	6.4	6.3	3.7	1.9	1.6	2.6
Provo	53,177	1.6	6.0	2.6	7.7	6.9	5.8	1.9	0.6	3.0
Salt Lake City	272,311	1.8	4.4	1.8	6.0	6.4	4.4	1.2	1.0	3.4
Vermont										
Burlington	139,474	2.8	5.0	1.6	9.6	4.8	2.1	2.6	2.5	1.6
Virginia										
Arlington	215,004	2.0	4.0	1.8	5.4	3.5	2.8	2.5	1.9	1.7
Charlottesville	116,978	2.1	4.5	1.8	7.0	4.5	2.9	1.5	1.5	1.7
Lynchburg	62,619	2.4	6.4	2.0	8.1	3.8	3.2	1.6	1.3	2.5
Newport News	99,508	2.5	6.7	2.2	6.3	5.0	5.3	2.6	3.1	2.3
Norfolk	224,337	2.5	6.6	2.3	7.3	4.6	4.1	3.5	3.0	1.2
Richmond	311,176	2.5	6.7	2.2	6.3	4.6	4.1	3.2	2.7	2.6
Roanoke	191,194	2.5	5.6	2.1	7.1	3.5	3.1	2.8	2.6	1.7
Winchester	79,661	2.4	5.6	1.9	6.8	4.1	3.1	1.7	1.5	1.4
Washington										
Everett	85,624	2.5	5.1	1.5	7.6	5.0	3.9	3.4	2.2	2.5
Olympia	69,634	2.2	4.5	2.4	7.4	5.3	3.7	3.4	2.2	2.3
Seattle	412,894	2.0	5.2	2.0	6.5	4.7	3.8	2.6	2.1	2.3
Spokane	295,612	2.2	5.7	2.4	8.5	5.4	4.2	2.8	1.8	3.0
Tacoma	117,556	2.1	4.9	1.6	7.0	5.0	4.2	2.5	3.1	2.4
Yakima	57,309	2.4	4.4	2.4	6.0	5.0	3.7	1.9	1.4	2.9
West Virginia										
Charleston	254,663	2.6	7.9	2.3	10.9	3.5	1.7	3.9	2.2	1.3
Huntington	100,539	2.7	5.8	2.0	8.9	3.0	2.0	3.1	1.3	1.9
Morgantown	114,348	2.5	5.1	2.4	9.8	5.0	1.9	3.6	2.1	1.3
Wisconsin										
Appleton	77,275	2.8	4.8	2.6	10.5	6.3	2.7	2.2	2.1	2.7
Green Bay	131,486	2.7	4.2	3.1	10.0	6.7	3.4	2.8	2.2	3.0
La Crosse	96,859	2.6	6.5	3.0	5.5	5.5	1.4	1.2	1.3	2.8
Madison	226,087	2.7	5.2	2.4	8.2	6.4	2.3	2.2	1.3	2.0
Marshfield	108,057	2.0	5.5	1.8	7.2	6.8	2.4	2.2	1.4	2.6
Milwaukee	574,223	2.6	6.9	2.5	8.5	5.6	2.5	2.7	2.0	1.8
Neenah	60,100	3.0	6.0	3.9	12.6	7.5	2.6	2.3	2.0	3.0
Wausau	53,614	2.6	5.2	2.3	10.2	6.0	2.4	3.2	2.1	2.8
Wyoming										
Casper	43,835	2.1	5.4	2.4	6.7	5.9	5.0	3.1	2.0	2.4
United States										
United States	58,796,484	2.5	5.7	2.2	8.5	4.6	2.9	3.0	2.1	2.0

Illness, Resources and Utilization

Illness, Resources and Utilization

What role does illness play in determining the variation in the allocation of resources and the use of medical care? It is true that people living in some areas are simply sicker than others; they have higher mortality rates, and have a higher incidence of self-reported "poor" or "fair" health. It comes as no surprise that such areas also have heavier than average demands for health care services. For example, Georgia, Tennessee, Alabama, and Mississippi are among the bottom ten states in the nation in self-reported health status, and among the top six states in Medicare's average adjusted per capita costs (AAPCCs), suggesting that variations in Medicare spending are an appropriate response to variations in the underlying reservoir of disease.

But how much of the variation in the distribution and utilization of health care resources is explained by underlying variations in health status? The evidence suggests that variations in resources and utilization are not strongly related to underlying disease.

■ The pattern of variation in surgical procedures used to treat cardiovascular disease bears little apparent relationship to the underlying incidence of the disease, as measured by hospitalizations for strokes and heart attacks.

■ While sick people do indeed use health care services more often than the less sick, the rates of use of health care for all members of society — the sick and the not so sick — are higher in regions with more resources and higher spending.

■ Self-reported health status explains only a small part of the higher-than-average hospitalization rates in regions with higher-than-average per capita supplies of hospital beds.

■ The need for medical care, as estimated by community health status, has very little to do with the level of Medicare spending.

Coronary Artery Bypass Grafting, Percutaneous Transuliminal Coronary Angioplasty, and the Incidence of Acute Myocardial Infarction

Acute myocardial infarction (AMI) is a serious complication of coronary artery disease; the incidence of AMI in defined populations is, therefore, a reasonable measure of the prevalence of coronary artery disease. By extension, the rates of use of coronary artery bypass grafting (CABG) and percutaneous transluminal coronary angioplasty (PTCA), which are procedures used to treat coronary artery disease, should correspond to higher incidence of AMI — and more heart disease — in local populations.

But there is, in fact, no relationship between the incidence of heart attacks and CABG among the nation's 306 hospital referral regions (Figure 6.1) There is also little relationship between the incidence of heart attacks and rates of PTCA (Figure 6.2).

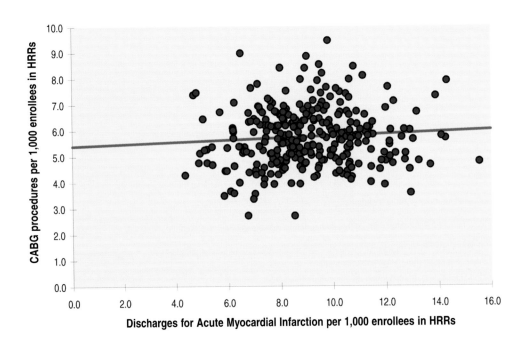

Figure 6.1. The Association Between CABG Procedures and Discharges for Acute Myocardial Infarction (1994-95)
The rates of hospitalizations for acute myocardial infarction and the rates of CABG are uncorrelated (R^2 = .005).

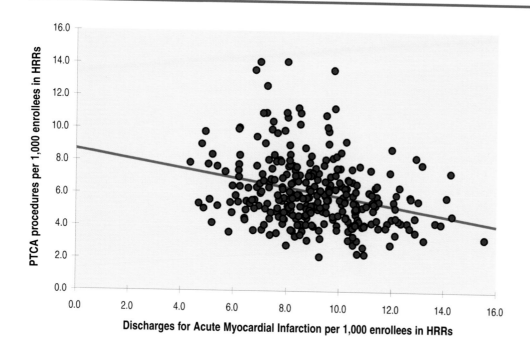

Figure 6.2. The Association Between Discharges for Acute Myocardial Infarction and PTCA Procedures (1994-95)
Very little of the variation in the rates of balloon angioplasty is associated with the incidence of coronary artery disease as measured by the rates of hospitalizations for AMI (R^2 = .07).

Carotid Endarterectomy, Lower Extremity Bypass, and the Incidence of Stroke and Related Illnesses

Carotid endarterectomy and lower extremity bypass procedures are undertaken to treat degenerative vascular disease, which is primarily due to atherosclerosis. Strokes are a common manifestation of this illness. If illness rates are an important determinant of the use of carotid endarterectomy and lower extremity bypass procedures, then communities with higher hospitalization rates for stroke should have a higher incidence of these procedures.

Figure 6.3 illustrates the relationship between the rates of hospitalizations for strokes and the rates of carotid endarterectomy in 1994-95. According to this measure of the prevalence of vascular disease, about 22% of the variation in carotid endarterectomy was associated with illness rates.

The association between hospitalization rates for stroke and lower extremity bypass procedures (Figure 6.4) was even weaker. Only 5% of the variation in these procedures was associated with hospitalization rates for stroke.

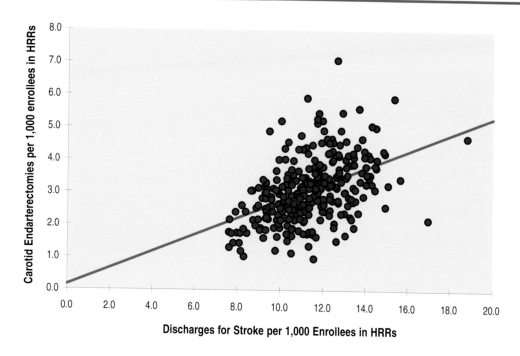

Figure 6.3. The Association Between Discharges for Stroke and Carotid Endarterectomy (1994-95) (R^2=.22).

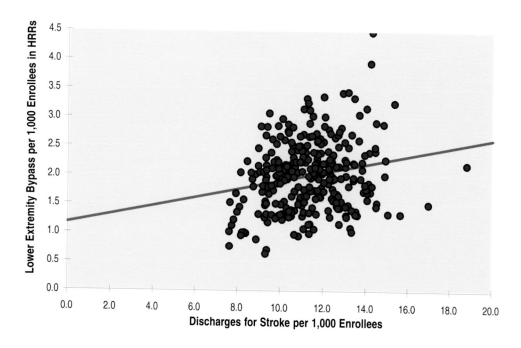

Figure 6.4. The Association Between Rates of Discharges for Stroke and Rates of Lower Extremity Bypass Procedures (1994-95) (R^2=.05)

Cardiovascular Disease and the Surgical Signature

Chapter Three explored the idiosyncratic patterns of rates of surgery that create communities' "surgical signatures," focusing particularly on seven hospital referral regions in Southwest Florida. The contrast between the prevalence of vascular disease in these seven hospital referral regions — as measured by the rates of hospitalizations for myocardial infarction and stroke — and the rates of surgical treatment of these conditions further illustrates that the prevalence of illness is not an important determinant of the rates of treatment for cardiovascular disorders.

In the Tampa Bay area of Florida in 1994-95, there was little variation in the rates of hospitalization for stroke among hospital referral regions. The rates ranged from a low of 1% below the national average in the St. Petersburg hospital referral region to a high of 12% above the national average in the Clearwater hospital referral region. The incidence of carotid endarterectomy, however, was highly variable among the regions, and was not related to the incidence of stroke. The highest rate of carotid endarterectomy was in the St. Petersburg hospital referral region (which was two times higher than the national average), the lowest rate was in Tampa (which was 1% below the national average). The rates of lower extremity bypass were 57% higher than the national average among the Medicare residents of the St. Petersburg hospital referral region, and 5% lower than the national average in among Medicare residents of the neighboring Tampa hospital referral region (Figure 6.5).

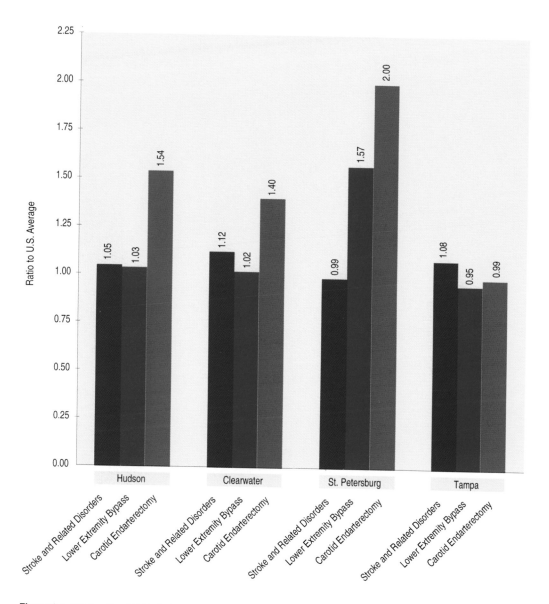

Figure 6.5. Stroke, Carotid Endarterectomy and Lower Extremity Bypass Among Selected Florida Hospital Referral Regions (1994-95)

The figure gives the ratio to the national average of the discharge rate for stroke and related diseases, lower extremity bypass procedures and carotid endarterectomy in selected Florida hospital referral regions. Although the rates of stroke were relatively uniform among the selected regions, rates of treatment varied from 5% below the national average to 100% above it.

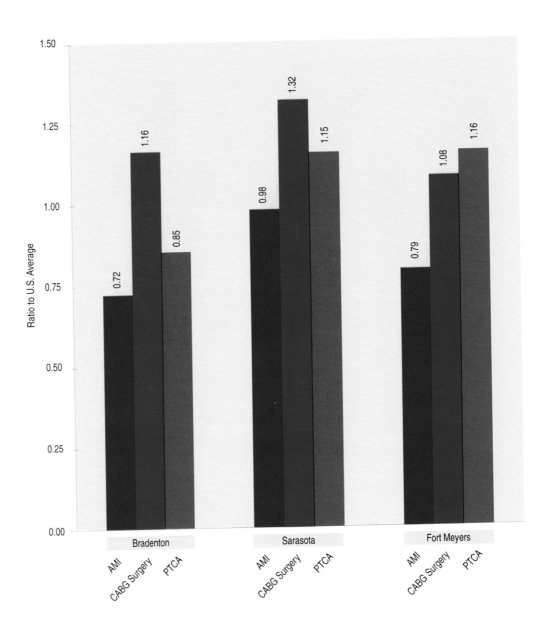

Figure 6.6. Acute Myocardial Infarction, CABG And PTCA Among Selected Florida Hospital Referral Regions (1994-95)

The figure gives the ratio of the rates of discharge for acute myocardial infarction, coronary artery bypass surgery (CABG) and percutaneous transluminal coronary angiography (PTCA) in selected Florida hospital referral regions to the national average. Rates of AMI ranged from 28% below the national average among residents of the Bradenton hospital referral region to 2% below the national average among residents of the Sarasota hospital referral region. Rates of the procedures used to treat heart disease were more variable than the rates of AMI. Rates of PTCA ranged from 15% below the national average among residents of the Bradenton hospital referral region to 16% above the national average among residents of the Fort Myers hospital referral region.

The three hospital referral regions south of Tampa Bay had widely differing rates of surgery for heart disease in 1994-95 (Figure 6.6). The incidence of acute myocardial infarction among Medicare residents of the Bradenton hospital referral region was 28% lower than the national average, but the rate of CABG surgery in the same population was 16% higher than the national average. The incidence of acute myocardial infraction among Medicare residents of Fort Myers was 21% lower than the national average, but the incidence of PTCA in the same population was 16% higher than the national average. Medicare residents of the Sarasota hospital referral region, whose rate of AMI was close to the national average, had the highest rate of CABG procedures in the region (32% above the national average).

Sicker People Use More Health Care

Common sense dictates and scientific evidence confirms that, on average, sicker people use more care than those who are less sick. Traditional economic theory about supply and demand would predict that much of the difference among hospital referral regions in local supply — the per capita number of hospital beds — could be explained by differences in demand — the illness level of the local population. If local hospital capacity were created in response to illness among the elderly in the region, we would expect populations in sicker regions to have more hospital beds per thousand residents, and we would expect that differences in hospitalization rates would be explained by differences in illness.

Health service researchers have long recognized that one of the best predictors of use of health care is self-reported health status. The Medicare Current Beneficiary Survey (MCBS) provides information about self-reported health status and hospitalizations among a sample of approximately 8,800 people over age 65 who were not members of risk-bearing health maintenance organizations at the time of the survey. Details about the MCBS are provided in the Appendix on Methods.

The survey data show that, in the Medicare population, enrollees who reported themselves in "excellent health" spent an average of only 1.5 days in hospitals in 1993. Those with "poor" self-reported health status spent an average of 4.2 days as inpatients. The likelihood that an enrollee would spend more days in the hospital increased in a step-wise fashion according to reported health status (Figure 6.7). Clearly, self-reported health status is a powerful indicator of "demand" for hospital care.

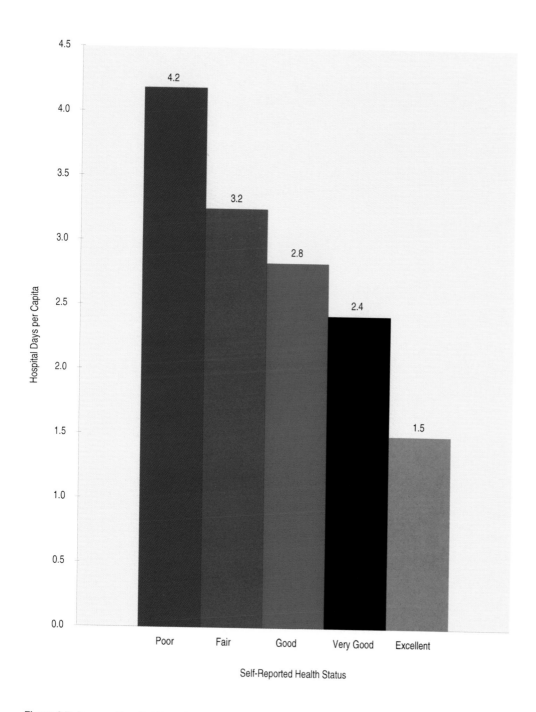

Figure 6.7. Average Hospital Days Stratified by Self-Reported Health (1993)

The average number of hospital days used corresponds to Medicare enrollees' self-reported health status, with enrollees who report themselves to be in better health using fewer days of hospital care. The data are adjusted for differences in age and sex.

Differences in Average Illness Do Not Explain Differences in Utilization of Hospital Beds

To what extent are the differences in the supply and utilization of hospital beds among hospital referral regions explained by differences in population health status? One common theory is that the numbers of hospital beds per thousand residents are determined by the illness level of the population. The relationship between hospital beds per thousand residents and utilization, documented by variation studies, would thus reflect underlying differences in health needs, rather than the "thermostat" effect of the supply of hospital beds on clinical decision making described in Chapter Three.

In research conducted in conjunction with this edition of the Atlas, the Medicare Current Beneficiary Survey (MCBS) was used to test the theory that illness explains the association between hospital beds and hospital utilization. According to this theory, populations living in regions with fewer beds per capita would be healthier than average, and those living in regions with more beds per capita would be sicker than average.

To test the relationship between illness and the bed supply, we divided the MCBS sample into five roughly equal groups, according to the number of hospital beds per thousand residents in the 306 hospital referral regions. The information on use of hospitals according to self-reported health status (Figure 6.7) was used to predict hospitalization rates for residents living in each quintile. (See the Appendix on Methods for further details.) The actual use of hospitals, measured in patient days per person, was also calculated.

The research confirmed the expected relationship between supply and utilization: residents of regions with higher per capita supplies of hospital beds had higher observed rates of hospitalization than residents of regions with lower per capita supplies of hospital beds. Residents of the region with the lowest per capita supply of hospital beds used, on average, 1.6 hospital bed days per year; those living in the region with the highest per capita supply of beds used 2.6 hospital bed days per person per year (Table 6.1).

Table 6.1. Actual and Predicted Days in Hospitals (1993)

(1) Quintile of Beds	(2) Beds/1,000 (Range)	(3) Actual Hospital Days	(4) Hospital Days as Predicted by Health Status
1 Bottom 20%	<2.9	1.6	2.2
2 Second 20%	2.9–3.2	1.8	2.1
3 Middle 20%	3.2–3.5	2.0	2.2
4 Fourth 20%	3.5–3.9	2.6	2.2
5 Highest 20%	>3.9	2.6	2.2

Data Source: Medicare Current Beneficiary Survey, Atlas Data

The research failed to find evidence that greater numbers of hospital beds (and the associated increase in hospitalization rates) occurred because residents of high rate areas were sicker. Predicted demand for hospital days based on self-reported health status was the same in the regions in the lowest quintile of per capita supply of hospital beds as in the region in the highest quintile — about 2.2 days per person per year.

While health needs (at least those reflected by self-reported illness) are a powerful predictor of the demand for health care at the level of the individual patient, health needs do not explain the distribution of hospital beds, nor are they an important factor in determining variations in the rate of hospital utilization among hospital referral regions.

Both the Sick and the Less Sick, If They Live in Regions With Higher Supplies of Hospital Beds, Use More Hospital Care

While there is little difference among hospital referral regions in illness rates ("demand for hospital beds"), as predicted by self reported health status, it is possible that regions with higher per capita supplies of hospital beds provide more intensive treatment for sicker patients. Figure 6.8 illustrates the influence of self-reported health status on per capita hospital days, considering separately individuals living in areas with lower supplies of hospital beds (the bottom 50%) and individuals living in areas with higher supplies of hospital beds (the top 50%). In other words, the figure is examining whether clinicians practicing in regions with higher hospital bed capacity allocate their excess beds to people in the poorest health, or whether the effect of the excess supply of beds affects all segments of the population (the sick and the less sick) more or less equally.

There is evidence that the local per capita supply of hospital beds exercises an across-the-board effect on clinical decision making. The likelihood of being hospitalized increases across all levels of health status when the per capita supply of hospital beds increases. An enrollee with the same "good" self-reported health status who lived in a region in the bottom 50% of local per capita bed supply would have expected to spend just 2.3 days in the hospital each year, or about one-third fewer days than a person with "good" self-reported status who lived in a region with a high per capita supply of beds.

A similar gap exists between enrollees in "excellent" self-reported health and those in "poor" self-reported health. In some cases, the per capita hospital bed supply matters more than health status: people in "fair" self-reported health in regions with low per capita supplies of hospital beds spent, on average, fewer days in hospitals than people in "good" or "very good" self-reported health who lived in regions where the per capita bed supply was high. The threshold effect of capacity is similar in each group.

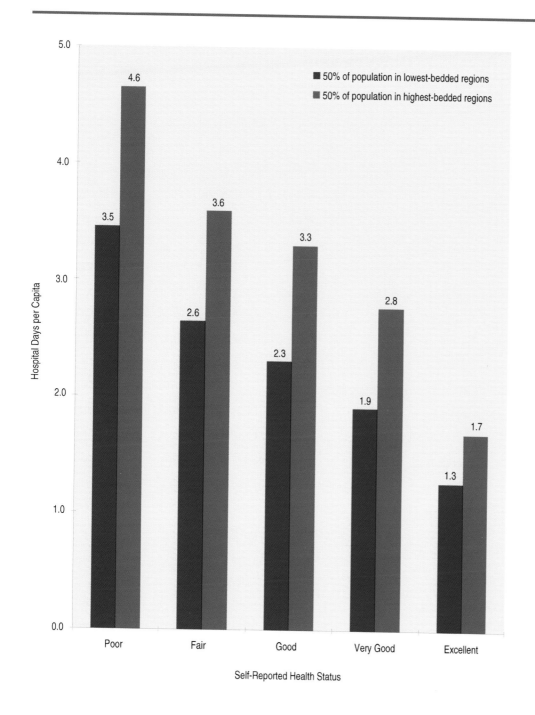

Figure 6.8. Self-Reported Health Status and Hospital Days Segmented by Regions With High and Low Supplies of Hospital Beds (1993)

The left-hand (blue) bars represent the population living in the hospital referral regions with low per capita supplies of hospital beds; the right hand (red) bars represent those in hospital referral regions with high per capita supplies of hospital beds. The vertical axis is the average number of days spent in hospitals; the horizontal axis is self reported health status. Medicare enrollees living in regions with higher per capita supplies of hospital beds had higher hospital use, independent of reported health status.

Differences in Health Status Do Not Explain Differences in Medicare Spending

How much of the overall variations in Medicare spending across hospital referral regions is explained by regional differences in health status? We used the Medicare claims data to develop a measure of health status for the populations of the 306 hospital referral regions. These measures comprise the region-specific mortality rate as well as the incidence of heart attacks, strokes, gastrointestinal hemorrhage, cancer of the colon and lung, and hip fracture. The measures were used to adjust spending for differences in underlying health of the regions. The Appendix on Methods considers in more detail the specification and justification of the illness index.

Figure 6.9 displays the distributions for total Medicare spending (Part A and Part B) for the 306 hospital referral regions. The distribution on the left is actual per person spending, calculated by dividing Medicare spending for residents of each region by the number of residents of the region. Next is the distribution for spending adjusted for age, sex and race. Third is the distribution adjusted for age, sex, race and illness. The distribution on the right in Figure 6.9 is fully adjusted for age, sex, race, illness and price.

The distributions in Figure 6.9 give the impression that age, sex, and race adjustment have little effect on the distribution in Medicare spending. Standard statistics bear this out (Table 6.2). The coefficient of variation shows little change after the adjustment; the range of variation is hardly changed, and the numbers of regions with high and low rates remain about the same. Further adjustment for illness reduces variation to a degree: the coefficient of variation is reduced by 13% over the unadjusted rate; the ratio of the highest to the lowest region is reduced from 3.27 to 3.10; and the number of regions with Medicare spending more than 20% above the na-

Table 6.2. Measures of Variation in Medicare Spending (Part A and B) 1995 by Strategies for Adjustment

	Unadjusted Medicare Spending	Adjusted for Age, Sex and Race	Adjusted for Age, Sex, Race and Illness	Adjusted for Age, Sex, Race, Illness and Price
Index of Variation				
Coefficient of variation	21.2	20.4	18.5	15.1
Ratio to unadjusted rate	1.00	0.96	0.87	0.71
Range of variation				
Extremal ratio	3.27	3.21	3.10	2.98
Interquartile ratio	1.32	1.32	1.25	1.21
Number of regions with high and low rates				
Rates more than 20% higher than national average	31	32	26	23
Rates less than 20% lower than national average	77	72	54	16

tional average is reduced from 31 to 26 regions. Illness adjustment reduced number with spending more than 20% below the national average from 77 to 54 regions.

The addition of price adjustment further reduces variation; of the three adjustments, price has the largest effect. Compared to unadjusted spending, age, sex, race, and illness adjustment results in a 31% reduction in variation (measured by the coefficient of variation). Yet a great deal of variation remains unexplained: the rate in the region with the highest Medicare spending (the McAllen, Texas hospital referral region) is 2.98 times higher than the rate in the region with the lowest Medicare spending (the Lynchburg, Virginia hospital referral region). Twenty-three regions have spending rates 20% or more above the national average; 16 are more than 20% below it.

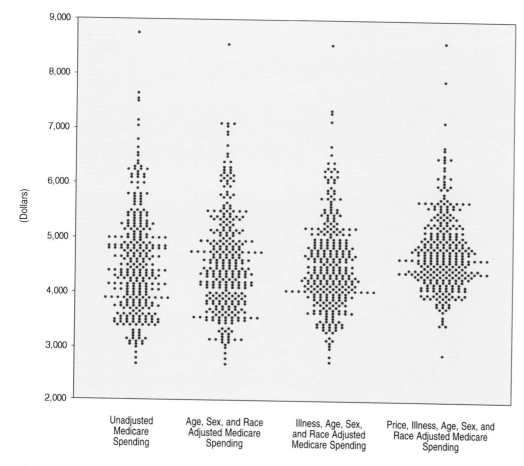

Figure 6.9. Distribution of Medicare Spending Rates (1995) Unadjusted and Adjusted for Various Factors
Medicare spending varied substantially among hospital referral regions, even after adjustment for age, sex, race, illness and price.

Chapter Six Table   Rates are age, sex and race adjusted and are expressed in dollars per enrollee. Additional adjustments were made for price and for illness and for price and illness, as described in the Appendix on Methods. Data exclude Medicare enrollees who were members of risk bearing health maintenance organizations.

CHAPTER SIX TABLE

Actual, Price Adjusted, Illness Adjusted and Price and Illness Adjusted Total Medicare Reimbursements Among Non-HMO Medicare Enrollees for All Services by Hospital Referral Region (1995)

Hospital Referral Region	Medicare Enrollees (1995)	Reimbursements for Non-Capitated Medicare	Price Adjusted Reimbursements for Non-Capitated Medicare	Price & Illness Adjusted Reimbursements for Non-Capitated Medicare
Alabama				
Birmingham	264,920	5,092	5,650	4,900
Dothan	44,420	4,644	5,390	4,641
Huntsville	51,660	4,455	4,842	4,534
Mobile	80,880	4,958	5,606	4,808
Montgomery	46,840	4,585	5,153	4,655
Tuscaloosa	27,660	4,487	5,103	4,605
Alaska				
Anchorage	26,620	5,616	4,739	4,798
Arizona				
Mesa	51,640	4,701	4,717	5,360
Phoenix	178,580	4,627	4,763	4,993
Sun City	45,580	3,946	3,950	4,437
Tucson	72,620	4,523	4,856	5,367
Arkansas				
Fort Smith	44,660	5,047	6,026	5,659
Jonesboro	29,360	4,578	5,766	5,206
Little Rock	189,560	4,306	5,137	4,779
Springdale	45,460	3,526	4,328	4,355
Texarkana	33,960	5,106	6,143	5,257
California				
Orange Co.	127,960	6,400	5,564	5,625
Bakersfield	58,280	5,829	5,826	5,554
Chico	33,920	4,179	4,452	4,355
Contra Costa Co.	56,760	4,844	4,204	4,398
Fresno	75,840	4,086	4,164	4,564
Los Angeles	448,600	7,006	5,900	5,671
Modesto	56,760	5,139	5,209	5,128
Napa	35,220	5,346	5,365	5,196
Alameda Co.	93,540	5,209	4,444	4,389
Palm Spr/Rancho Mir	28,960	6,261	5,982	5,967
Redding	42,160	4,882	5,142	5,220
Sacramento	168,680	4,719	4,523	4,635
Salinas	30,820	5,558	5,263	5,660
San Bernardino	83,660	6,141	5,868	5,696
San Diego	156,340	6,018	5,685	5,986
San Francisco	104,260	4,978	4,085	4,146
San Jose	86,520	5,105	4,140	4,439
San Luis Obispo	21,260	4,130	3,919	4,131
San Mateo Co.	54,680	4,475	3,603	3,811
Santa Barbara	30,360	4,500	4,130	4,297

Hospital Referral Region	Medicare Enrollees (1995)	Reimbursements for Non-Capitated Medicare	Price Adjusted Reimbursements for Non-Capitated Medicare	Price & Illness Adjusted Reimbursements for Non-Capitated Medicare
Santa Cruz	21,400	4,907	4,472	4,817
Santa Rosa	37,800	4,886	4,461	4,576
Stockton	36,180	5,357	5,264	5,096
Ventura	41,920	5,352	4,735	4,799
Colorado				
Boulder	14,220	4,263	4,408	4,884
Colorado Springs	57,580	3,687	4,074	4,478
Denver	145,020	4,661	4,830	5,205
Fort Collins	24,540	4,075	4,502	4,815
Grand Junction	29,380	3,169	3,756	4,527
Greeley	28,680	4,190	4,721	5,276
Pueblo	17,720	4,301	4,905	5,271
Connecticut				
Bridgeport	83,600	5,294	4,395	4,796
Hartford	187,880	4,907	4,282	4,883
New Haven	171,220	5,240	4,396	4,805
Delaware				
Wilmington	74,880	4,410	4,110	4,283
District of Columbia				
Washington	203,960	4,727	4,330	4,371
Florida				
Bradenton	46,860	4,410	4,671	5,021
Clearwater	89,560	5,322	5,586	5,355
Fort Lauderdale	313,740	5,773	5,500	5,914
Fort Myers	168,540	4,928	5,311	5,647
Gainesville	47,640	5,146	5,746	5,580
Hudson	83,640	5,384	5,638	5,602
Jacksonville	117,200	5,147	5,533	5,302
Lakeland	42,700	4,732	5,241	5,309
Miami	214,520	8,537	7,955	7,874
Ocala	81,220	4,420	5,032	5,429
Orlando	349,420	5,086	5,351	5,395
Ormond Beach	44,900	4,435	4,848	4,875
Panama City	22,560	5,500	6,288	5,586
Pensacola	71,500	5,028	5,689	5,202
Sarasota	95,980	4,821	5,115	5,483
St Petersburg	66,980	5,573	5,859	5,723
Tallahassee	69,920	4,593	5,161	4,859
Tampa	86,240	5,443	5,720	5,428
Georgia				
Albany	20,980	4,424	4,962	4,587
Atlanta	352,220	4,733	4,822	4,516
Augusta	62,940	4,397	4,750	4,426
Columbus	33,420	3,668	4,183	3,983
Macon	69,460	4,588	5,119	4,756
Rome	30,300	4,237	4,977	4,313
Savannah	69,860	4,702	5,253	4,704
Hawaii				
Honolulu	86,860	3,631	3,332	3,570
Idaho				
Boise	69,800	3,512	3,980	4,596
Idaho Falls	17,220	3,215	3,776	4,097
Illinois				
Aurora	16,920	4,053	3,755	3,759
Blue Island	90,560	5,724	5,302	4,821
Chicago	221,300	5,717	5,280	5,050
Elgin	41,400	4,855	4,498	4,419
Evanston	111,200	4,893	4,534	4,669
Hinsdale	31,620	5,313	4,923	4,870
Joliet	46,680	5,219	5,116	4,827
Melrose Park	128,440	5,068	4,695	4,619
Peoria	95,480	4,003	4,567	4,646
Rockford	82,740	3,692	4,096	4,240
Springfield	123,540	3,913	4,532	4,355
Urbana	54,800	3,579	4,267	4,369
Bloomington	19,520	3,501	3,930	4,081
Indiana				
Evansville	96,560	4,135	4,737	4,461
Fort Wayne	98,700	3,529	3,938	4,126
Gary	54,860	5,524	5,852	5,433
Indianapolis	283,160	4,383	4,717	4,608
Lafayette	22,320	3,653	4,253	4,186
Muncie	21,700	4,101	4,783	4,639
Munster	38,760	5,187	5,397	5,002
South Bend	80,100	3,843	4,204	4,515
Terre Haute	25,100	4,129	4,739	4,556
Iowa				
Cedar Rapids	33,380	3,126	3,511	3,651
Davenport	68,960	3,483	3,946	3,915
Des Moines	137,620	3,431	3,974	3,983
Dubuque	21,380	3,108	3,524	3,465
Iowa City	40,820	3,401	4,038	4,039
Mason City	27,160	3,145	3,896	4,185
Sioux City	39,620	3,060	3,691	4,069
Waterloo	31,800	3,165	3,627	3,532
Kansas				
Topeka	54,880	3,317	3,823	3,933
Wichita	174,560	4,180	4,960	5,025
Kentucky				
Covington	35,560	4,314	4,430	4,114
Lexington	152,400	4,190	4,872	4,463
Louisville	184,080	4,626	5,105	4,769

Hospital Referral Region	Medicare Enrollees (1995)	Reimbursements for Non-Capitated Medicare	Price Adjusted Reimbursements for Non-Capitated Medicare	Price & Illness Adjusted Reimbursements for Non-Capitated Medicare
Owensboro	17,840	4,381	5,146	5,021
Paducah	55,220	4,267	5,131	4,709
Louisiana				
Alexandria	32,780	6,078	7,178	6,464
Baton Rouge	66,340	6,506	7,227	6,494
Houma	23,580	5,997	6,959	6,117
Lafayette	58,240	4,947	5,739	5,684
Lake Charles	24,400	5,398	6,032	5,550
Metairie	40,740	6,692	7,013	6,329
Monroe	33,080	6,250	7,385	6,458
New Orleans	79,100	7,055	7,205	6,638
Shreveport	82,800	5,404	6,167	6,037
Slidell	15,600	6,390	7,019	6,126
Maine				
Bangor	55,000	3,598	4,022	4,287
Portland	127,580	3,870	4,094	4,630
Maryland				
Baltimore	270,160	5,500	5,240	4,867
Salisbury	53,520	4,532	4,820	5,085
Takoma Park	61,700	5,373	4,697	4,752
Massachusetts				
Boston	536,340	6,222	5,564	5,832
Springfield	97,520	4,382	4,322	4,762
Worcester	67,820	6,041	5,377	5,590
Michigan				
Ann Arbor	129,920	5,451	5,079	5,084
Dearborn	72,500	6,014	5,372	5,095
Detroit	225,400	5,931	5,321	5,026
Flint	57,500	5,760	5,460	5,265
Grand Rapids	112,560	3,861	3,989	4,306
Kalamazoo	75,620	4,324	4,477	4,674
Lansing	62,540	4,716	4,858	5,120
Marquette	32,880	3,863	4,284	4,341
Muskegon	35,320	3,759	3,850	4,117
Petoskey	25,200	3,639	4,009	4,152
Pontiac	36,160	6,477	5,792	5,600
Royal Oak	80,860	6,103	5,452	5,379
Saginaw	92,200	4,342	4,489	4,671
St Joseph	19,780	4,363	4,611	4,646
Traverse City	31,660	3,579	3,938	4,124
Minnesota				
Duluth	54,520	3,040	3,369	3,401
Minneapolis	276,540	3,300	3,528	3,722
Rochester	54,480	3,525	3,881	4,159
St Cloud	24,380	3,146	3,539	3,926
St Paul	73,160	3,820	3,771	3,974
Mississippi				
Gulfport	18,880	6,244	7,023	6,442
Hattiesburg	30,960	4,563	5,595	5,218
Jackson	117,660	4,588	5,354	4,979
Meridian	25,840	4,547	5,574	4,933
Oxford	17,480	4,177	5,121	4,310
Tupelo	45,080	4,239	5,202	4,796
Missouri				
Cape Girardeau	36,760	3,499	4,383	4,271
Columbia	86,360	4,700	5,776	5,626
Joplin	49,340	4,396	5,432	4,817
Kansas City	231,380	4,795	5,205	4,994
Springfield	106,080	3,635	4,389	4,417
St Louis	404,240	4,478	4,809	4,535
Montana				
Billings	61,040	3,713	4,351	4,640
Great Falls	20,000	3,639	4,349	4,274
Missoula	41,000	4,000	4,809	5,128
Nebraska				
Lincoln	76,160	2,859	3,550	4,074
Omaha	150,640	3,603	4,328	4,592
Nevada				
Las Vegas	78,240	5,451	5,278	5,118
Reno	61,400	4,131	4,155	4,554
New Hampshire				
Lebanon	52,420	3,548	3,819	4,385
Manchester	81,120	3,806	3,583	3,938
New Jersey				
Camden	349,480	5,006	4,562	4,532
Hackensack	152,200	4,926	4,107	4,323
Morristown	104,380	4,659	3,914	4,193
New Brunswick	98,200	4,907	4,140	4,468
Newark	165,940	4,949	4,183	4,283
Paterson	40,080	4,945	4,123	4,047
Ridgewood	42,460	4,697	3,946	4,266
New Mexico				
Albuquerque	106,580	3,940	4,382	4,973
New York				
Albany	231,580	4,101	4,079	4,459
Binghamton	56,320	3,452	3,626	3,920
Bronx	95,280	6,865	5,473	5,758
Buffalo	202,440	3,905	3,997	4,213
Elmira	53,840	3,828	4,126	4,372
East Long Island	458,840	6,067	4,806	5,109
New York	422,100	7,067	5,649	6,118
Rochester	146,540	3,947	3,944	4,332

Hospital Referral Region	Medicare Enrollees (1995)	Reimbursements for Non-Capitated Medicare	Price Adjusted Reimbursements for Non-Capitated Medicare	Price & Illness Adjusted Reimbursements for Non-Capitated Medicare
Syracuse	128,300	3,809	3,940	4,352
White Plains	120,940	5,550	4,551	4,818
North Carolina				
Asheville	90,640	3,501	4,051	4,229
Charlotte	194,000	4,095	4,466	4,302
Durham	143,580	3,733	4,176	4,076
Greensboro	62,220	3,527	3,862	3,763
Greenville	81,940	3,989	4,698	4,409
Hickory	30,060	3,790	4,313	4,232
Raleigh	132,340	4,225	4,669	4,370
Wilmington	40,360	4,751	5,290	4,683
Winston-Salem	119,000	3,991	4,436	4,067
North Dakota				
Bismarck	31,220	3,752	4,577	4,912
Fargo Moorhead -Mn	69,360	3,123	3,713	3,987
Grand Forks	24,980	3,666	4,404	4,897
Minot	19,260	3,477	4,384	4,732
Ohio				
Akron	86,120	4,887	5,003	4,631
Canton	84,480	3,843	4,261	4,380
Cincinnati	183,500	4,289	4,453	4,316
Cleveland	274,040	5,079	5,084	4,871
Columbus	294,480	4,070	4,451	4,403
Dayton	137,400	4,185	4,479	4,623
Elyria	29,360	4,717	4,682	4,248
Kettering	46,600	4,143	4,302	4,430
Toledo	126,200	4,835	5,099	4,998
Youngstown	118,500	4,712	5,218	5,168
Oklahoma				
Lawton	23,380	4,705	5,558	5,660
Oklahoma City	198,700	4,799	5,488	5,208
Tulsa	141,720	4,738	5,406	5,209
Oregon				
Bend	20,360	3,509	4,014	4,486
Eugene	83,260	3,134	3,533	3,907
Medford	59,100	3,468	3,815	4,312
Portland	149,800	3,503	3,680	3,871
Salem	26,840	3,089	3,410	3,829
Pennsylvania				
Allentown	149,240	4,802	4,802	4,996
Altoona	45,500	4,443	5,073	5,115
Danville	74,020	4,120	4,566	4,717
Erie	113,240	4,338	4,870	4,714
Harrisburg	124,380	4,263	4,517	4,712
Johnstown	42,540	4,903	5,704	5,419
Lancaster	69,460	4,152	4,254	4,672
Philadelphia	458,740	5,900	5,402	5,252
Pittsburgh	509,880	5,305	5,545	5,266
Reading	81,060	4,348	4,510	4,711
Sayre	27,540	3,629	4,053	4,216
Scranton	55,400	4,386	4,779	4,526
Wilkes-Barre	44,620	5,064	5,495	5,062
York	49,380	3,446	3,683	3,910
Rhode Island				
Providence	145,220	4,861	4,511	4,843
South Carolina				
Charleston	81,400	4,251	4,707	4,636
Columbia	111,640	3,580	4,000	4,029
Florence	39,820	4,332	4,966	4,422
Greenville	85,700	3,785	4,192	4,137
Spartanburg	43,160	3,861	4,297	3,967
South Dakota				
Rapid City	21,920	3,497	4,335	4,683
Sioux Falls	113,760	3,272	4,081	4,351
Tennessee				
Chattanooga	74,520	5,488	6,012	5,460
Jackson	45,660	4,615	5,408	4,935
Johnson City	30,680	4,566	5,222	4,952
Kingsport	66,780	4,663	5,343	4,928
Knoxville	148,520	4,782	5,431	4,831
Memphis	179,440	4,598	5,176	4,726
Nashville	240,580	5,312	6,000	5,484
Texas				
Abilene	43,860	4,825	5,735	5,141
Amarillo	51,560	4,785	5,465	5,909
Austin	77,080	4,289	4,476	4,646
Beaumont	58,680	6,941	7,444	6,508
Bryan	17,760	3,999	4,703	4,752
Corpus Christi	48,020	6,177	6,875	6,293
Dallas	280,940	5,400	5,546	5,541
El Paso	79,140	4,614	5,215	5,714
Fort Worth	126,140	5,468	5,783	5,681
Harlingen	42,320	6,115	7,264	7,140
Houston	325,460	6,188	6,216	6,097
Longview	23,360	4,695	5,319	5,004
Lubbock	76,480	5,143	6,039	5,671
Mcallen	32,800	7,091	8,384	8,599
Odessa	31,000	5,276	5,791	5,984
San Angelo	21,680	4,516	5,445	5,686
San Antonio	163,060	5,779	6,434	6,686
Temple	30,360	3,858	4,345	4,720
Tyler	70,720	5,464	6,294	6,166

Hospital Referral Region	Medicare Enrollees (1995)	Reimbursements for Non-Capitated Medicare	Price Adjusted Reimbursements for Non-Capitated Medicare	Price & Illness Adjusted Reimbursements for Non-Capitated Medicare
Victoria	18,340	5,186	5,818	5,597
Waco	41,020	3,248	3,761	3,952
Wichita Falls	28,560	4,532	5,415	4,927
Utah				
Ogden	27,380	3,649	3,980	4,639
Provo	25,700	3,826	4,474	4,889
Salt Lake City	134,000	3,740	4,165	4,774
Vermont				
Burlington	68,420	3,766	4,035	4,385
Virginia				
Arlington	100,640	4,442	3,871	3,978
Charlottesville	58,780	3,874	4,185	4,118
Lynchburg	30,060	2,657	2,929	2,887
Newport News	50,760	3,759	3,961	3,982
Norfolk	108,020	4,227	4,539	4,491
Richmond	152,100	4,057	4,072	3,842
Roanoke	94,860	3,744	4,234	4,086
Winchester	38,040	3,994	4,133	3,797
Washington				
Everett	40,520	3,983	4,072	4,298
Olympia	35,020	3,798	4,021	4,427
Seattle	198,460	4,082	4,060	4,422
Spokane	144,880	3,673	4,018	4,449
Tacoma	56,160	4,137	4,256	4,504
Yakima	27,800	3,941	4,298	4,582
West Virginia				
Charleston	125,280	4,422	5,085	4,553
Huntington	49,920	4,164	4,701	4,223
Morgantown	57,720	4,335	5,156	4,951
Wisconsin				
Appleton	37,000	2,984	3,323	3,721
Green Bay	66,920	3,283	3,671	3,881
La Crosse	47,560	2,783	3,215	3,442
Madison	110,940	3,465	3,812	4,064
Marshfield	53,320	3,271	3,768	4,306
Milwaukee	280,300	4,150	4,231	4,390
Neenah	28,400	3,901	4,339	4,298
Wausau	27,340	3,505	3,988	4,158
Wyoming				
Casper	21,060	4,286	4,889	4,934
United States				
United States	28,341,260	4,790	4,878	4,878

Which Rate is Right?
How Much is Enough?
and What is Fair?

Which Rate is Right? How Much is Enough? and What is Fair?

Ideally, the use of health care services by a given population would depend on local levels of illness, and would comprise an efficient mix of preventive, acute and chronic care. Resource allocation decisions would be guided at the patient level by need and knowledge of outcomes, and by the tradeoffs patients made between the costs, risks and benefits of care. At the population level, resource allocation decisions would be made based on society's beliefs about cost-effectiveness and social justice. Ideally, spending by the Medicare program would also reflect the goals of efficiency and equity.

Unfortunately, the Atlas provides little evidence that these ideals are being achieved — that the quantities of health services and resources consumed by Americans are determined by patient needs and preferences, or by knowledge about the outcomes of care, much less by consensus about society's needs and priorities. On the contrary, the Atlas demonstrates that:

■ There is wide variation in Medicare spending, and in the supply of acute care hospital resources and physicians among the nation's hospital referral regions (Chapter Two).

■ Hospital capacity has a dominating influence on hospital utilization rates, particularly for medical conditions (Chapter Three).

■ There is wide variation in the intensity of hospital care Americans receive during the last six months of their lives, and the variation is closely associated with local supplies of hospital resources (Chapter Four).

■ Discretionary surgical procedures have idiosyncratic patterns which result in regional "surgical signatures," a phenomenon which can be traced to scientific uncertainty about what works and the failure to involve patients in a meaningful way in the surgical decision making process (Chapter Five).

■ Variations in illness rates do not explain the patterns of variation in hospital resource supply and Medicare spending (Chapter Six).

The reality of health care in the United States is that geography is destiny. The amount of care consumed by Americans depends more on where they live — the local supply of resources and the prevailing practice style — than on their needs or preferences.

Practice variations challenge basic assumptions about the nature of the health care economy and theories as to how it should be reformed. While it is beyond the scope of the Atlas to consider the question of how policies for addressing unwanted variations in health care delivery might be specifically designed or implemented, the Atlas can help frame the debate over what should be done.

Surgical variations point to the need for better science at the patient level and the need to bring the patient into the decision process through shared decision making. Through the diligent application of outcomes research, much can be learned about what works in medicine, particularly in those examples of care where a discrete intervention, such as a drug or a surgical procedure, is hypothesized to improve outcomes in specific ways. By bringing patients into the decision process through shared decision making, health care markets can be improved so that the use of care reflects the preferences of patients, rather than the preferences of providers or payers. Part I of this chapter addresses these opportunities for improving health care delivery.

The struggle for rationality at the patient level of care is both never-ending and fated to only partial success. New medical ideas and technologies will constantly challenge, and often outstrip, our best efforts to evaluate the end results of care. Moreover, much of clinical decision making is not driven by discrete, testable hypotheses, but by the need to help solve the myriad and complex sets of problems patients bring to physicians. When problem solving decisions are made under the assumption that more is better, as is common in the United States, the supply of medical resources will always be used up to the point of exhaustion, regardless of how much is available. Rational reform requires a policy for setting limits.

Part II of this chapter considers the problem of variation in hospital capacity and the inevitable association between having more resources and providing more services. How should the debate over whether more is better be framed? The first step is to understand the impact of increased supply on population-based utilization and outcomes. Most of the marginal resources in the acute care hospital sector appear to be invested in admitting patients to medical wards in the hope of reducing mortality. The most important outcome question, then, is population mortality: Do patient populations destined to receive more care in hospitals on the basis of their residence live longer than their counterparts in regions with fewer resources who receive less?

Part III of this chapter examines variations in the physician supply. The impact of an increase in physician supply on rates of delivery of specific services depends on the physicians' specialties, their incentives to work and, ultimately, on the idiosyncratic nature of the individual physician's "practice style." The complexities of the impact of physician supply on utilization make it impossible to base workforce planning on either patient level need and outcomes or on patient demand. In planning federal subsidies to medical education, or in recruiting physicians into a system of care, we suggest that the better planning alternative is to use benchmarking. Benchmarking allows us to compare specific regional workforces to other workforces and to health plans that have been successful in competitive markets, are low cost, and where global outcomes, measured at the population level, are good.

Part IV of this chapter raises questions about the equity of current federal policy determining reimbursements to health care markets, particularly with regard to the amount paid to managed care companies. These amounts vary among the regions according to historical spending levels under fee-for-service medicine. The policy is unfair because it penalizes individual Medicare enrollees who live in regions where spending has historically been low. In such areas, enrollees have less opportunity for an expanded benefit package under capitation than managed care companies can provide to those living in regions where spending has historically been high. It is also unfair because Medicare enrollees living in regions where spending is low subsidize through their taxes the expanded benefits received by those living in regions where spending is high. The policy can also result in windfall profits to managed care companies that achieve the efficiencies now being realized in regions where spending is low.

Part V of this chapter summarizes the policy steps we recommend for resolving unwanted variations in health care delivery.

I. Islands of Rationality

The tradition of decision making based on professional paternalism does not deal well with the complex tradeoffs created by modern technology. Rates of elective surgery and other discretionary interventions, which now are determined in large part by practice style and geographic variations in resources, should be determined by the choices informed patients make. To accomplish this "right rate," patients must participate in the decision making process; to do so, patients must understand what is known, as well as what is not known, about the outcomes that matter to them. Further, patients must be enabled to choose according to their own preferences, even if they ultimately decide to let their doctors decide for them.

This reform will require a new model of clinical decision making. Fortunately, the time is ripe; the escalation in medical spending over the past three decades has created an environment in which it has become possible for patients to challenge the paternalistic role of physicians as agents and sole decision makers. Employers, as payers, have promoted the growth of managed care, which challenges the autonomy of physicians, imposes rules on clinical medicine, and substitutes the managed care company as the decision maker. This transfer of agency power to third parties — payers, insurance companies, and health maintenance organizations — has opened a national debate about the role of the patient in the choice of medical care.

A new model of the doctor-patient relationship is emerging in response to paternalism and third party intrusion into health care. Shared decision making recognizes the complex tradeoffs that patients must make in the choice of medical care, and addresses the ethical requirement to fully inform patients about the risks and benefits of treatments as well as the need to ensure that patients' values and preferences play a prominent role in medical decision making.

The shared decision making model holds promise for establishing health care markets in which the right rate of service is determined by the choices made by informed and empowered patients. Shared decision making has been implemented in several clinical studies, some of which are discussed here. The studies provide evidence about both patients' willingness to participate in decisions about their own care, and the rates at which patients choose certain procedures when they are fully informed about the risks and benefits of their choices. Most patients willingly participate in shared decision making, even when, as in case of early stage prostate cancer, decisions are complicated and difficult because medical science provides no clear evidence that invasive treatment extends life expectancy. The studies of shared decision making also provide initial benchmarks for addressing the question, Which rate is right? The preliminary evidence indicates that the amount of discretionary invasive care now prescribed in the United States might substantially exceed the amount that informed patients actually want.

Shared Decision Making: The Treatment of Benign Prostatic Hyperplasia

Benign prostatic hyperplasia (BPH) is a common disease in men over the age of 50, and there is considerable debate about how — and whether — the condition should be treated. Traditionally, men with BPH have relied on their physicians to decide on the course of treatment for them, assuming that "the doctor knows best." Outcomes research has done much to clarify the theoretical reasons for undertaking treatment. The primary reason for treatment in most men is to improve the quality of life by reducing the intensity of symptoms. For most men, surgery does not increase the length of life and, in fact, may shorten life expectancy slightly because of operative mortality. The need for the patient's active involvement in the choice of treatment is elucidated by these outcomes studies. The most important consideration for the patient is the tradeoff between surgery, which is superior in improving urinary tract symptoms, and the avoidance of surgical complications associated with foregoing surgery. Individual patients differ substantially in how they assess their own situations; and there is nothing in the physical examination, the clinical history, or the results of laboratory tests that allows physicians to forecast which treatment a given patient will prefer.

A recently published observational study of treatment choice for BPH in two health maintenance organizations showed that under shared decision making, treatment choice was determined by the individual patient's own assessment of how much his symptoms bothered him and his concern about the side effects, particularly the possible negative impact of surgery on sexuality. These subjective factors mattered even more to patients than the severity of their symptoms (as measured objectively by a standardized questionnaire).

When the study began, the rates of surgery for BPH among men in both health maintenance organizations were already substantially lower than the national average. When shared decision making was adopted, the rates fell even lower — more than 40% below the baseline rate for men in the health maintenance organizations. No reduction occurred among men enrolled in a control group. The results were highly significant statistically, clinically and economically. A subsequent randomized clinical trial showed a similar result, but the trial was underpowered and the result was not statistically significant.

The experience of the health maintenance organization in implementing shared decision making provides a benchmark for addressing the question, Which rate is right? In 1992-93, the last years of the shared decision making observational study, the rates of surgery for BPH among men participating in shared decision making were comparable to the rates in the hospital referral regions with the lowest rates in the United States (Figure 7.1). If the preferences about surgical treatment of BPH of the men who participated in the shared decision making study reflect the preferences of most men, then the amount of surgery for BPH provided in the United States in those years substantially exceeded the amount that informed men would actually want. The health maintenance organization benchmark suggests that in 1992-93, 160,000 more prostate operations were performed in the United States than would have been the case had shared decision making been in use throughout the country.

See the endnote for references and further reading.

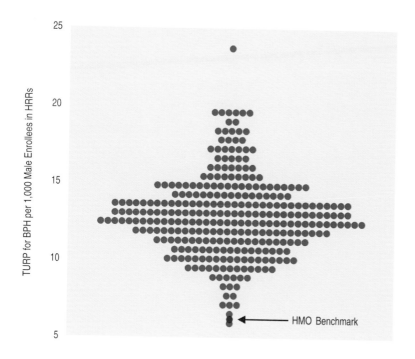

Figure 7.1. Distribution of Transurethral Prostatectomies for Benign Prostatic Hyperplasia Among Hospital Referral Regions (1992-93) Compared to Shared Decision Making Benchmark in Two Staff Model HMOs

The rate of surgery under shared decision making was substantially lower than the rates in most hospital referral regions.

Shared Decision Making: The Treatment of Coronary Artery Disease

The rates of revascularization procedures for coronary artery disease in Ontario, Canada in 1995 were substantially lower than in any of the 306 hospital referral regions in the United States (Figure 7.2). If the rate of invasive treatments in Ontario had prevailed in the United States in 1994-95, 481,000 fewer procedures would have been performed among the Medicare population. Which rate is right?

Researchers in Ontario conducted a randomized clinical trial to evaluate the impact of shared decision making on the choice of treatment among patients with coronary artery disease. Patients who were randomized to shared decision making were informed about their treatment options, using a standardized interactive video, and encouraged to participate in their own treatment decisions. The control group received usual care. The group of patients who participated in shared decision making chose coronary revascularization with either coronary artery bypass surgery or percutaneous transluminal coronary angioplasty 22% less often than the control group. This suggests that even the low prevailing rate in Ontario might be more than informed patients actually want.

If the rate of surgery chosen by the participants in the Ontario study reflects the average preferences of patients in the United States, then the amount of surgery now provided in the United States exceeds by a wide margin the amount that informed patients want. While it is unlikely that preferences about revascularization operations of patients with coronary artery disease in the United States and in Ontario are the same, the Ontario study provides further evidence that in order to find the "right" American rate (which will vary from region to region) it will be necessary to strengthen the American patient's role in choosing the care that best fits their individual preferences and needs.

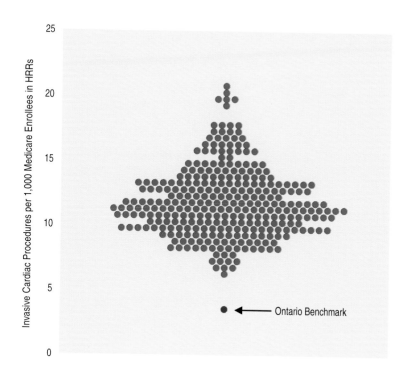

Figure 7.2. Distribution of Rates of Coronary Artery Revascularization Procedures (CABG and PTCA) for Coronary Artery Disease Among Hospital Referral Regions (1994-95) Compared to the Ontario, Canada Benchmark (1995)

The rates of invasive treatments in Ontario were substantially lower than in the United States. The rates in Ontario were determined by studies of the population over age 64 conducted by Ontario's Institute for Clinical Evaluative Sciences. In a clinical trial in Toronto, patients who were randomized to shared decision making elected invasive treatment 22% less often than the controls, suggesting that fully informed Canadians might want less surgery than the amount now being performed in Ontario.

Shared Decision Making: The Diagnosis of Prostate Cancer

Shared decision making also has an important role in the decision about whether to be screened for certain conditions, including prostate cancer. The development of the prostate-specific antigen (PSA) test has resulted in a surge in the number of American men who have been diagnosed with early stage cancer of the prostate. The PSA test is effective at finding cancer, but there is a great deal of scientific uncertainty about the value of active treatment for the disease (Chapter Five).

The American College of Physicians has issued guidelines for the use of PSA, emphasizing the importance of informed patient choice in the decision about screening. It is far from clear that most men, given the choice, would prefer to know that they have a condition — prostate cancer — for which medical science has not validated the efficacy of invasive treatment.

Experience with shared decision making underscores the importance of the College's guidelines. The treatment dilemmas that men must face when diagnosed with prostate cancer are not well understood by the average patient undergoing diagnostic testing. Some men are even tested without their knowledge, as part of routine annual examinations. Yet preferences about knowing one's cancer status clearly differ from one individual to another. In one study, about half of men who were fully informed about the choices they would face if they learned they had cancer preferred not to be screened. Even if these results are atypical, it is clear that public health programs should focus on efforts to inform men about all the risks and benefits of screening and treatment, rather than working to persuade men to be screened.

Shared Decision Making: The Treatment of Prostate Cancer

A community-based study of shared decision making for men with prostate cancer was conducted in Hartford, Connecticut. Each participant viewed a video about the options for treating the disease. The video presented the possible advantages of invasive treatments, but included a careful explanation of the limits of current scientific knowledge as to whether these advantages would actually occur. It also included information about the possible complications associated with treatment.

Prior to seeing the videotape, 44% of the participants felt that they were well-informed about prostate cancer; after seeing the video, 94% felt that they had a "good" or "excellent" understanding about their choices. Although few of the participants were pleased to learn that there was so much scientific uncertainty, more than 75% of men in the study participated actively in the choice of treatment. Of the men who chose treatment, about 37% chose surgery, 38% chose radiation therapy, and 25% chose watchful waiting.

Shared decision making, if widely adopted, offers a significant opportunity for improving the scientific basis of clinical medicine. The careful follow up of patients who choose different treatments makes it possible to learn more about the outcomes of care and the effects of shared decision making on such measures as satisfaction and functional status. Shared decision making could also expand the opportunity to conduct randomized clinical trials: men with prostate cancer who do not have a strong preference for one treatment over another might be willing to be randomized to treatment. Twenty-five percent of the men in the Hartford study were uncertain about their own choices and asked their physicians to decide for them.

Linking shared decision making to outcomes research will improve the knowledge base for decision making by those who will face the same decision in the future. Shared decision making can create islands of rationality — areas of clinical medicine where uncertainty is reduced by patient-level outcomes research, where choice is based on the best available information, and where patients choose according to their own values and preferences.

II. Setting Limits on Hospital Capacity

While shared decision making and patient-level outcomes research hold promise for creating more rational approaches to making choices among available treatments, these strategies do not effectively address global variations in the supply of resources and medical spending. Much of medicine is not driven by well articulated medical theories that are (at least conceptually) testable by randomized clinical trials or other forms of outcomes research. Hospitalization is often an effort — sometimes a desperate effort — to hold the tide against the inevitable. The quantity of care provided under these circumstances is often limited only by supply. Judgments about how much care is enough must be grounded in an understanding of the relationship between health care capacity and utilization — on how available resources are used. Decisions about how much is enough must also focus on global outcomes. In the case of the supply of acute care hospital resources, the size of the physician workforce, and the level of Medicare spending, the primary focus should be on the marginal effects of resources and spending (and the services they purchase) on the health outcomes of populations.

The nation is already moving to reduce hospital capacity (Chapter Two). In the section that follows, we concentrate on the benchmarks provided by two hospital service areas which have been studied extensively: Boston, Massachusetts, and New Haven, Connecticut. We ask whether more is better. The nature of the relationship between hospital supply and utilization, and the failure to find evidence that more is better, are indications of the validity of using low-resource, low-utilization areas to define reasonable limits. Using such areas as benchmarks, it is possible to estimate the magnitude of potential savings which could be realized if high-resource, high-utilization regions were constrained to the level of low-resource, low-utilization regions.

We also evaluate the range of allocations of acute hospital care in hospital referral regions throughout the United States. The estimates we provide for resource savings assume that all regions with higher levels of resources and utilization than the benchmark are reduced to the benchmark level, but that regions with resources and utilization lower than the benchmark remain constant — that is, their resources and utilization are not increased.

Acute Care Hospital Resources Allocation: The New Haven, Connecticut Benchmark

Most of the care in Boston and New Haven is delivered by clinicians affiliated with some of the nation's finest medical schools. The communities are remarkably similar demographically. But thanks to a strong certificate of need program, hospital capacity in New Haven (and throughout Connecticut) is among the lowest in the nation. Over time, the dynamics that foster hospital construction projects in Boston have created many more beds and resulted in the hiring of many more hospital employees and hospital-based nurses per thousand residents than in the New Haven hospital service area.

The first question to ask about this difference in resources is, What is the impact on utilization? The clinicians caring for residents of Boston work with fewer resource constraints on their decisions about hospitalization. How do they use these "extra" beds in Boston? The major "product" purchased by the greater investment in acute care in Boston, in the end, is simply more admissions and more frequent readmissions for treatment of medical conditions.

The second question is, Why does Boston have so many "extra" beds? The higher rates of admissions and readmissions of Bostonians, compared to residents of New Haven, are not the result of higher illness rates in Boston. Hospital managers and boards of trustees did not decide to construct more beds in response to higher levels of illness; a more likely explanation is that the excess beds were constructed in response to local social, religious, political and economic factors, most of which were unrelated to population health.

What would it mean for Boston to achieve a level of resource allocation at least as efficient as New Haven's? (Table 7.1) If Bostonians had used resources and services at the same level as the residents of the New Haven hospital service area in 1995,

residents of Boston would have required 585 fewer beds, 9,335 fewer hospital employees, and 1,574 fewer hospital-based registered nurses. Medicare enrollees who
lived in Boston would have spent 72,450 fewer days in hospitals for the treatment
of medical conditions.

If the resources allocated to regions which had higher per capita numbers of hospital
resources than New Haven in 1995 were reduced to New Haven's level, nationally
there would have been 205,000 fewer hospital beds (a 26% reduction); 598,000
fewer hospital employees (a 17% reduction); and 185,000 fewer hospital-based registered nurses (a 21% reduction). Had all areas with higher hospital utilization than
New Haven in 1995 been reduced to the level of the New Haven hospital service
area, the Medicare population of the United States would have spent 13.9 million
fewer days in acute care hospitals.

Table 7.1. Estimated Excess Resources Allocated to Bostonians Compared to the New Haven, Connecticut Benchmark (For Hospital Service Areas, 1995)

	Resources Allocated per 1,000 to Residents of Hospital Service Area (1995)		Excess Resources Used by Bostonians According to New Haven Benchmark
	Boston	**New Haven**	
Acute Care Beds	3.2	2.4	585
Hospital Personnel	25.5	12.7	9,335
Hospital-Based Nurses	5.3	3.2	1,574
Medical Bed Days	1,644	1,199	72,450

Is More Acute Hospital Care Better?

The Boston and New Haven hospital service areas provide useful natural
laboratories for examining this question. In New Haven (and throughout
Connecticut) sick patients are more often treated outside the hospital than similarly
sick patients who live in Boston. If the resources now spent on acute hospital care
in areas with higher levels of resources were reduced to the level of New Haven,
money available for other sectors of care — providing ambulatory care to the
underserved, for example — could be increased. But do patients who live in areas
with lower acute care hospital capacity receive adequate levels of care? Are the
constraints on supply of the New Haven hospital service area harmful to patients?

There are three arguments that suggest that patients living in New Haven are not harmed.

First, New Haven clinicians do not appear to be aware of constraints that lower levels of resources impose on their practice styles. Before they were informed about comparative levels of hospital resources in their hospital service area, clinicians in New Haven were asked if they were aware of differences between themselves and their colleagues at Boston's teaching hospitals. Similar interviews were held with clinicians in Boston and in other areas. These discussions made it clear that clinicians are generally unaware of the per capita supply of beds in their own areas, and cannot identify their own areas' absolute or relative supplies of beds. Indeed, physicians who had at some time in their careers practiced in both New Haven and Boston were unaware of the differences in practice styles between the two communities.

Second, clinicians practicing in areas with low per capita supplies of acute care hospital beds are not aware of danger, harm, or even scarcity. When asked, clinicians in New Haven did not believe they were withholding valued and necessary hospital care because of a lack of resources. Indeed, they did not profess to have more conservative treatment theories or to exercise conscious choice that it was better to treat seriously ill patients outside of the hospital.

Third, subliminal adaptation of the theory and practice of medicine to the constraints of capacity is further evidenced by the fact that occupancy rates (the average proportion of available beds that are actually occupied by patients) are not closely correlated with per capita bed capacity. If the low bed supply in New Haven created scarcity, one would expect more crowding of hospital beds — that the occupancy rate in New Haven would be higher than the rate in Boston. But historically the occupancy rates in both cities' hospitals have been about the same.

There is a bottom line to this comparison: outcomes, in terms of life expectancy, are not different for patients in Boston and New Haven. Arguably life expectancy is the most important outcome; it is, inarguably, measurable. In the years since these studies began, the mortality rates of residents of Boston and New Haven have been essentially the same. Research performed in conjunction with the Atlas confirms this pattern across all hospital referral regions in the United States; areas with greater hospital capacity, and with more inpatient days per capita, do not have lower mortality rates, even after controlling for a wide variety of health indicators. In other words, the United States might be on the "flat of the curve" in terms of mortality, and, if so, a reduction in overall bed capacity would not affect life expectancy.

Acute Hospital Care: Benchmarking the American Experience

New Haven is but one of the many available benchmarks against which to profile the American experience of hospital care. This section provides a report card profiling the pattern of resource allocation in seven hospital referral regions in the United States. The report displays the potential savings in health care resource use if the level in each of the seven regions represented the upper limit for resource allocation. The estimates for hospital beds have been adjusted for age and sex, as well as for illness, using a community-based index of illness. Figure 7.3 gives the adjusted numbers of hospital beds per thousand residents in seven selected areas. The table at the end of this chapter provides illness, age, and sex adjusted rates per 1,000 residents for each of the 306 hospital referral regions in the United States.

The rates range from a low of 1.8 beds per thousand residents of the Seattle, Washington hospital referral region, to a high of 4.4 beds per thousand residents in the Chicago hospital referral region. Two hundred ninety-four of the nation's 306 hospital referral regions had more hospital beds per thousand residents than Seattle. If hospital capacity in all regions with higher rates were reduced to the Seattle benchmark (on an illness, age and sex adjusted basis), then hospital capacity in the United States would be reduced more than 28%, or by more than 223,000 hospital beds. If the Atlanta rate (2.9 beds per thousand residents) prevailed throughout the country, capacity would be reduced by more than 116,000 hospital beds.

On the other hand, only five regions in the United States have more beds per thousand residents than the Manhattan hospital referral region, and reducing those five regions to the Manhattan benchmark would result in a reduction in the national supply of only about 1,000 hospital beds.

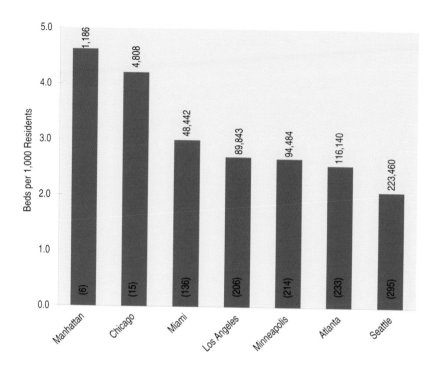

Figure 7.3. Illness and Age and Sex Adjusted Acute Care Hospital Beds per 1,000 Residents in Selected Hospital Referral Regions and Cumulative Number of Hospital Beds in Excess of Benchmark in Regions with Higher Rates

The age, sex and illness adjusted numbers of hospital beds per 1,000 residents varied substantially. For each benchmark, the figure gives the region's rank (in parentheses) and estimates the excess number of hospital beds, had the benchmark region's rate prevailed in higher regions in 1995. Seattle ranked 295th. The Seattle benchmark estimates an excess of 223,000 hospital beds in regions with higher rates.

III. Setting Limits on the Physician Workforce

The size of the physician workforce in the United States has been determined by factors that have little to do with patient demand for health care, and much to do with federal policy and the needs of training institutions as they are currently structured. In the 1970s it was widely assumed that the United States faced a physician shortage, which led to policy which encouraged an increase in the number of medical schools and the enlargement of medical school class sizes.

The federal government, through the Medicare program, is the primary source of funding for the training of physicians in residency programs, providing an estimated $70,000 for every resident in training in 1992. The number of specialty residency positions, however, has been determined by the training institutions themselves, aided by an accreditation process that focuses on academic standards, not the numbers of specialists needed by the population outside the training institutions.

From 1970 to 1996, the per capita supply of clinically active physicians in the United States grew by about 67%, from 113.1 per 100,000 residents to 188.9. During this period, the number of specialists almost doubled, increasing from 63 specialists per 100,000 residents to 123 per 100,000. The supply of generalist physicians increased from 49 to 65 per 100,000 residents. By 1996, about 66% of the physician workforce were specialists.

But how many physicians are really needed? Traditionally, workforce requirements have been forecast on the basis of either needs-based or demand-based planning models, both of which are seriously flawed.

Needs-based planning relies on experts to estimate the correct number of physicians to meet need and produce optimal outcomes. Unfortunately, the uncertainties inherent in clinical medicine, rapid changes in technology, and the inevitable failure of outcomes research to keep up with innovation mean that even "experts" are unable to accurately predict the need for physicians.

Demand based planning assumes that the utilization of care is driven by patient demand; the trends in prevailing rates of service are therefore assumed to be the right rate and are used to project the need for physicians. The evidence that the supply of resources and provider preferences influence the rates of use of care for discretionary services is evidence of the futility of using utilization as a measure of patient demand, and consequently its failure as a method by which to project workforce requirements.

Benchmarking provides a pragmatic alternative for estimating the requirements for a reasonably sized workforce. Elsewhere, we have argued that the hiring practices of large, stable, staff model health maintenance organizations or the population-based physician supply in regions with efficient delivery systems should be used as benchmarks for estimating the nation's resource and workforce requirements. Benchmarks provide a useful measure of the level of need for several reasons:

■ Benchmarks provide working examples of the actual deployment of the workforce, realistic guidelines drawn from successful health care plans or regions. In the case of staff model health maintenance organizations, workforce configurations have succeeded in competition with fee-for-service in markets, often in places such as San Francisco (Figure 7.5) where the numbers of physicians per 100,000 residents serving the fee-for-service market is among the highest in the nation. Regions with efficient health care markets are also useful as benchmarks because their workforce configurations serve entire populations, not just the part of the population enrolled in health maintenance organizations.

■ There is little or no evidence that patients are harmed because they are served by health plans with constrained workforces, or live in regions with fewer physicians per capita. Indeed, there is some evidence that the current surgical workforce is more than sufficient to meet patient demand for discretionary surgery. Figure 7.1 shows that even with the relatively low per capita numbers of urologists employed by health maintenance organizations, the supply was more than adequate to meet the demand for prostate surgery, once patients were engaged in shared decision making to select the treatments they preferred.

■ Finally, while studies of the global impact of marginal increases in physician supply on population mortality have not been done and should be encouraged, when it is unclear that spending more is beneficial, common sense argues against the status quo (continuing to produce physicians at a rate which increases the nation's per capita supply) particularly when the trend in the market is toward managed care.

The Physician Workforce: The Health Maintenance Organization Benchmark

The employment practices of well-established staff model health maintenance organizations such as Kaiser-Permanente indicate that the physician workforce requirements under fully integrated managed care systems are considerably less than the numbers of physicians now in practice in the United States. In research related to the Atlas, the staffing patterns of a large West Coast staff model health maintenance organization were used to provide a quantitative measure of the excess in capacity predicted for the United States, should the workforce requirements of that health maintenance organization become the standard for the nation.

On an age and sex adjusted basis, the number of clinically active physicians practicing in the United States in 1996 was substantially in excess of the health maintenance organization benchmark. The supply of specialists exceeded the workforce requirements of the staff model health maintenance organization by 35%. Had the number of specialists per hundred thousand residents represented by this health maintenance organization's staffing level been used to determine the size of the employed workforce throughout the United States in 1996, 74,267 full time equivalent specialists would have been unemployed. (This comparison is restricted to "selected specialists — those specialists actually employed by the health maintenance organization — and therefore does not include such specialties as forensic pathology. See the endnote and the Appendix on the Physician Workforce for further information.)

The health maintenance organization's per capita employment rate of generalists was also below the national average: the supply of generalists in the United States was 1.41 times higher than in the health maintenance organization, indicating a national excess of 49,334 full time equivalent generalist physicians.

Excess capacity existed for virtually every major category of specialists (Figure 7.4). For example, if the health maintenance organization's staffing level of specialists had prevailed throughout the United States in 1996, the estimated excess supply of cardiologists would have been 61% of the cardiology workforce, or 9,436 physicians; and the excess supply of pathologists 55% of the pathology workforce, or 6,561 physicians. The sole specialty for which the health maintenance organization benchmark predicted underservice elsewhere in the United States was emergency care physicians.

The Physician Workforce: Benchmarking the American Experience

The health maintenance organization benchmark for workforce planning is useful to the extent that it reliably forecasts the demand for physicians, should capitated managed care become the prevailing method of organizing health care delivery in the United States. There are currently no regions, however, where health maintenance organizations serve the entire population of a region, and benchmarks based on the managed care experience fail to take into account the health care of special populations, such as the uninsured, those who are covered by Medicaid, or those with illnesses that make them unlikely candidates for enrollment in managed care. The experiences of regions, however, are valid benchmarks for entire populations.

This section provides a "report card" profiling the pattern of physician resource allocation in eight hospital referral regions in the United States. Figures 7.5 and 7.6 show the age and sex adjusted numbers of generalist and selected specialist physicians per 100,000 residents in the eight selected hospital referral regions (see the endnote for the definition of "selected specialists"). The figures display the ranks of these areas, compared to all others in the United States, and give the surplus in physician supply if the level in each of the eight regions represented the upper limit for physician resource allocation in the United States. The Appendix on the Physician Workforce in the United States provides the same information for each of the 306 hospital referral regions, as well as maps showing how each region compares to the Minneapolis, Wichita, and health maintenance organization benchmarks. Rates of physicians per 100,000 residents and maps are also provided for each of the 12 specialists listed in Figure 7.4.

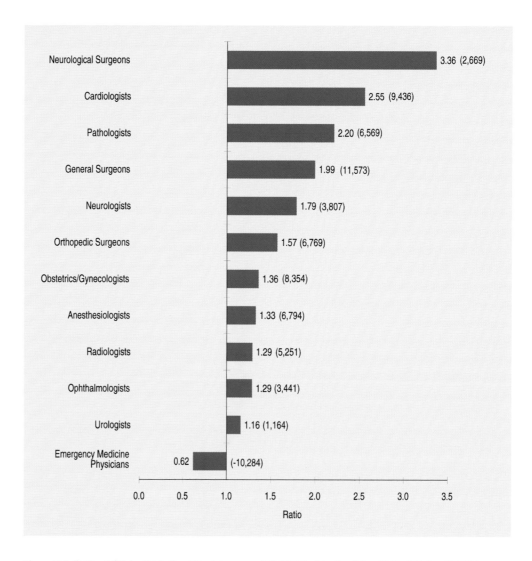

Figure 7.4. Ratio of Clinically Active Physicians per 100,000 Residents of the United States (1996) to Physicians per 100,000 Enrollees in a Large Staff Model HMO (1993)
The figure gives the ratio of the U.S. physician supply to the numbers employed or contracted for by a large West Coast health maintenance organization. The numbers in parentheses are the excess supply of physicians that would have existed in 1996, had the employment practices of the health maintenance organization been the standard for the nation.

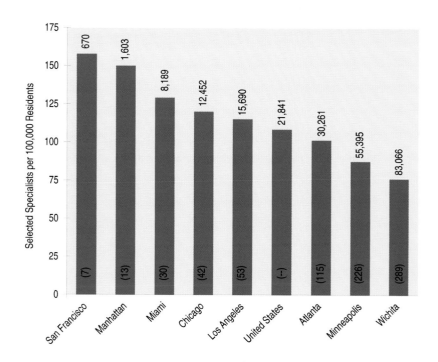

Figure 7.5. Selected Specialist Physicians per 100,000 Residents in Selected Hospital Referral Regions and Cumulative Number of Physicians in Excess of Benchmark in Regions with Higher Rates
The full time equivalent numbers of selected specialist physicians (those employed by the benchmark HMO) varied substantially. For each benchmark, the figure gives the region's rank in terms of the physicians per 100,000 residents (in parentheses) and estimates the excess number of physicians, had the benchmark region's rate prevailed in regions with larger per capita supplies of specialists in 1996. Wichita ranked 289th. The benchmark estimates an excess of 83,066 full time equivalent clinically active physicians in regions with higher rates.

San Francisco, with 158 selected specialists per 100,000 residents, had the seventh-highest age and sex adjusted supply of physicians among the nation's 306 hospital referral regions. Minneapolis, a hospital referral region with a long history of managed care, ranked 226th. It had only about half as many selected specialists per 100,000 residents as the San Francisco hospital referral region, and was well below the United States average. If the level of physician supply of the Minneapolis benchmark prevailed in the 225 hospital referral regions with higher rates, the estimated excess number of selected specialists would have been 20% of the selected specialist workforce, or 55,395 physicians. Wichita provides an interesting benchmark because it represents a model of low physician supply in a market where managed care has not had strong penetration. The Wichita benchmark, however, estimates an even lower supply of selected specialists than the Minneapolis benchmark. Wichita ranked 289th in numbers of selected specialists per 100,000 residents; had this benchmark prevailed in 1996 in regions with higher rates, the estimated excess number of specialists would have been 29% of the selected specialist workforce, or 83,066 physicians.

The Minneapolis hospital referral region benchmark for generalist physicians was higher than the national average, but the Wichita region's supply was below it. Had the Wichita level of supply prevailed in 1996 in regions with higher rates, the estimated excess number of generalists would have been 10% of the generalist workforce, or 17,704 physicians.

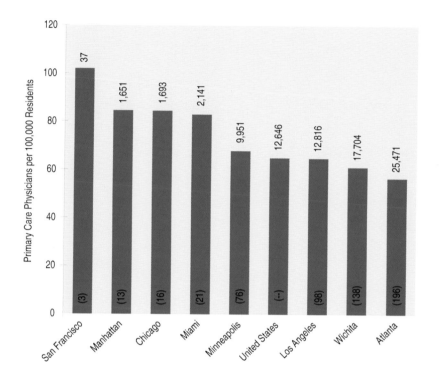

Figure 7.6. Generalist Physicians per 100,000 Residents in Selected Hospital Referral Regions and Cumulative Numbers of Physicians in Excess of Benchmark in Regions with Higher Rates

The full time equivalent numbers of generalist physicians varied substantially. For each benchmark, the figure gives the region's rank in terms of generalist physicians per 100,000 residents (in parentheses) and estimates the excess number of generalist physicians, had the benchmark region's rate prevailed in regions with higher rates in 1996. Wichita ranked 138th. The benchmark estimates an excess of 17,704 full time equivalent clinically active generalist physicians in regions with higher rates.

IV. Medicare Spending and Equity

What does greater Medicare spending buy? Just as Boston and New Haven provide a useful lesson on the effects of hospital capacity, the health care experience of Medicare residents of two retirement communities — Miami Beach, Florida, and Sun City, Arizona — provide a remarkable contrast in Medicare spending and insight into the "benefits" that greater spending buys. Both Miami Beach and Sun City are prosperous communities, with average household incomes well above the national average; and both are magnets for retirees, attracting large numbers of Americans, principally from the Northeast and the Midwest and, in the case of Sun City, from the Mountain States.

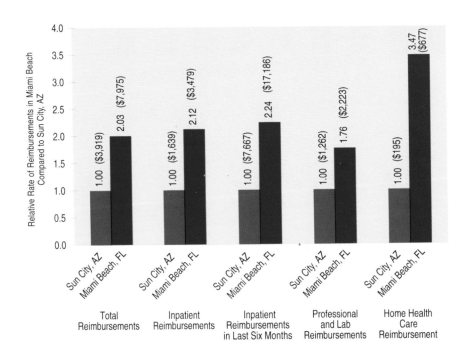

Figure 7.7. Medicare Spending for Enrollees Living in Miami Beach, Florida and Sun City, Arizona by Program Component (1995)
The figure gives the ratio of per enrollee Medicare spending in Miami Beach to spending in Sun City, as well as the amount spent per enrollee (in parentheses). Per enrollee spending was higher for residents of Miami Beach across all components of the Medicare program.

Although the populations are similar in many respects, the average price adjusted reimbursement for fee-for-service Medicare enrollees living in the Miami Beach hospital service area in 1995 was $8,655, about 2.2 times higher than for Medicare enrollees living in Sun City ($3,918). Residents of Miami Beach received substantially more from the Medicare program in all categories of spending than residents of Sun City (Figure 7.7). Price adjusted spending for physician and laboratory services was 76% higher; for inpatient care was 112% higher; and for home health care was more than 240% higher. During the last six months of life, more than $17,000 per enrollee was spent on inpatient care for residents of Miami Beach — 2.24 times as much as the $7,559 per enrollee spent for Medicare enrollees in Sun City.

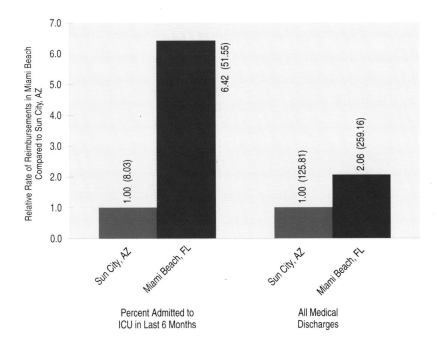

Figure 7.8. Admissions to Intensive Care During the Last Six Months of Life and Acute Care Hospital Utilization for Medical Conditions and Among Medicare Enrollees Living in Miami Beach, Florida and Sun City, Arizona (1994-95)

The figure gives the ratio of rates of acute care hospital services for enrollees living in Miami Beach to the rate among residents of Sun City, as well as the actual rate (in parentheses). Residents of Miami Beach received much more inpatient care for all medical conditions per 1,000 residents, and the percent of enrollees admitted to intensive care during the last 6 months of life was more than 6 times higher among residents of Miami Beach than among residents of Sun City.

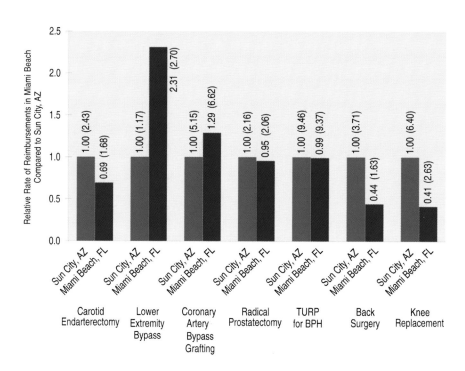

Figure 7.9. Selected Surgical Procedures for Medicare Enrollees Living in Miami Beach, Florida and Sun City, Arizona (1994-95)

The figure gives the ratio of the use of selected surgical procedures among enrollees living in Miami Beach to rates for residents of Sun City, as well as the rates per 1,000 residents (in parentheses). The patterns of use of surgery varied in an idiosyncratic way; Miami Beach had higher rates of some procedures (e.g., lower extremity bypass) than Sun City, while rates for other procedures (e.g., back surgery and knee replacement) were lower among Medicare enrollees in Miami Beach than among enrollees in Sun City.

The increased spending on inpatient care purchased more than twice as many discharges for medical conditions per thousand Medicare residents of Miami Beach than per thousand Medicare residents of Sun City. The higher level of spending also purchased much more intensive care: 52% of Miami Beach enrollees spent one or more days in intensive care during the last six months of their lives, compared to 8% of enrollees in Sun City (Figure 7.8).

By contrast, varying rates of specific surgical procedures demonstrated a typical "surgical signature" phenomenon. Rates were sometimes higher, and sometimes lower, for Medicare residents of Miami Beach than for Medicare residents of Sun City (Figure 7.9). For example, the rate of lower extremity bypass surgery among Medicare enrollees in Miami Beach was 2.3 times higher than the rate among enrollees in Sun City; but the rates of knee replacement and back surgery among Medicare enrollees in Miami Beach were less than half the rates of those procedures among Medicare residents of Sun City.

Medicare Spending: Is More Better?

In Sun City, and in many other parts of the country, the Medicare program spends considerably less per enrollee than in Miami Beach and other regions with similarly high rates. Should something be done about this? The argument for "doing something" about the differences in spending has several facets. We have already seen that differences in spending relate to differences in supply of resources and physician practice styles (Chapter Four), and that illness explains only a small proportion of the differences in spending among regions (Chapter Six). We also know that the differences are not explained by differences in regional prices (Chapter Six).

The differences are unfair, because residents living in regions with low rates of reimbursement are subsidizing, through their contributions to Medicare, the care received by enrollees with similar health needs who live in high cost regions. And the transfer payments (subsidies) flowing from low reimbursement to high reimbursement regions are economically unwise, because they reward inefficient providers and sustain excess capacity.

But what should the policy goal be? Is it better to increase spending in regions with low rates, in order to equalize them with high rate regions? Should all regions be equalized at the national average? Or should the overall level of spending be reduced to the level of less costly regions, such as Sun City — or even lower?

A comparison of spending by the Medicare program in Miami Beach and in Sun City illustrates what is bought with an increase in Medicare reimbursements: an increase in the intensity of treatment of sick people; an increase in the rates of hospitalization for medical conditions; an increase in the use of intensive care; and an increase in the level of spending on diagnostic tests, physician services and home health care. The increase is not in specific discretionary surgical procedures aimed at improving enrollees' quality of life, and the investment is not simply monetary. The incremental investment in medical interventions for enrollees living in Miami Beach purchases more time spent in hospitals and intensive care, more encounters with physicians, and more diagnostic tests. Yet evidence of benefit, at least in terms of life expectancy, has not been found in studies of areas with similar disparities of resource allocation and utilization.

The lack of evidence that more is better argues in favor of adopting the patterns of practice and reimbursements now in effect in low reimbursement regions. The case for lower spending can also be based on national priorities: if the level of spending in high reimbursement hospital referral regions, such as Miami Beach, were reduced to the levels in hospital referral regions with low reimbursement rates, total Medicare spending would be considerably reduced, at least for a few years (Figure 1.4). The opposite policy, increasing spending to the level of Miami, would result in fiscal calamity.

Medicare's AAPCC: Equity, Managed Care and the Minneapolis Benchmark

The history of health care in Minneapolis is the history of managed care itself. Frugal in every sector of Medicare spending (Chapter Three), the Minneapolis hospital referral region provides a cogent example of the economies that can be realized in health care delivery. The per capita size of the physician workforce, the numbers of hospital resources, and Medicare spending (on a price and illness adjusted basis) are all substantially lower in the Minneapolis hospital referral region than the national average, and much lower than in the Miami hospital referral region (which includes the Miami Beach hospital service area).

Ironically, the government's strategy for promoting managed care imposes a stiff penalty on Medicare enrollees living in regions, like Minneapolis, with historically efficient health care systems, because the capitation rate for Medicare enrollees who join managed care organizations is based on the historical per capita Medicare spending in the county where the enrollee lives. The Adjusted Average Per Capita Cost (AAPCC, Medicare's method of determinating capitation payments) for enrollees living in the Miami hospital referral region in 1997 was set at $8,690; for enrollees living in the Minneapolis hospital referral region it was set at $4,108. On a price adjusted basis, the AAPCC for Miami is 86% higher than for Minneapolis ($8,180 versus $4,403); and on an illness and price adjusted basis, it is 81% higher: $8,117 versus $4,478.

In order to attract Medicare participants, managed care companies can elect to expand their benefit packages to include services not available under fee-for-service reimbursements: prescription drugs, hearing aids, and exercise programs, for example. But these additional benefits cost money, and the ability to provide them depends on the capitated rate paid to the managed care company by the Medicare program. The substantial differences in AAPCC for Miami and Minneapolis can result in far different benefit packages that can profitably be offered in the two regions.

The 1997 AAPCC predicts that if managed care plans in Miami achieve the Minneapolis benchmark of spending for the benefits provided under tradition fee-for-service medicine, the companies would realize savings of about $4,353 (the difference between 95% of $8,690 and 95% of $4,108) per enrollee. This saving would then be available for additional benefits such as prescriptions and eyeglasses, while still allowing the managed care companies a comfortable profit (a low "medical loss ratio"). By contrast, for enrollees living in Minneapolis to receive even a nearly similar package of additional benefits (and for managed care companies providing such benefits to make a profit), spending on traditional Medicare benefits would have to drop to an impossible zero.

The value of Medicare's AAPCC thus raises yet another issue in the Which rate is right? debate. If the Minneapolis hospital referral region's level of efficiency is widely adopted as the standard for managed care, enrollees (and managed care companies) in some parts of the country stand to win, while other regions — those with lower spending — stand to gain little. The equity implications of the variations in the AAPCC in six hospital referral regions are displayed in Figure 7.10. The figure examines the "surplus" in dollars that under current policy would be available in each region for additional benefits for each enrollee, if the historical model of efficiency of the Minneapolis hospital referral region prevailed. The Chapter Seven Table provides estimates for each of the 306 hospital referral regions in the United States.

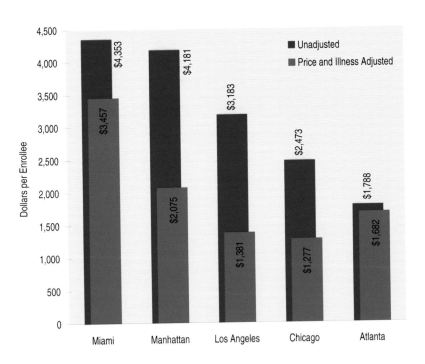

Figure 7.10. Estimated Dollars per Enrollee Available Under Medicare Risk Contracts for New Benefits and/or Managed Care Company Profit if Managed Care Companies in Selected Regions Achieved the Minneapolis Benchmark for Efficient Health Care Delivery (1997)
The figure gives the per enrollee dollars in excess of the amount predicted by the Minneapolis benchmark in each selected region based on the 1997 AAPCC. The price and illness adjusted amounts are also shown.

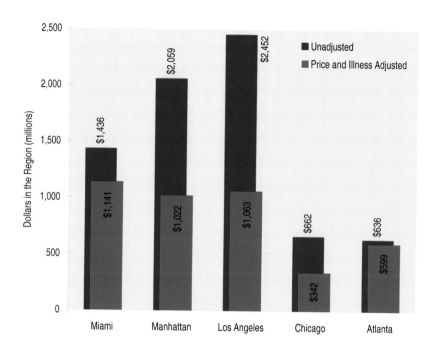

Figure 7.11. Estimated Revenues (in Millions of Dollars) Under Medicare Risk Contracts for New Benefits and/or Managed Care Company Profit in Selected Hospital Referral Regions (1997)
The figure gives the revenues, in millions, that would be attained if managed care companies enrolled the Medicare population living in the selected regions and achieved the Minneapolis benchmark for efficient health care delivery. The estimates are based on the 1997 AAPCC and are also given for the price and illness adjusted AAPCC.

The estimates in the figure include those based on the 1997 illness and price adjusted AAPCC among hospital referral regions (for a description of this calculation, see the Appendix on Methods).

Figure 7.11 looks at the situation from the perspective of the financial incentives to managed care companies to enter each market. The figure contains estimates of the Medicare dollars to be gained by converting the entire Medicare population from fee-for-service financing to risk bearing managed care. The estimate is based on the average number of enrollees living the region in 1994-95, and includes enrollees in fee-for-service as well as current members of risk bearing health maintenance organizations. For example, the Miami estimate for dollars based on illness and price adjusted AAPCC was obtained by multiplying the per enrollee surplus by the number of enrollees living in the Miami region: $3,457 x 330,001 = $1.14 billion.

Maps 7.1 and 7.2 show the location of hospital referral regions with AAPCCs lower and higher than the Minneapolis hospital referral region, and indicate the excess per enrollee amount paid to managed care companies, compared to the Minneapolis benchmark. Map 7.1 is based on the actual 1997 AAPCC, unadjusted for illness or price. Thirty-two regions, primarily in the Upper Midwest and parts of Oregon, Idaho and Montana (light green) had AAPCCs lower than the rate in the Minneapolis hospital referral region. Sixty-two regions had AAPCCs of less than $500 more than the rate in Minneapolis (cream). One hundred forty-two regions had AAPCCs of $1,000 or more (oranges and reds). Fifty-one regions, primarily in Massachusetts, New York, Pennsylvania, the Washington-Baltimore area, parts of Florida, Louisiana, Texas and California, had per enrollee payments more than $2,000 higher than the Minneapolis benchmark (blue).

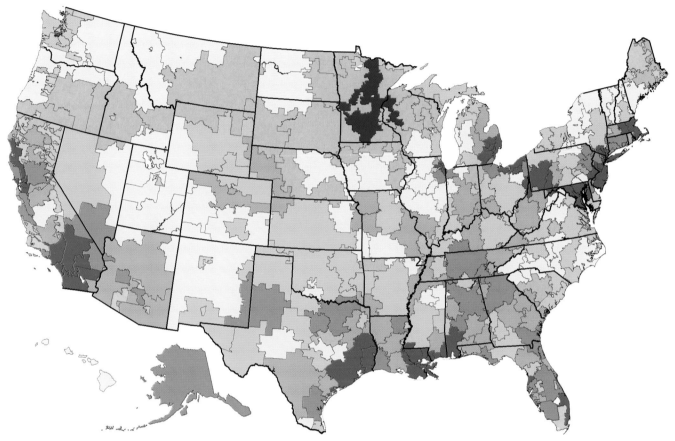

Map 7.1. Per Enrollee Annual Payment to Managed Care Companies in Excess of the Amount for Enrollees Living in the Minneapolis Hospital Referral Region (1997)

There were 32 hospital referral regions (light green) with per enrollee AAPCCs lower than the Minneapolis region (blue). The AAPCC exceeded the Minneapolis rate by $2,000 or more in 51 regions (red); and by $1,000 or more in 142 regions.

Managed Care Payments in Excess of Minneapolis Benchmark ($4,108 for 1997)
by Hospital Referral Region

- 2,000 to 4,582   (51)
- 1,500 to 2,000   (40)
- 1,000 to 1,500   (51)
- 500 to 1,000   (69)
- 1 to 500   (62)
- All Others   (32)
- Minneapolis
- Not Populated

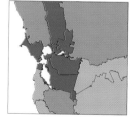

San Francisco

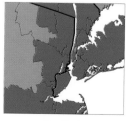

Chicago

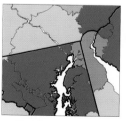

New York

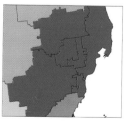

Washington-Baltimore

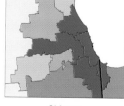

Detroit

When the estimates are price and illness adjusted (Map 7.2), only 17 regions had AAPCCs lower than the rate in the Minneapolis hospital referral region. One hundred fifty-three regions had AAPCCs more than $1,000 higher than the Minneapolis hospital referral region. The main effect of price adjustment is to reduce estimates for hospital referral regions in the Northeast and California, where prices are particularly high.

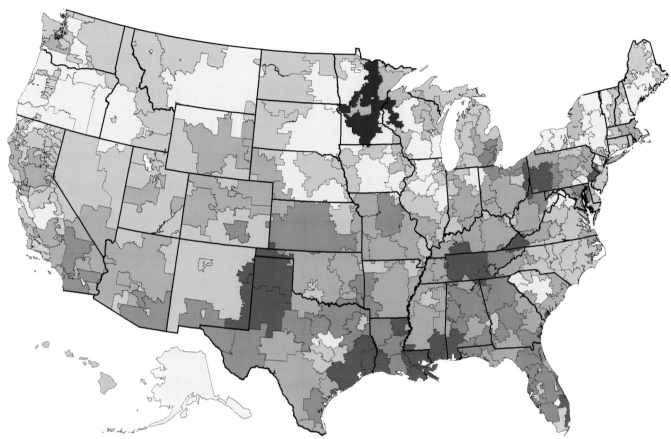

Map 7.2. Price and Illness Adjusted Per Enrollee Annual Payment to Managed Care Companies in Excess of the Amount for Enrollees Living in the Minneapolis Hospital Referral Region (1997)

Seventeen hospital referral regions with price and illness adjusted per enrollee AAPCCs equal to or lower than the Minneapolis region (light green). The adjusted AAPCC exceeded the Minneapolis rate by $2,000 or more in 25 regions (red); and by $1,000 or more in 153 regions (medium orange to red). The principal effect of price adjustment is to reduce the estimates for regions with higher prevailing prices, and to increase the estimates for regions with lower prevailing prices.

Price Adjusted and Illness Adjusted Managed Care Payments in Excess of Minneapolis Benchmark ($4,478 for 1997)
by Hospital Referral Region

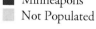

- 2,000 to 3,639   (25)
- 1,500 to 2,000   (49)
- 1,000 to 1,500   (79)
-   500 to 1,000   (83)
-     1 to   500   (52)
- All Others   (17)
- Minneapolis
- Not Populated

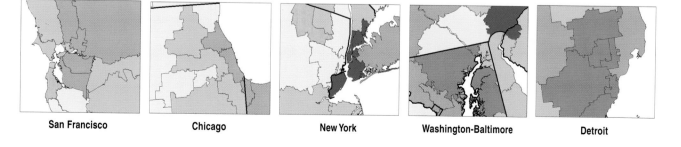

San Francisco   Chicago   New York   Washington-Baltimore   Detroit

V. Focusing the Debate: A Summary Statement

Health care markets in the United States are characterized by wide variations in the supply of hospital beds and physicians, in illness and price adjusted Medicare spending, in rates of hospitalization and surgery, and in the intensity of care during the last six months of life. Practice variations challenge basic assumptions about the nature of the health care economy and theories about how it should be reformed. For decades, the health care debate has taken place against the background assumption that more is better, and that constraint leads inevitably to the rationing of efficacious health care. It is time to re-frame the debate over health care reform to address the fundamental issue of value itself: Which rate is right? How much is enough? and What is fair?

This Atlas suggests certain conclusions and important hypotheses that bear on the debate:

1. Patients should be fully informed about what is known and what is not known about the outcomes of available treatment options, and should be encouraged to choose among those options according to their own preferences.

2. Outcomes research should become part of the everyday practice of medicine, and routine follow up of patients according to treatment choice should be incorporated into strategies to improve the scientific basis for clinical decision making.

3. It is safe for patients and in the public interest to adopt the level of acute hospital capacity, physician supply, and Medicare spending of efficient benchmarks such as New Haven and Minneapolis.

4. In order to achieve fairness in Medicare, spending among regions should be equalized on an illness adjusted basis.

The impact on the health care economy of reform along these lines would be considerable. When informed patients actively participate in the choice of treatment, there is evidence that patients express less demand for invasive treatments than the amount now being provided. Extrapolations into the future show that if Medicare spending in regions with higher rates than Minneapolis were brought down to that benchmark, the depletion of the Medicare trust funds would be avoided or substantially delayed. Indeed, the Minneapolis configuration of resources suggests a level of illness adjusted health care spending for populations of all ages that is far less than the current average for the United States. Within the savings generated by the judicious reduction of resources and spending to the level of such benchmarks, the nation can find the resources to provide access to health care for all Americans.

Chapter Seven Table   The table provides age, sex, and illness adjusted estimates of acute care hospital beds per 1,000 residents as well as estimates of the price, the illness and the price and illness adjusted AAPCC. Estimates for hospital referral regions (HRRs) are a weighted average of each HRR's constituent counties (weighted according to the relative Medicare population). See Appendix on Methods for details. Estimates for projected surplus on a per enrollee and on an area-wide basis were made according to the formula described above. (See text associated with figures 7.10 and 7.11.)

CHAPTER SEVEN TABLE

Estimated 1997 Average Adjusted Per Capita Costs (AAPCC) and Related Statistics for Medicare by Hospital Referral Region (in dollars)

Hospital Referral Region	Age, Sex and Illness Adjusted Acute Care Hospital Beds	AAPCC (1997)	Price Adjusted AAPCC (1997)	Illness Adjusted AAPCC (1997)	Price and Illness Adjusted AAPCC (1997)	Unadjusted Projected Surplus / Deficit per Enrollee according to Minneapolis Benchmark (1997)	Price and Illness Adjusted Projected Surplus /Deficit per Enrollee acc. to Mpls. Benchmark (1997)	Unadjusted Projected Surplus /Deficit per Region acc. to Mpls. Benchmark (1997) in millions	Price and Illness Adjusted Projected Surplus /Deficit per Region acc. to Mpls. Benchmark (1997) in millions
Alabama									
Birmingham	3.48	5,835	6,526	5,624	6,290	1,727	1,812	468	491
Dothan	2.99	5,328	6,272	5,283	6,219	1,220	1,741	55	79
Huntsville	2.99	5,060	5,525	5,177	5,652	952	1,174	51	64
Mobile	3.09	6,156	7,032	5,679	6,488	2,047	2,010	172	169
Montgomery	3.23	5,312	6,032	5,233	5,942	1,203	1,465	59	72
Tuscaloosa	3.23	5,289	6,093	5,262	6,063	1,180	1,585	33	45
Alaska									
Anchorage	3.47	5,630	4,681	5,641	4,690	1,522	213	41	6
Arizona									
Mesa	2.07	5,921	5,962	6,346	6,389	1,813	1,912	158	167
Phoenix	2.83	5,425	5,618	5,711	5,915	1,316	1,437	318	347
Sun City	2.49	5,854	5,894	5,933	5,974	1,745	1,496	112	96
Tucson	2.64	5,373	5,841	5,676	6,171	1,265	1,693	152	203
Arkansas									
Fort Smith	3.02	4,711	5,674	5,049	6,081	603	1,604	27	71
Jonesboro	3.13	4,370	5,606	4,216	5,409	262	931	8	29
Little Rock	3.40	4,869	5,885	4,772	5,768	761	1,290	148	251
Springdale	2.31	3,941	4,918	4,091	5,106	-167	628	-8	30
Texarkana	3.31	5,409	6,611	5,095	6,227	1,300	1,749	45	61
California									
Orange Co.	2.39	6,841	5,850	6,819	5,832	2,733	1,354	639	316
Bakersfield	2.28	5,414	5,377	5,579	5,541	1,306	1,063	104	84
Chico	2.23	5,231	5,593	5,139	5,495	1,123	1,017	46	42
Contra Costa Co.	1.76	6,689	5,723	6,893	5,897	2,581	1,419	210	115
Fresno	2.42	4,580	4,652	4,794	4,870	472	392	42	35
Los Angeles	2.69	7,458	6,130	7,216	5,931	3,350	1,453	2,581	1,119
Modesto	2.47	5,442	5,495	5,314	5,365	1,334	887	98	65
Napa	2.60	6,118	6,126	5,844	5,851	2,010	1,373	78	53
Alameda Co.	2.07	6,722	5,657	6,631	5,580	2,614	1,103	346	146
Palm Spr/Rancho Mir	2.38	6,230	5,905	6,258	5,932	2,122	1,454	100	69
Redding	2.59	5,348	5,643	5,096	5,376	1,240	899	53	39
Sacramento	1.98	5,694	5,410	5,796	5,506	1,586	1,029	346	224
Salinas	2.19	5,692	5,352	5,711	5,370	1,584	892	54	30
San Bernardino	2.20	6,266	5,941	6,360	6,029	2,158	1,552	456	328
San Diego	2.25	6,119	5,724	6,418	6,004	2,011	1,526	609	462
San Francisco	2.27	6,281	5,071	6,196	5,003	2,172	525	335	81
San Jose	1.94	5,745	4,559	5,723	4,541	1,637	64	203	8
San Luis Obispo	2.35	4,647	4,372	4,566	4,295	539	-182	16	-5
San Mateo Co.	2.25	5,464	4,307	5,527	4,356	1,356	-121	116	-10
Santa Barbara	2.20	4,683	4,252	4,765	4,328	574	-150	27	-7

Hospital Referral Region	Age, Sex and Illness Adjusted Acute Care Hospital Beds	AAPCC (1997)	Price Adjusted AAPCC (1997)	Illness Adjusted AAPCC (1997)	Price and Illness Adjusted AAPCC (1997)	Unadjusted Projected Surplus / Enrollee according to Minneapolis Benchmark (1997)	Price and Illness Adjusted Projected Surplus / Enrollee according to Minneapolis Benchmark (1997)	Unadjusted Projected Surplus / Region according to Minneapolis Benchmark (1997) in millions	Price and Illness Adjusted Projected Surplus / Region according to Minneapolis Benchmark (1997) in millions
Santa Cruz	2.04	5,509	4,977	5,480	4,951	1,400	474	35	12
Santa Rosa	1.96	5,661	5,119	5,668	5,125	1,553	647	83	35
Stockton	2.23	5,327	5,210	5,183	5,069	1,219	591	53	26
Ventura	2.14	6,028	5,258	5,892	5,139	1,920	662	129	44
Colorado									
Boulder	2.09	5,141	5,326	5,631	5,834	1,033	1,356	18	24
Colorado Springs	2.69	4,598	5,111	4,920	5,469	490	991	30	61
Denver	2.81	5,281	5,476	5,703	5,914	1,173	1,436	233	285
Fort Collins	2.35	4,722	5,256	4,823	5,368	614	890	15	22
Grand Junction	2.68	4,254	5,085	4,752	5,679	146	1,202	4	36
Greeley	3.02	4,818	5,483	5,122	5,828	710	1,351	21	40
Pueblo	3.41	4,890	5,627	5,407	6,222	782	1,744	17	37
Connecticut									
Bridgeport	2.44	6,008	4,892	6,019	4,900	1,900	422	169	37
Hartford	2.50	5,623	4,836	5,836	5,019	1,514	541	288	103
New Haven	2.40	5,796	4,777	5,615	4,628	1,688	151	300	27
Delaware									
Wilmington	2.41	6,031	5,547	5,801	5,336	1,923	858	145	65
District of Columbia									
Washington	2.70	6,320	5,706	6,279	5,669	2,212	1,191	483	260
Florida									
Bradenton	2.75	5,124	5,533	4,941	5,336	1,016	858	51	43
Clearwater	2.38	6,001	6,387	5,713	6,080	1,893	1,603	206	174
Fort Lauderdale	2.78	7,054	6,787	7,231	6,956	2,946	2,479	1,276	1,073
Fort Myers	2.69	5,765	6,370	5,710	6,310	1,657	1,832	275	304
Gainesville	2.58	5,556	6,317	5,627	6,398	1,448	1,920	80	106
Hudson	2.33	6,341	6,748	6,032	6,420	2,232	1,942	219	191
Jacksonville	3.00	6,042	6,583	5,877	6,403	1,934	1,926	257	256
Lakeland	2.72	4,755	5,371	4,787	5,408	646	930	29	42
Miami	2.99	8,690	8,180	8,623	8,117	4,582	3,639	1,512	1,201
Ocala	2.46	5,085	5,957	5,119	5,997	977	1,519	84	130
Orlando	2.55	5,734	6,122	5,715	6,102	1,625	1,624	634	633
Ormond Beach	3.02	5,130	5,724	5,083	5,673	1,021	1,195	69	80
Panama City	2.86	5,658	6,592	5,055	5,889	1,550	1,412	34	31
Pensacola	3.16	5,521	6,346	5,215	5,995	1,412	1,518	107	114
Sarasota	2.31	5,548	6,010	5,607	6,073	1,440	1,596	139	154
St Petersburg	2.88	6,001	6,387	5,809	6,182	1,893	1,705	158	142
Tallahassee	3.27	4,915	5,607	5,122	5,843	807	1,366	59	100
Tampa	2.59	5,944	6,325	5,665	6,029	1,835	1,552	218	184
Georgia									
Albany	3.62	4,931	5,597	5,309	6,027	822	1,549	18	34
Atlanta	2.55	5,990	6,107	6,128	6,248	1,882	1,771	670	630
Augusta	3.66	5,140	5,584	5,086	5,525	1,032	1,047	64	65
Columbus	4.26	4,615	5,334	4,730	5,466	507	989	17	33
Macon	3.40	5,360	6,046	5,408	6,100	1,252	1,622	91	118
Rome	2.78	5,201	6,210	5,344	6,381	1,092	1,903	33	58

Hospital Referral Region	Age, Sex and Illness Adjusted Acute Care Hospital Beds	AAPCC (1997)	Price Adjusted AAPCC (1997)	Illness Adjusted AAPCC (1997)	Price and Illness Adjusted AAPCC (1997)	Unadjusted Projected Surplus / Enrollee according to Minneapolis Benchmark (1997)	Price and Illness Adjusted Projected Surplus / Enrollee according to Minneapolis Benchmark (1997)	Unadjusted Projected Surplus / Region according to Minneapolis Benchmark (1997) in millions	Price and Illness Adjusted Projected Surplus / Region according to Minneapolis Benchmark (1997) in millions
Savannah	3.10	5,545	6,256	5,111	5,766	1,436	1,288	102	91
Hawaii									
Honolulu	2.29	4,458	4,089	4,443	4,076	349	-402	47	-54
Idaho									
Boise	2.74	3,855	4,411	4,192	4,796	-253	318	-18	22
Idaho Falls	3.48	3,957	4,705	4,223	5,022	-152	544	-3	9
Illinois									
Aurora	2.73	4,898	4,516	4,874	4,494	789	16	13	0
Blue Island	2.55	6,650	6,131	5,938	5,475	2,541	998	270	106
Chicago	4.21	6,711	6,188	6,314	5,822	2,603	1,344	696	360
Elgin	2.19	5,598	5,162	5,423	5,000	1,490	523	66	23
Evanston	2.49	6,563	6,051	6,303	5,811	2,455	1,334	296	161
Hinsdale	1.93	5,569	5,135	5,084	4,688	1,461	210	48	7
Joliet	3.10	5,748	5,636	5,309	5,205	1,640	728	81	36
Melrose Park	2.65	6,250	5,762	5,834	5,379	2,141	901	311	131
Peoria	3.16	4,396	5,072	4,287	4,947	287	469	27	45
Rockford	3.10	4,143	4,645	4,175	4,681	35	203	3	18
Springfield	2.98	4,377	5,147	4,281	5,034	268	557	35	72
Urbana	2.97	4,139	5,038	4,075	4,960	31	483	2	27
Bloomington	2.47	4,139	4,704	4,328	4,919	31	442	1	8
Indiana									
Evansville	3.17	4,642	5,350	4,596	5,297	534	819	53	81
Fort Wayne	2.86	4,108	4,609	4,284	4,806	0	328	0	32
Gary	4.22	5,982	6,333	5,215	5,521	1,873	1,043	108	60
Indianapolis	2.88	5,151	5,540	5,197	5,590	1,042	1,113	304	324
Lafayette	2.39	4,260	5,004	4,265	5,010	152	532	4	12
Muncie	2.82	4,689	5,513	4,639	5,454	580	977	13	22
Munster	4.02	6,479	6,715	5,723	5,932	2,371	1,454	99	61
South Bend	3.15	4,422	4,855	4,564	5,011	313	534	26	45
Terre Haute	3.06	4,827	5,572	4,759	5,494	718	1,017	20	28
Iowa									
Cedar Rapids	3.72	3,916	4,453	3,772	4,289	-192	-188	-7	-7
Davenport	3.05	4,394	5,026	4,381	5,011	286	533	20	37
Des Moines	3.26	4,115	4,839	4,051	4,763	7	286	1	40
Dubuque	3.00	3,896	4,446	3,760	4,291	-212	-187	-5	-4
Iowa City	2.97	3,995	4,831	3,965	4,795	-113	318	-5	13
Mason City	3.37	3,742	4,730	4,011	5,070	-366	593	-10	16
Sioux City	3.42	3,838	4,732	4,045	4,987	-270	510	-11	21
Waterloo	2.97	4,181	4,837	4,231	4,896	72	418	2	13
Kansas									
Topeka	2.86	4,375	5,138	4,530	5,321	266	843	15	47
Wichita	3.56	4,784	5,808	5,008	6,079	676	1,602	119	283
Kentucky									
Covington	2.51	5,274	5,419	5,067	5,207	1,165	729	43	27
Lexington	2.94	4,670	5,493	4,661	5,482	562	1,005	85	153
Louisville	3.03	5,359	5,946	5,269	5,846	1,251	1,368	237	259

Hospital Referral Region	Age, Sex and Illness Adjusted Acute Care Hospital Beds	AAPCC (1997)	Price Adjusted AAPCC (1997)	Illness Adjusted AAPCC (1997)	Price and Illness Adjusted AAPCC (1997)	Unadjusted Projected Surplus / Enrollee according to Minneapolis Benchmark (1997)	Price and Illness Adjusted Projected Surplus / Enrollee according to Minneapolis Benchmark (1997)	Unadjusted Projected Surplus / Region according to Minneapolis Benchmark (1997) in millions	Price and Illness Adjusted Projected Surplus / Region according to Minneapolis Benchmark (1997) in millions
Owensboro	2.98	4,559	5,443	4,735	5,653	450	1,176	8	21
Paducah	3.43	4,849	5,942	4,558	5,585	741	1,108	42	63
Louisiana									
Alexandria	3.83	5,378	6,448	5,061	6,068	1,270	1,590	43	54
Baton Rouge	2.93	6,576	7,377	6,259	7,021	2,468	2,544	177	183
Houma	3.11	6,444	7,574	5,696	6,694	2,335	2,217	54	51
Lafayette	4.03	5,368	6,309	5,225	6,141	1,260	1,663	74	98
Lake Charles	3.88	5,923	6,681	5,752	6,488	1,815	2,011	48	53
Metairie	3.38	7,591	7,971	7,254	7,617	3,483	3,140	165	149
Monroe	4.22	5,995	7,201	5,967	7,167	1,887	2,689	64	92
New Orleans	4.35	7,591	7,790	7,089	7,275	3,483	2,797	317	254
Shreveport	3.91	5,197	6,014	5,259	6,085	1,089	1,607	92	136
Slidell	3.08	7,143	7,874	6,610	7,286	3,035	2,808	49	45
Maine									
Bangor	2.66	4,058	4,581	4,210	4,754	-51	276	-3	15
Portland	2.76	4,371	4,653	4,606	4,903	263	425	34	55
Maryland									
Baltimore	2.47	6,729	6,375	6,394	6,057	2,621	1,580	731	440
Salisbury	2.98	4,911	5,248	5,010	5,354	803	877	42	46
Takoma Park	2.29	6,459	5,535	6,403	5,487	2,351	1,009	157	68
Massachusetts									
Boston	2.46	6,537	5,798	6,479	5,747	2,429	1,269	1,443	754
Springfield	2.89	5,130	5,060	5,305	5,233	1,022	755	105	78
Worcester	2.18	6,329	5,585	6,542	5,773	2,221	1,295	214	125
Michigan									
Ann Arbor	2.55	6,696	6,275	6,576	6,162	2,588	1,685	344	224
Dearborn	3.23	7,660	6,884	7,043	6,330	3,551	1,852	263	137
Detroit	3.46	7,237	6,504	6,631	5,959	3,129	1,482	731	346
Flint	3.36	7,094	6,720	6,830	6,470	2,986	1,992	173	116
Grand Rapids	2.48	4,519	4,718	4,807	5,019	410	541	46	61
Kalamazoo	3.04	4,893	5,116	4,925	5,150	785	672	61	52
Lansing	3.02	5,431	5,659	5,463	5,693	1,322	1,216	89	82
Marquette	3.56	4,754	5,349	4,843	5,450	645	972	21	32
Muskegon	2.88	4,482	4,639	4,908	5,080	374	602	13	21
Petoskey	2.93	4,620	5,198	4,507	5,072	512	594	13	15
Pontiac	2.61	7,229	6,497	7,013	6,303	3,120	1,825	114	67
Royal Oak	2.53	7,219	6,488	6,916	6,216	3,110	1,738	256	143
Saginaw	3.32	5,273	5,507	5,181	5,410	1,165	933	110	88
St Joseph	3.05	4,995	5,350	4,695	5,029	887	551	17	11
Traverse City	2.84	5,068	5,703	4,732	5,324	960	847	30	27
Minnesota									
Duluth	2.96	3,889	4,334	3,806	4,242	-219	-236	-12	-13
Minneapolis	2.67	4,108	4,403	4,178	4,478	0	0	0	0
Rochester	2.92	4,066	4,501	4,129	4,571	-43	94	-2	5
St Cloud	3.05	3,583	4,068	3,720	4,223	-525	-255	-13	-7
St Paul	2.54	4,677	4,596	4,928	4,843	569	365	54	35

Hospital Referral Region	Age, Sex and Illness Adjusted Acute Care Hospital Beds	AAPCC (1997)	Price Adjusted AAPCC (1997)	Illness Adjusted AAPCC (1997)	Price and Illness Adjusted AAPCC (1997)	Unadjusted Projected Surplus / Enrollee according to Minneapolis Benchmark (1997)	Price and Illness Adjusted Projected Surplus / Enrollee according to Minneapolis Benchmark (1997)	Unadjusted Projected Surplus / Region according to Minneapolis Benchmark (1997) in millions	Price and Illness Adjusted Projected Surplus / Region according to Minneapolis Benchmark (1997) in millions
Mississippi									
Gulfport	3.55	6,746	7,625	6,542	7,394	2,638	2,916	50	55
Hattiesburg	4.05	5,388	6,733	5,494	6,867	1,280	2,389	41	77
Jackson	4.11	4,904	5,817	4,947	5,867	796	1,389	95	166
Meridian	3.82	4,728	5,908	4,547	5,682	619	1,205	17	32
Oxford	3.89	4,604	5,753	4,348	5,433	495	956	9	16
Tupelo	3.67	4,378	5,465	4,560	5,691	270	1,214	12	55
Missouri									
Cape Girardeau	3.25	3,945	5,067	3,989	5,123	-163	646	-6	25
Columbia	3.02	4,859	6,095	4,796	6,016	751	1,538	67	137
Joplin	3.04	4,552	5,743	4,527	5,711	444	1,233	23	65
Kansas City	2.97	5,422	5,951	5,346	5,866	1,314	1,389	337	356
Springfield	3.16	4,334	5,340	4,551	5,609	225	1,131	24	122
St Louis	3.27	5,474	5,924	5,308	5,745	1,365	1,267	576	534
Montana									
Billings	3.36	4,092	4,867	4,181	4,973	-16	495	-1	31
Great Falls	3.56	4,561	5,527	4,357	5,280	453	802	9	16
Missoula	3.23	4,188	5,119	4,313	5,272	79	795	3	34
Nebraska									
Lincoln	3.85	3,405	4,327	3,610	4,588	-704	111	-56	9
Omaha	3.63	4,320	5,273	4,391	5,359	212	882	33	137
Nevada									
Las Vegas	2.41	6,059	5,845	5,753	5,549	1,951	1,072	231	127
Reno	3.50	5,015	5,053	5,373	5,414	906	937	57	59
New Hampshire									
Lebanon	3.36	4,315	4,669	4,713	5,100	207	622	11	34
Manchester	2.58	4,765	4,466	4,894	4,587	657	109	56	9
New Jersey									
Camden	2.93	6,183	5,564	5,941	5,346	2,075	868	757	317
Hackensack	3.48	6,199	5,038	6,088	4,948	2,091	470	337	76
Morristown	2.88	5,773	4,723	5,777	4,726	1,664	248	177	26
New Brunswick	2.92	6,125	5,049	6,274	5,172	2,017	694	201	69
Newark	4.93	6,350	5,201	6,049	4,954	2,241	477	398	85
Paterson	3.66	5,830	4,733	5,434	4,411	1,722	-66	72	-3
Ridgewood	3.07	6,165	5,071	6,113	5,028	2,057	550	92	25
New Mexico									
Albuquerque	3.22	4,183	4,686	4,834	5,416	74	938	10	130
New York									
Albany	3.26	4,708	4,668	4,662	4,623	600	145	145	35
Binghamton	2.83	4,337	4,563	4,511	4,745	229	267	13	15
Bronx	4.96	8,472	6,645	8,704	6,827	4,363	2,349	488	263
Buffalo	3.48	4,743	4,843	4,698	4,796	635	319	137	69
Elmira	3.44	4,199	4,559	4,206	4,566	91	88	5	5
East Long Island	3.34	7,240	5,614	7,130	5,529	3,132	1,051	1,695	569
New York	4.62	8,510	6,673	8,496	6,662	4,402	2,184	2,167	1,075
Rochester	2.99	4,653	4,633	4,787	4,766	545	289	86	45

Hospital Referral Region	Age, Sex and Illness Adjusted Acute Care Hospital Beds	AAPCC (1997)	Price Adjusted AAPCC (1997)	Illness Adjusted AAPCC (1997)	Price and Illness Adjusted AAPCC (1997)	Unadjusted Projected Surplus / Enrollee according to Minneapolis Benchmark (1997)	Price and Illness Adjusted Projected Surplus / Enrollee according to Minneapolis Benchmark (1997)	Unadjusted Projected Surplus / Region according to Minneapolis Benchmark (1997) in millions	Price and Illness Adjusted Projected Surplus / Region according to Minneapolis Benchmark (1997) in millions
Syracuse	3.17	4,282	4,437	4,317	4,474	174	-4	23	-1
White Plains	3.28	6,534	5,262	6,472	5,212	2,426	734	325	98
North Carolina									
Asheville	2.62	4,201	4,920	4,702	5,507	93	1,029	9	94
Charlotte	2.69	4,574	5,008	4,815	5,273	466	795	90	153
Durham	2.83	4,410	4,964	4,653	5,237	302	759	44	110
Greensboro	2.56	4,564	5,016	4,751	5,222	456	744	29	47
Greenville	2.72	4,550	5,428	4,511	5,381	442	903	37	76
Hickory	2.93	4,398	5,049	4,833	5,549	289	1,072	9	33
Raleigh	2.37	4,780	5,310	4,911	5,456	671	978	89	130
Wilmington	2.57	4,969	5,567	4,854	5,438	860	960	35	39
Winston-Salem	2.46	4,649	5,194	4,714	5,266	541	789	67	97
North Dakota									
Bismarck	4.97	4,221	5,245	4,239	5,269	112	791	4	25
Fargo Moorhead -Mn	3.08	3,693	4,461	3,787	4,574	-416	97	-30	7
Grand Forks	4.20	3,823	4,659	4,106	5,003	-285	525	-7	13
Minot	5.40	4,146	5,346	4,215	5,434	38	957	1	19
Ohio									
Akron	2.47	6,222	6,378	5,946	6,096	2,113	1,618	192	147
Canton	2.94	4,530	5,092	4,617	5,190	422	713	37	62
Cincinnati	2.70	5,503	5,729	5,362	5,582	1,395	1,104	258	204
Cleveland	3.07	6,244	6,244	6,086	6,085	2,136	1,608	647	487
Columbus	2.82	5,016	5,538	4,975	5,493	908	1,015	273	306
Dayton	3.19	5,041	5,433	5,106	5,503	933	1,026	132	145
Elyria	2.77	5,813	5,758	5,191	5,141	1,705	664	51	20
Kettering	2.75	5,278	5,503	5,394	5,624	1,170	1,147	55	54
Toledo	2.90	6,063	6,442	6,034	6,412	1,954	1,934	246	243
Youngstown	3.11	5,937	6,645	5,974	6,686	1,829	2,208	213	257
Oklahoma									
Lawton	4.07	4,415	5,258	4,598	5,475	307	998	7	24
Oklahoma City	3.25	4,770	5,490	4,807	5,533	662	1,055	138	220
Tulsa	3.00	4,825	5,540	5,121	5,879	717	1,402	110	216
Oregon									
Bend	3.09	4,066	4,703	4,111	4,755	-42	278	-1	6
Eugene	2.19	4,136	4,716	4,351	4,961	28	483	3	44
Medford	2.53	3,917	4,341	4,132	4,580	-191	103	-12	7
Portland	2.12	4,470	4,705	4,617	4,860	362	382	91	96
Salem	2.15	3,827	4,257	3,965	4,411	-281	-67	-10	-2
Pennsylvania									
Allentown	2.72	6,037	6,024	5,894	5,881	1,929	1,404	302	220
Altoona	2.86	5,551	6,388	5,561	6,399	1,443	1,921	69	92
Danville	2.78	4,930	5,504	5,064	5,654	822	1,176	65	93
Erie	2.96	4,996	5,659	4,920	5,573	887	1,096	101	124
Harrisburg	2.24	5,021	5,341	5,165	5,494	913	1,017	116	130
Johnstown	3.34	6,155	7,214	6,105	7,155	2,047	2,677	91	119
Lancaster	2.72	4,592	4,717	4,731	4,860	484	382	34	27

Hospital Referral Region	Age, Sex and Illness Adjusted Acute Care Hospital Beds	AAPCC (1997)	Price Adjusted AAPCC (1997)	Illness Adjusted AAPCC (1997)	Price and Illness Adjusted AAPCC (1997)	Unadjusted Projected Surplus / Enrollee according to Minneapolis Benchmark (1997)	Price and Illness Adjusted Projected Surplus / Enrollee according to Minneapolis Benchmark (1997)	Unadjusted Projected Surplus / Region according to Minneapolis Benchmark (1997) in millions	Price and Illness Adjusted Projected Surplus / Region according to Minneapolis Benchmark (1997) in millions
Philadelphia	3.00	7,327	6,644	7,192	6,522	3,219	2,044	1,754	1,114
Pittsburgh	2.98	6,644	6,935	6,336	6,613	2,536	2,136	1,334	1,123
Reading	2.76	5,207	5,408	5,124	5,322	1,098	844	95	73
Sayre	3.17	4,302	4,846	4,473	5,039	194	561	5	16
Scranton	2.58	5,713	6,267	5,327	5,843	1,605	1,366	93	79
Wilkes-Barre	2.67	5,757	6,271	5,479	5,968	1,649	1,490	81	73
York	2.23	4,489	4,821	4,495	4,828	380	350	19	17
Rhode Island									
Providence	2.37	5,539	5,128	5,477	5,071	1,430	594	233	97
South Carolina									
Charleston	3.34	5,096	5,663	5,017	5,576	988	1,099	80	89
Columbia	3.05	4,063	4,556	4,243	4,758	-45	280	-5	31
Florence	3.27	4,842	5,598	5,112	5,909	734	1,432	29	57
Greenville	2.72	4,139	4,594	4,370	4,851	31	373	3	33
Spartanburg	3.07	4,186	4,673	4,497	5,019	78	542	3	23
South Dakota									
Rapid City	4.22	3,783	4,774	4,256	5,371	-326	894	-7	20
Sioux Falls	3.85	3,671	4,681	3,667	4,676	-437	198	-51	23
Tennessee									
Chattanooga	2.82	6,024	6,613	5,967	6,550	1,916	2,072	144	156
Jackson	3.26	5,052	5,987	4,951	5,867	944	1,389	44	64
Johnson City	3.42	4,806	5,521	5,129	5,892	698	1,415	22	44
Kingsport	3.20	5,178	5,949	5,765	6,624	1,069	2,147	71	143
Knoxville	2.76	5,268	6,012	5,366	6,123	1,160	1,646	177	250
Memphis	3.61	5,158	5,855	4,937	5,604	1,050	1,126	194	208
Nashville	3.04	5,797	6,587	5,837	6,633	1,688	2,156	411	524
Texas									
Abilene	3.04	4,982	5,992	5,025	6,044	874	1,566	39	70
Amarillo	5.01	4,898	5,639	5,720	6,585	790	2,107	42	111
Austin	2.05	4,763	4,993	5,005	5,245	655	768	53	62
Beaumont	3.84	6,900	7,456	6,143	6,638	2,792	2,161	167	129
Bryan	2.26	4,495	5,379	4,477	5,357	387	879	7	17
Corpus Christi	3.14	5,784	6,471	5,621	6,288	1,676	1,810	94	101
Dallas	2.95	5,784	5,948	5,930	6,098	1,675	1,621	495	479
El Paso	3.23	4,915	5,589	5,290	6,015	807	1,537	66	126
Fort Worth	2.59	5,762	6,118	6,091	6,467	1,654	1,989	233	281
Harlingen	2.73	4,667	5,594	4,750	5,693	559	1,215	23	50
Houston	3.48	6,688	6,734	6,726	6,772	2,580	2,295	959	853
Longview	2.61	4,698	5,376	4,737	5,421	590	943	14	22
Lubbock	4.43	5,747	6,839	6,060	7,211	1,639	2,734	126	210
Mcallen	2.52	4,564	5,427	4,793	5,699	456	1,221	16	42
Odessa	4.01	5,088	5,611	5,686	6,270	980	1,792	32	58
San Angelo	4.24	4,245	5,205	4,585	5,622	137	1,145	3	24
San Antonio	3.09	5,111	5,732	5,314	5,960	1,003	1,482	211	312
Temple	2.40	4,358	4,950	4,553	5,171	250	694	8	22
Tyler	3.17	5,233	6,101	5,215	6,080	1,124	1,602	78	111

Hospital Referral Region	Age, Sex and Illness Adjusted Acute Care Hospital Beds	AAPCC (1997)	Price Adjusted AAPCC (1997)	Illness Adjusted AAPCC (1997)	Price and Illness Adjusted AAPCC (1997)	Unadjusted Projected Surplus / Enrollee according to Minneapolis Benchmark (1997)	Price and Illness Adjusted Projected Surplus / Enrollee according to Minneapolis Benchmark (1997)	Unadjusted Projected Surplus / Minneapolis Region according to Minneapolis Benchmark (1997) in millions	Price and Illness Adjusted Projected Surplus Region according to Minneapolis Benchmark (1997) in millions
Victoria	3.48	5,181	5,847	4,916	5,549	1,072	1,071	21	21
Waco	2.86	3,656	4,292	3,865	4,538	-453	60	-19	3
Wichita Falls	3.00	4,611	5,599	4,689	5,694	503	1,216	15	35
Utah									
Ogden	3.01	4,228	4,614	4,691	5,119	120	641	3	18
Provo	2.67	4,387	5,170	4,797	5,653	279	1,175	7	31
Salt Lake City	3.22	4,361	4,872	4,833	5,399	253	921	35	126
Vermont									
Burlington	2.74	4,286	4,614	4,471	4,814	178	336	12	23
Virginia									
Arlington	2.07	5,023	4,304	5,319	4,558	915	80	99	9
Charlottesville	2.44	4,515	4,896	4,830	5,237	407	759	24	44
Lynchburg	2.82	3,651	4,039	3,834	4,242	-458	-235	-14	-7
Newport News	2.69	4,675	4,915	4,718	4,961	567	483	29	24
Norfolk	2.85	5,073	5,450	5,123	5,504	965	1,027	109	116
Richmond	2.84	5,072	5,049	5,002	4,980	964	502	150	78
Roanoke	3.10	4,738	5,397	4,860	5,535	630	1,058	60	101
Winchester	2.34	4,370	4,522	4,338	4,489	262	12	10	0
Washington									
Everett	1.68	4,735	4,845	4,749	4,859	627	381	34	21
Olympia	2.66	4,801	5,105	5,170	5,498	693	1,020	27	40
Seattle	2.08	4,934	4,902	5,125	5,092	825	614	207	154
Spokane	2.99	4,519	4,980	4,866	5,363	410	885	62	133
Tacoma	2.09	4,772	4,916	5,084	5,238	663	761	42	48
Yakima	2.32	4,231	4,654	4,209	4,631	122	153	4	4
West Virginia									
Charleston	2.91	5,312	6,171	5,123	5,952	1,204	1,474	153	188
Huntington	3.04	4,872	5,568	4,714	5,387	764	910	38	46
Morgantown	2.59	5,243	6,321	5,281	6,367	1,135	1,889	65	108
Wisconsin									
Appleton	2.81	3,651	4,123	3,669	4,144	-458	-334	-18	-13
Green Bay	2.66	3,709	4,207	3,680	4,174	-399	-303	-26	-20
La Crosse	3.08	3,424	4,021	3,426	4,022	-684	-456	-33	-22
Madison	2.79	4,185	4,653	4,192	4,660	77	183	9	21
Marshfield	3.48	3,886	4,567	4,177	4,909	-222	431	-12	23
Milwaukee	3.04	4,825	4,935	4,667	4,772	717	295	207	85
Neenah	2.80	3,949	4,447	3,674	4,137	-159	-341	-5	-10
Wausau	2.75	3,950	4,579	3,757	4,356	-159	-121	-4	-3
Wyoming									
Casper	4.31	4,648	5,335	4,840	5,555	540	1,077	12	24

Appendices

Appendix on Methods

1. The Geography of Health Care in The United States

1.1 Files Used in the Atlas

The Atlas depends on the integrated use of databases provided by the American Hospital Association (AHA), the American Medical Association, the American Osteopathic Association, and several federal agencies, including the Agency for Health Care Policy and Research, the Bureau of the Census, the Health Care Financing Administration, the National Center for Health Statistics, and the Department of Veterans Affairs. Table 1 lists these files and provides a short description of the uses made of them in the Atlas.

TABLE 1.

Data Files Used in Analysis

File	Year Used (Sample)	Source / Provider	Description and Use in Analyses
Medicare Files			
Denominator File	1994 & 1995 (100%)	HCFA	Contains one record for each Medicare beneficiary, and includes demographic information (age, sex, race), residence (ZIP Code), program eligibility and mortality. Used to determine denominators for utilization rates and to determine mortality.
MEDPAR File	1994 & 1995 (100%)	HCFA	One record for each hospital stay by Medicare beneficiaries. Includes data on dates of admission / discharge, diagnoses, procedures and Medicare reimbursements to the hospital. Used for (1) allocation of acute care resources and physicians and (2) numerators for utilization rates.
Continuous Medicare History Sample File	1995 (5%)	HCFA	Includes a record for each beneficiary in a 5% sample for each year. Includes summary expenditure data. Used to estimate Medicare spending by program component.
Medicare Provider of Services File	1995	HCFA	Includes a record for each hospital eligible to provide inpatient care through Medicare. Includes location and resource data. Used in measuring acute care resource investments.
Medicare Cost Reports	1994	HCFA	Includes a record for each hospital and provides detailed accounting data for the specified year. Used in measuring acute care resource investments.

TABLE 1. (CONTINUED)

File	Year Used	Source/Provider	Description and Use in Analyses
Resource Files			
American Hospital Association Annual Survey of Hospitals	1995	American Hospital Association	Includes a record for each hospital registered with the AHA. Used in measuring acute care resources (beds, personnel).
Physician File	1995	American Medical Association	Includes one record for each allopathic physician with practice ZIP Code, self-designated specialty, major professional activities, and federal / non-federal status. Used to determine specialty-specific counts of physicians in each health care market.
Osteopath File	1995	American Osteopathic Association	Includes one record for each osteopathic physician with practice ZIP Code, self-designated specialty, major professional activities, and federal / non-federal status. Used to determine specialty-specific counts of physicians in each health care market.
Federal hospital utilization and resources	1993-1994	U.S. Medicine Directory 1993-94 ISSN 0890-6637	Provides location, counts and occupancy rates of federal hospital beds.
VA patient travel pattern file	1989	VA Outcomes Group, White River Jct VA	ZIP Code level patient origin file for veterans using VA hospitals in 1989. Used to allocate VA physicians to appropriate HSAs.
Other Files			
Geographic Practice Cost Index	1993	HCFA	Records for each MSA and non-MSA area of each state. Records include area-level values for each of the components of the GPCI (physician work, practice cost, malpractice) and summary index value. Used for price adjustment.
National Hospital Discharge Survey	1989	NTIS	Provides age-sex specific hospital discharge rates for the U.S. as a whole, which were used as the basis for the age-sex adjustment of acute care resources.
National Ambulatory Medical Care Survey (NAMCS)	1989-1994	NTIS	Ambulatory services from samples of patient records selected from a national sample of office-based physicians. Allows estimation of age-sex specific use rates by specialty. Used for age-sex adjustment of physician workforce.
Population files	1995	Claritas, Inc., Arlington, VA	1990 STF3 data from the U.S. Bureau of the Census was adapted by Claritas, Inc. to 1995 ZIP Code geography; includes 1995 age-sex specific estimated counts of residents in the ZIP Code. Used (1) for age-sex adjustment, (2) as denominator for rates of allocated and adjusted resources.
ZIP Code boundary files	1995	Geographic Data Technology, Lebanon, NH	Includes records for each ZIP Code with the coordinates of the boundary precisely specified. Used as basis for mapping HSAs and HRRs and for assigning ZIP Codes appropriately.

1.2 Defining Hospital Service Areas

Hospital Service Areas (HSAs) represent local health care markets for community-based inpatient care. The definitions of HSAs used in the 1996 edition of the Atlas were retained in the 1998 edition. HSAs were originally defined in three steps using 1993 provider files and 1992-93 utilization data. First, all acute care hospitals in the 50 states and the District of Columbia were identified from the American Hospital

Association Annual Survey of Hospitals and the Medicare Provider of Services files and assigned to a location within a town or city. The list of towns or cities with at least one acute care hospital (N=3,953) defined the maximum number of possible HSAs. Second, all 1992 and 1993 acute care hospitalizations of the Medicare population were analyzed according to ZIP Code to determine the proportion of residents' hospital stays that occurred in each of the 3,953 candidate HSAs. ZIP Codes were initially assigned to the HSA where the greatest proportion (plurality) of residents were hospitalized. Approximately 500 of the candidate HSAs did not qualify as independent HSAs because the plurality of patients resident in those HSAs were hospitalized in other HSAs.

The third step required visual examination of the ZIP Codes used to define each HSA. Maps of ZIP Code boundaries were made using files obtained from Geographic Data Technologies (GDT) and each HSA's component ZIP Codes were examined. In order to achieve contiguity of the component ZIP Codes for each HSA, "island" ZIP Codes were reassigned to the enclosing HSA, and/or HSAs were grouped into larger HSAs (See the Appendix on the Geography of Health Care in the United States for an illustration). Certain ZIP Codes used in the Medicare files were restricted in their use to specific institutions (e.g., nursing homes) or post offices. These "point ZIPs" were assigned to their enclosing ZIP Code based on the ZIP Code boundary map.

This process resulted in the identification of 3,436 HSAs, ranging in total 1995 population from 627 (Turtle Lake, North Dakota) to 2,949,506 (Houston) in the 1998 edition of the Atlas. Thus, the HSA boundaries remained the same but the HSA populations might have changed between the two editions of the Atlas. In most HSAs, the majority of Medicare hospitalizations occurred in a hospital or hospitals located within the HSA. See the Appendix on the Geography of Health Care in the United States for further details.

1.3 Defining Hospital Referral Regions

Hospital referral regions (HRRs) represent health care markets for tertiary medical care. As defined in the 1996 Atlas, each HRR contained at least one HSA that had a hospital or hospitals that performed major cardiovascular procedures and neuro-surgery in 1992-93. Three steps were taken to define HRRs.

First, the candidate hospitals and HRRs were identified. A total of 862 hospitals performed at least 10 major cardiovascular procedures (DRGs 103-107) on Medicare enrollees in both years. These hospitals were located within 458 HSAs, thereby defining the maximum number of possible HRRs. Further checks verified that all 458 HSAs included at least one hospital performing the specified major neurosurgical procedures (DRGs 1-3 and 484).

Second, we calculated in each of the 3,436 HSAs in the United States the proportion of major cardiovascular procedures performed in each of the 458 candidate HRRs in 1992-93. Each HSA was then assigned provisionally to the candidate HRR where most patients went for these services.

Third, HSAs were reassigned or further grouped to achieve (a) geographic contiguity, unless major travel routes (e.g., interstate highways) justified separation (this occurred in only two cases, the New Haven, Connecticut, and Elmira, New York, HRRs); (b) a minimum population size of 120,000; and (c) a high localization index. Because of the large number of hospitals providing cardiovascular services in California, several candidate California HRRs met the above criteria but were found to perform small numbers of cardiovascular procedures. These HRRs were further aggregated according to county boundaries to achieve stability of cardiovascular surgery rates within the areas.

The process resulted in the definition of 306 hospital referral regions which ranged in total 1995 population from 124,656 (Minot, North Dakota) to 9,230,785 (Los Angeles) in the 1998 edition of the Atlas. See the Appendix on the Geography of Health Care in The United States for further details.

1.4 Populations of HSAs and HRRs
Total population counts were estimated for residents of all ages in each HSA using 1995 ZIP Code level files obtained from Claritas, Inc. The Claritas file is based on

the latest U.S. Census STF3B ZIP Code file, updated to account for changes in ZIP Code definitions. Population counts for HRRs are the sum of the counts of the constituent HSAs. These serve as denominators for estimating rates for hospital resource and physician workforce allocations (Chapter Two and the Appendix on the Physician Workforce in the United States).

For rates that apply to the Medicare population for the years 1994-95, enrollee counts were obtained from the Medicare Denominator file. The 1994 and 1995 Medicare enrollee population included those alive and age 65 to age 99 on June 30, 1994 and 1995, respectively, and were summed to give person-years. For Medicare reimbursement rates, the enrollee counts are based on a 5% sample of 1995 enrollees (selected on the basis of Social Security numbers) who were enrolled in both Part A and Part B of the Medicare program. For all rates presented in the Atlas, the numerator and the denominator counts exclude those who were enrolled in risk bearing HMOs on June 30.

2. Variations in Hospital Resources

Acute care hospital resources consist of hospital beds and personnel. Three tasks were required to estimate the rates presented in Chapter Two. First, the resources for each hospital were determined; second, resources were allocated to populations, proportionate to their rates of use; third, rates were computed and adjusted to take into account differences in age and sex among regions.

2.1 Measuring Hospital Resources

Hospitals were eligible for inclusion if they were located within the 50 states or the District of Columbia and were classified either by Medicare or the AHA as short term general medical and surgical hospitals (AHA service code = 10), specialty hospitals listed as obstetrics and gynecology (code 44), eye, ear, nose and throat (code 45), orthopedic (code 47), or other specialty (code 49); and children's hospitals (codes 50, 59). For inclusion in this study, hospitals must have been open on June 30, 1995. Certain specialty hospitals were excluded if additional information gathered from external sources (e.g., telephone calls) indicated they did not meet the inclusion criteria, or if they fell into the following categories: Shriners' hospitals, crippled children's hospitals, hospital units of institutions (prisons, colleges, etc.), institutions for mental retardation, psychiatric facilities, rehabilitation or chronic disease facilities, addiction treatment facilities, communication disorders facilities, podiatry facilities, small surgery centers, obstetrics and gynecology clinics, and hospices. Department of Veterans' Affairs hospitals were excluded from this edition of the Atlas because of the non-comparability of expenditure and personnel data.

The American Hospital Association Annual Survey file and the Medicare Provider file were searched to identify all non-federal hospitals (AHA control code = 12-33) and federal PHS Indian Service hospitals (control code = 47) that met the criteria for inclusion. Short term general hospitals (N= 5,004), children's hospitals (N=47), and specialty hospitals (N=56) located in the 50 states or the District of Columbia as of June 30, 1995 were identified.

The resources for each hospital were determined as follows:

Hospital beds were ascertained primarily from the AHA file. The field selected was "hospital beds (including cribs, pediatric and neonatal bassinets) that were set up and staffed at the end of the reporting period." Our measure of intensive care beds included both "medical/surgical intensive care" and "cardiac intensive care" beds. For the 60 hospitals completely lacking AHA data, and for 607 of the 635 hospitals that were non-reporting in 1995, we used data from the Medicare Cost Reports for "total beds available in the hospital" and "intensive care" plus "coronary care beds" as the measure of intensive care beds. The remaining 28 non-reporting hospitals (all PHS Indian Service hospitals) also lacked cost report data, so AHA data were used to measure all resources, even though the data came from a prior year's Annual Survey.

Full time equivalent hospital personnel were defined as the sum of full time employees and 1/2 of the part time employees. Hospital employees do not include medical or dental interns or residents or trainees. For the 60 hospitals lacking AHA data completely and for 607 of the 635 hospitals that were non-reporting in 1995, the Medicare Cost Report value for "average number of employees, hospital total" was used to estimate hospital personnel at these hospitals.

Full time equivalent registered nurses were defined as the sum of full time nurses and 1/2 of the part time nurses. For the 60 hospitals lacking AHA data completely and for 607 of the 635 hospitals that were non-reporting for 1995, the Medicare Provider of Services file count of "licensed registered nurses" was used to estimate the number of registered nurses at these hospitals.

2.2 Allocation of Hospital Resources

In order to account for the use of care by patients who live in one HSA but obtain care in another, hospital resources for acute care short-term hospitals have been allocated to the HSAs in proportion to the actual patterns of use. This was accomplished using the proportion of all Medicare patient days (1994-95) provided by each specific hospital to each HSA. For example, if 60% of total Medicare inpatient days at a hospital were used by residents of the HSA where the hospital was located, then 60% of that hospital's resources would be assigned to its HSA. If 20% of the Medicare patient days provided by that hospital were used by a neighboring HSA, 20% of the hospital's resources would be assigned to that neighboring HSA.

Children's hospitals and specialty hospitals were found to have too little actual utilization data in the Medicare files to allow their allocation based on hospital-specific proportionate utilization. These hospitals were allocated according to the utilization patterns of all Medicare enrollees residing in the HSA. In other words, if 80% of the patient days in an HSA were provided by hospitals within the HSA, then 80% of the resources of any specialty or children's hospital located within that HSA would be assigned to it.

The use of Medicare data to estimate resources allocated to populations of all ages is justified by studies which show that the geographic patterns of use of hospital care by patients under and over sixty-five years of age are similar. Our own analyses of data from both New York and New England revealed that travel patterns for those under age 65 are nearly identical to those over age 65. Radany and Luft (1993) found similar results in California.

Once each of the hospital resources had been allocated to HSAs, the allocated resources were summed. For example, the allocated beds of each HSA were equal to the sum of allocated acute short-term beds and allocated specialty/children's beds. For the HSAs located in a given HRR, resources were further summed to obtain the total for the HRR. Crude rates were then calculated for HRRs using the 1995 population for all ages described in Section 1.4.

2.3 Calculation of Adjusted Per Capita Hospital Resource Rates

The resource allocation rates presented in Chapter Two of the Atlas were adjusted for differences in age and sex using the indirect method and the 1995 U.S. population as the standard (Breslow and Day, 1987). Since indirectly standardized rates cannot be "rolled up" from HSAs to HRRs, we computed observed and expected counts at the HSA level and summed these to the HRR levels. The expected counts within HSAs are weighted averages of the stratum-specific crude rates in the standard population. These observed and expected counts were then used to compute HRR-level indirectly standardized rates.

Since the national age-sex specific bed supply rates are not available, these were estimated using the national age and sex specific patient day rates obtained from the 1989 National Hospital Discharge Survey. These estimates were used to calculate the expected bed supply in each HRR. Under the assumption that employee allocations across age and sex groups are also proportionate to patient days, a similar strategy was used to adjust employees.

3. Medicare Program Reimbursement Rates

The numerators for Medicare reimbursement rates are from the 1995 Continuous Medicare History Sample (CMHS), which documents reimbursements by calendar year for each component of the Medicare program. The data are for a 5% sample of Medicare enrollees selected on the basis of the terminal digits in the Social Security number. The denominator for rates is the corresponding 5% sample of the enrollment file (see Section 1.4).

3.1 Categories of Medicare Reimbursement Examined in Chapter Two

Categories of Medicare reimbursement in the Atlas are listed in Table 2 with their definitions from the CMHS file.

TABLE 2.

Definitions for Categories of Reimbursement

Category of Reimbursement	For each service, the specified components were selected from the file and summed as indicated. All fields refer to packed-decimal, variable length, EBCDIC, mainframe record layout locations.
All Services	File: Annual Data trailer Part A Reimb, incl. passthru amts. cols. 14-17 Part B Reimb, incl. passthru amts. cols. 18-21 Total Reimb. = Part A + Part B Reimb.
Professional and Laboratory Services	File: Payment trailer 1. Total Reimb., cols. 9-11 2. Medical line items, cols. 12-13 (TOS=1, 3, Y, Z) 3. Medical Reimb., cols. 17-19 4. Surgical line items, cols. 20-21 (TOS=2, 8) 5. Surgical Reimb., cols. 25-27 6. Lab/X-ray line items, cols. 28-29 (TOS=4, 5) 7. Lab/X-ray Reimb., cols. 33-35 Professional and Lab. reimb. = 3+5+7
Acute Care Hospital Services	File: Short Stay trailer Stays, cols. 4-5 LOS, cols. 8-9 Reimbursement, cols.18-21 Passthrough amount, cols. 62-65
Outpatient Hospital Services	Outpatient trailer Total bills, cols. 4-5 Total Reimb., cols. 9-11 Outpatient POS bills, cols. 12-13 Outpatient POS Reimb., cols. 17-19 Inpatient POS bills, cols. 20-21 Inpatient POS bills, cols. 25-27 Total Reimb. = Outpatient POS Reimb. + Inpatient POS Reimb.
Home Health Care Services	HHA trailer Part A Reimb., cols. 9-11 Part B Reimb., cols. 17-19 Total Reimb. = Part A + Part B

3.2 Calculation of Adjusted Medicare Program Reimbursement Rates

Rates were adjusted using the indirect method for the following strata: sex, race (black, non-black) and age (65-69, 70-74, 75-79, 80-84, 85-99), with the 1995 Medicare population as the standard, as described in Section 2.3.

Medicare program rates were further adjusted to account for regional differences in price. Two different price adjustors were used, depending on the category of Medicare spending: the Dartmouth Price Index and the HCFA Part B Index, both of which are based on the Geographic Practice Cost Index (GPCI) developed by Pope, Welch, Zuckerman, and Henderson (1989). These price indexes are described below.

The Dartmouth (Modified GPCI) Price Index. Seeking to avoid a price adjustment that depended on physician or hospital market conditions, we focused on cost of living indices using non-medical regional price measures. We relied on the Geographic Practice Cost Index (GPCI), which uses the weighted sum of three components: the relative cost of non-physician professional labor across areas, the relative cost of physician practice inputs (principally rents and wages to office employees) and the relative cost of malpractice. The weights are based on the national proportions of these costs in physician services. We re-weighted the index, excluding the malpractice costs. We also used the full professional labor component in our revised index (HCFA used only one-quarter of the professional labor component). While not perfectly exogenous to health care (as it includes physician office expenses), this modified GPCI index is available at the level of geographic analysis needed in this study, and is preferable to the major alternative, Medicare's hospital wage index. (The hospital wage index is based on actual wages paid to hospital employees in each area and is thus distorted by differences in occupational mix and market conditions. Hospitals that hire more highly paid staff have those costs reflected in the wage index.) The Dartmouth index was available for each metropolitan statistical area (MSA) and for non-MSA areas of each state. The values for the area-specific modified GPCI were assigned to each HSA according to the location of the principal city or town of each HSA.

HCFA Part B Index. Because Medicare Part B payments compensate for only one-quarter of the difference in professional wage adjustments across areas and include an adjustment for malpractice insurance costs, these adjustments were made in reverse to recover the original value of the Part B billings.

For both indexes, HRR-level modified GPCIs were calculated as weighted sums of the HSA-specific indexes, using the number of Medicare enrollees in the HSA as the weight. The Dartmouth Price Index was used to adjust all components of Medicare expenditures except professional and laboratory services. This latter component was adjusted using the HCFA Part B regional price measure.

To implement the adjustment, each component of the Medicare program was first age sex and race adjusted at the HSA level. Observed and expected dollars were then summed to the HRR level and indirectly standardized rates were computed. HRR-specific Medicare expenditures were then divided by the index for that HRR to adjust for regional differences in price. Total noncapitated Medicare reimbursement rates were computed as the sum of the component rates.

3.3 Precision of the Medicare Reimbursement Rates

The precision of the HRR-specific Medicare reimbursement rates varies according to the population of the HRR but, in general, these rates are precisely determined. For all HRRs with at least 12,000 Medicare enrollees, the width of the approximate 95% confidence interval for the reimbursement rate is +/- 20% of the corresponding national rate. For HRRs with a minimum Medicare population of 48,000 enrollees, it is +/- 10% of the national average.

4. Physician Workforce Rates

The methods for allocating and estimating the per capita rates of physicians serving HSAs and HRRs are analogous to the methods used for estimating and allocating hospital resources described in Sections 2.2 and 2.3. The sources of information on physicians are the American Medical Association (AMA; January 1, 1996) and the American Osteopathic Association (AOA; June 1, 1996) Physician Masterfiles. These files have been used extensively to study physician supply and are the only comprehensive data available on physician location, specialty and level of effort devoted to clinical practice. Both the AMA and the AOA physician files classify physicians according to self-reported level of effort devoted to clinical practice. In this study, we excluded physicians who reported that they worked the majority of the time in medical teaching, administration or research, and part time physicians working fewer than 20 hours a week in clinical practice. Both files also list ZIP Code fields indicating the physician's primary place of practice, which was complete in more than 90% of records. When this information was not available, we used the physician's preferred professional address to indicate location. Based on these criteria, 495,510 physicians resident in the 50 states and District of Columbia constituted the clinically active physician workforce for 1996. There were also 99,972 physicians in residency or fellowship programs. See the Appendix on the Physician Workforce in the United States for more details.

4.1 Physician Specialties Considered in Chapter Two and the Appendix on the Physician Workforce in the United States of the Atlas

The AMA and AOA physician files include the physician's primary self-designated specialty from a list of 243 specialties. We grouped these into the categories in Table 3.

TABLE 3.

Categories of Clinically Active Physicians

Classification of physician specialties and type of utilization used for allocation and age adjustment

Dartmouth Specialty	AMA or AOA Specialty	AMA/AOA Code	Allocation	Age Adjustment
All Physicians	All except Unspecified (Codes US, T)			
Primary Physicians	Adolescent Medicine-GP	AGP	Medical	Family Practice
	Family Practice	FP		
	Geriatrics Medicine (Family Practice)	FPG		
		FSM		
	General Practice	GP		
	Sports Medicine-GP	SGP		
	Internal Medicine-Emergency Medicine	IEM	Medical	Internal Medicine
	Internal Medicine	IM		
	Internal Medicine-Pediatrics	IPD		
	Pediatrics	PD	Medical	Pediatrics
Specialty Physicians	All except Primary Physicians and Unspecified (Codes US, T)			
Anesthesiology	Anesthesiology	AN	Surgical	Surgery
	Cardiothoracic Anesthesiology	CAN		
	Obstetrics Anesthesiology	OBA		
	Pediatric Anesthesiology	PAN		
Cardiology	Cardiology	C	Medical	Cardiology
	Cardiovascular Diseases	CD		
		CVD		
	Cardiac Electrophysiology	ICE		
General Surgery	Abdominal Surgery	AS	Surgical	General Surgery
	Colon and Rectal Surgery	CRS		
	General Surgery	GS		
	Surgery-General	S		
Obstetrics/ Gynecology	Gynecological Oncology	GO	Surgical	Ob/Gyn
	Gynecological Surgery	GS		
	Gynecology	GYN		
	Maternal & Fetal Medicine	MFM		
	Obstetrics & Gynecology	OBG		
	Obstetrics	OBS		
	Obstetrics/Gynecology Surgery	OGS		
	Reproductive Endocrinology	RE		
	Reproductive Endocrinology	REN		
Ophthalmology	Ophthalmology	OPH	Surgical	Ophthalmology

TABLE 3. (CONTINUED)

Dartmouth Specialty	AMA or AOA Specialty	AMA/AOA Code	Allocation
Orthopedic Surgery	Hand Surgery (Ortho Surgery)	HSO	Surgical
	Adult Reconstructive Orthopedics	OAR	
	Pediatric Orthopedics	OP	
	Orthopedics	OR	
	Orthopedic Surgery	ORS	
	Sports Medicine (Orthopedic Surgery)	OSM	
	Orthopedic Surgery - Spine	OSS	
	Orthopedic Trauma	OTR	
Psychiatry	Child Psychiatry	CHP	Medical
	Psychiatry	P	
	Pediatric Psychiatry	PDP	
	Psychoanalysis	PYA	
	Geriatric Psychiatry	PYG	
	Psychosomatic Medicine	PYM	
Radiology	Angiography/Interventional Radiology	ANG	All
	Diagnostic Radiology	DR	
	Diagnostic Ultrasound	DUS	
	Nuclear Medicine	NM	
	Nuclear Radiology	NR	
	Neuroradiology	NRA	
	Pediatric Radiology	PDR	
	Radiology	R	
	Diagnostic Roentgenology	RTD	
Urology	Urological Surgery	U	Surgical
	Urology	URS	

4.2 Allocation of Clinically Active Physicians

Clinically active physicians were assigned to the HSA of their primary place of practice or preferred professional address. Since physicians, like hospitals, provide services to patients residing outside of the HSA in which their practices are located, the physician workforce was allocated to adjust for patient migration. Unfortunately, allocations could not be based on information about the travel patterns of the patients of individual physicians or information about the use of care outside acute hospitals. For clinically active non-federal physicians (N = 480,761), the adjustments are closely analogous to the method used for hospital resources, with an important exception. Since the hospital affiliations of the physicians were not determined, the physicians were allocated on the basis of the patterns of inpatient care of all the hospitals located in their HSAs. The 1994-95 MEDPAR records selected for allocation, which depended on the physician's specialty, are given in Table 3. For example, primary physicians were allocated on the basis of medical DRGs. If an HSA had 4 primary care physicians and if 25% of the medical DRG patient days at the local hospital(s) in 1994-95 were for residents of a neighboring HSA, then the four primary physicians would be estimated to contribute 1.0 FTE primary care physician to the neighboring HSA.

We included clinically active federal physicians (N = 14,749) in the study, since these physicians serve populations counted by the U.S. census, such as veterans, residents of Indian reservations, medically underserved areas, and military personnel and their dependents. Federal physicians were assigned to either the Department of Defense/Public Health Service (DoD/PHS) or the Department of Veterans Affairs (VA) in proportion to the mix of staffed federal beds within each HSA (U.S. Medicine; DoD technical document). All federal pediatricians and obstetrician/gynecologists were assigned to the DoD/ PHS. DoD/PHS physicians were allocated to HSAs in the same proportion as the non-federal physicians. Since VA utilization data were available that were analogous to the Medicare Part A data, VA physicians were allocated to areas in proportion to VA inpatient utilization (e.g., if 25% of the patient days of VA hospitals in Manhattan were provided to veterans residing in the Bronx, then 25% of the VA physicians in New York were assigned to the Bronx). If no federal inpatient facility (DoD, VAH, PHS, Indian Health Service) was present within the HSA, then the physicians were assumed to represent primary care and were allocated in the same proportion as non-federal primary care physicians (using inpatient medical days).

When all physician specialty groups had been allocated to HSAs, their allocated FTEs were summed. The physicians allocated to an HSA represent the total of all federal and non-federal FTE physicians allocated from local as well as remote HSAs. For the HSAs in a given HRR, physician resources were further summed to obtain the total for the HRR. Crude rates were then calculated for HRRs using the 1995 population for all ages described in Section 1.4. Measures of physicians in residency training programs used in the Atlas were prepared separately using similar methods.

4.3 Calculation of Adjusted Rates

The allocated rates presented in Chapter Two and the Appendix on the Physician Workforce in the United States were adjusted for age and sex using the indirect method, as described in Section 2.3, using the 1995 U.S. population as the standard. As with hospital bed supply rates, the national age-sex specific physician workforce rates are not known. These were estimated using outpatient age, sex and specialty-specific physician visit rates from the combined 1989-1994 National Ambulatory Care Survey (NAMCS). These estimates were used to calculate the expected physician supply in each HSA, by specialty. Specialties that had too few visits to reliably estimate age-sex-specific visit rates (< 800 total NAMCS) used the visit rates of allied specialties, as indicated in Table 3. Four NAMCS specialty categories could not be age and sex adjusted because of the low frequency of ambulatory visits and the lack of allied specialties: pathology, radiology, critical care and "unspecified." Expected counts of resident physicians were prepared separately using similar methods. The expected counts were summed to the HRR level and were used to calculate indirectly standardized rates. Rates for combined generalists, combined specialists and combined total physicians were obtained by first summing expected counts of the component specialties to the HRR level.

5. The Distribution Graph

The distribution graphs used in the Atlas provide a simple way to show the dispersion in particular rates of health care resources and utilization across the 306 hospital referral regions. For example, Figure 2.2 shows the distribution of hospital employees per thousand residents for each of the 306 hospital referral regions. The vertical axis shows the rate of hospital employees per thousand residents. The Bronx, which has 27.6 employees per thousand residents, is represented by the highest point on the graph. Chicago, which has 21.8, and Manhattan, which has 21.6 employees per thousand residents, are represented by the two next lowest points on the graph. Some areas which do not have exactly the same number of hospital employees per thousand residents are arrayed on a single line because their rates fall into a "bin" between two values.

This chart summarizes two features of the data. The first is a measure of dispersion; if the number of employees per thousand (or whatever measure is on the vertical axis) for the highest hospital referral region is two or three times higher than the number of employees per thousand for the lowest hospital referral region, it suggests substantial variation in health care resources. Second, the distribution graph shows whether the variation is caused by just a few outliers — hospital referral regions that for various reasons are very different from the rest of the country — or whether the variation is pervasive and widespread across the country. In the example above, there is widespread dispersion across the country, but one area, the Bronx, does stand apart from all other areas.

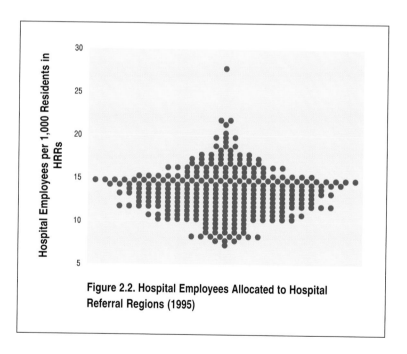

Figure 2.2. Hospital Employees Allocated to Hospital Referral Regions (1995)

6. Medicare Hospitalization Rates

Hospitalization rates represent counts of the number of discharges that occurred in a defined time period (the numerator) for a specific population (the denominator). The counts of discharges for specific conditions are based on the MEDPAR files for 1994-95. The denominator is the 1994-95 Medicare enrollee population (Section 1.4). In order to ensure that the events counted in the numerator correspond to the denominator population, certain records were excluded, including Medicare enrollees who were under age 65 or over age 99 on June 30, 1994 or 1995; Medicare enrollees who were enrolled in risk-bearing HMOs; MEDPAR records with a length of stay over 365 days; hospitalizations in psychiatric, rehabilitation or long term care units (provider codes = S, T, U or V; facility type not equal to S; third digit of Medicare provider number not equal to 0).

6.1 Procedures and Conditions Examined in the Atlas

The specific procedures and conditions, or "numerator events," and the codes used to identify the event in the file are given in Table 4. The "modified diagnosis-related group" (MDRG) Classification System used in Chapter Three to examine the pattern of variation in hospitalizations among the Medicare population is given in Table 5.

TABLE 4.

Condition	Codes used to define condition[1.]
All discharges	
Inhospital deaths	(Discharge status = 'B')
Medical discharges	
Low/moderate variation medical	DRGs 174, 175, 14, 121-123
High variation medical	DRGs 9-13, 15-35, 43-48, 64-74, 78-102, 124-145, 172-173, 176-190, 202-208, 235-256, 271-284, 294-301, 316-333, 346-352, 366-369, 372, 373, 376, 378-391, 395-399, 403-405, 409-414, 416-423, 425-437, 444-457, 460, 462-467, 473, 475, 487, 489, 490, 492
Surgical discharges	DRGs 1-8, 36-42, 49-63, 75-77, 103-108, 110-120, 146-171, 191-201, 209-234, 257-270, 285-293, 302-315, 334-345, 353-365, 370, 371, 377, 392-394, 400-402, 406-408, 415, 424, 439-443, 458, 459, 461, 468, 471-472, 476-486, 488, 491, 493, 494, 495
General Surgery	
cholecystectomy	Procedure code 51.2-51.23
resection for colorectal cancer	Procedure code 45.7-45.79, 45.8, 48.5, 48.6-48.69 <u>and</u> Diagnosis code 153-153.9, 154-154.1
mastectomy for cancer[f]	Procedure code 85.41, 85.43, 85.45, 85.47 <u>and</u> Diagnosis code 174-174.9 (but <u>not</u> 233.0)
partial mastectomy[f]	Procedure code 85.20 - 85.23 <u>and</u> Diagnosis code 174-174.9, <u>not</u> (233.0)
Vascular Surgery	
carotid endarterectomy	Procedure code 38.12
abdominal aortic aneurysm repair	Procedure code 38.44, 39.25 <u>and</u> Diagnosis code 441.3-441.9
lower extremity revascularization	Procedure code 39.25, 39.29 <u>and</u> Diagnosis codes <u>not</u> = 441.3-441.9
major leg amputation	Procedure code 84.15-84.17
Cardiothoracic Surgery	
Coronary artery bypass surgery	Procedure code 36.10-36.19
aortic / mitral valve replacement	Procedure code 35.20-35.24
lung resection	Procedure code 32.29-32.5 <u>and</u> Diagnosis code 162-162.9
PTCA	Procedure code 36.01, 36.02, 36.05
coronary angiography	Procedure code 37.22, 37.23, 88.55-88.57
Urology	
radical prostatectomy[m]	Procedure code 60.5
TURP for BPH[m]	Procedure code 60.2 <u>and</u> Diagnosis code (1-5) = 600-601.4, 601.8, 601.9, 602-602.1, 602.3, 602.8, 602.9, 788.2-788.29
radical nephrectomy	Procedure code 55.5-55.51 <u>and</u> Diagnosis code 189-189.1

TABLE 4. (CONTINUED)

Condition	Codes used to define condition[1.]
Orthopedic Surgery	
back surgery	Procedure code 03.0, 03.1, 03.2, 03.32, 03.39, 03.4, 03.5, 03.6, 03.93, 03.94, 03.96, 80.5-80.59, 81.0-81.09
hip replacement	Procedure code 81.51 <u>and</u> Diagnosis codes <u>not</u> = (820-821.39, 996.0-996.99)
knee replacement	Procedure code 81.54
hip fracture repair (by type) for*	
a) femoral neck fracture	Diagnosis code 820-820.19, 820.8-820.9 <u>and</u>
- total hip replacement	-Procedure code 81.51
- partial hip replacement	-Procedure code 81.52
- internal fixation	-Procedure code 78.55, 79.10, 79.15, 79.30, 79.35
- other treatment-	-None of the above procedure codes
b) other hip fracture	Diagnosis code 820.2-820.32 <u>and</u>
- total hip replacement	-Procedure code 81.51
- partial hip replacement	-Procedure code 81.52
- internal fixation	-Procedure code 78.55, 79.10, 79.15, 79.30, 79.35
- other treatment	-None of the above procedure codes

*Records were excluded if codes were present which indicated malunion or nonunion of fracture, aseptic necrosis of the hip, evidence of old fractures, or cancer in bone.

Fractures	
Hip	Primary diagnosis code 820-820.9
Shaft of femur	Primary diagnosis code 821-821.39
Patella	Primary diagnosis code 822.0-822.1
Tibia	Primary diagnosis code 823-823.92
Ankle	Primary diagnosis code 824-824.9
Foot	Primary diagnosis code 825-825.29
Proximal humerus	Primary diagnosis code 812-812.19
Elbow	Primary diagnosis code 812.4-812.59
Radius/ulna	Primary diagnosis code 813-813.93
Distal radius/ulna	Primary diagnosis code 813.4-813.55
Radius/ulna/wrist	Primary diagnosis code 813-813.93, 814-814.19

NOTES:

1. Unless otherwise specified, all codes are ICD-9-CM; up to 10 diagnoses and 6 procedures were coded on 1994-95 MEDPAR records, and all fields were searched for the presence of the conditions specified.

2. (f) refers to procedures for which counts of women served as the denominator; (m) refers to procedures for which counts of men served as the denominator.

TABLE 5.

MDRG	DRG Description	DRGs
Nervous System		
1	Craniotomy, Other Cranial and Nervous System Procedures	1-4, 7-8, 484
2	Extracranial Vascular Procedures (Carotid Endarterectomy)	5
3	Specific Cerebrovascular Disorders Except TIA	14
4	Transient Ischemic Attack (TIA)	15
5	Seizure and Headache	24-26
6	Coma and Concussion	27-33
7	Residual Nervous System Diagnoses	9-13, 16-23, 34-35
Eye		
8	Eye Procedures	36-42
112	Eye Diagnoses	43-48
Ear, Nose and Throat		
9	Tonsillectomy and/or Adenoidectomy	57-60
10	Sinus Procedures	53-55
11	Residual Ear-Nose-Throat Procedures	49-52, 56, 61-63, 168-169, 185-187
12	Ear-Nose-Throat Diagnoses	64-74
Respiratory System		
13	Major Chest and Other Respiratory Procedures	75-77
14	Respiratory Neoplasms	82
15	Pleural Effusion and Respiratory Failure	85-87
16	Adult Respiratory Infections	79-80
109	Adult Simple Pneumonia	89-90
17	Pediatric Respiratory Infections and Pneumonia	81, 91
18	Chronic Obstructive Pulmonary Disease	88
19	Adult Bronchitis and Asthma	96-97
20	Pediatric Bronchitis and Asthma	98
21	Residual Respiratory Diagnoses	78, 83-84, 92-95, 99-102
Circulatory System		
22	Valve Procedures Other Than CABG	104-105
23	Coronary Artery Bypass Graft	106-107
110	Other Heart Procedures	108
24	Major Vascular Procedures	110-111, 478-479
25	Vascular Procedures Other Than Major (PTCA)	112
26	Cardiac Pacemaker Procedures	115-118
27	Residual Circulatory System Procedures	109, 113-114, 119-120
28	Acute Myocardial Infarction	121-123
29	Cardiac Catheterization Except for AMI	124-125
30	Heart Failure and Shock (Congestive Heart Failure)	127
31	Peripheral Vascular Disorders	130-131

Table 5. (continued)

MDRG	DRG Description	DRGs
Circulatory System, Continued		
32	Cardiac Arrhythmia	138-139
33	Angina Pectoris	140
34	Syncope and Collapse	141-142
35	Chest Pain	143
36	Residual Circulatory System Diagnoses	126, 129, 132-137, 144-145
111	Deep Vein Thrombosis	128
Digestive System		
37	Major Small and Large Bowel Procedures	146-149
38	Stomach, Esophageal and Duodenal Procedures	154-156
39	Anal Procedures	157-158, 267
40	Inguinal and Femoral Hernia Procedures	159-163
41	Appendectomy	164-167
42	Residual Digestive System Procedures	150-153, 170-171
43	Gastro-Intestinal Hemorrhage	174-175
44	Gastro-Intestinal Obstruction	180-181
45	Adult Gastroenteritis	182-183
46	Pediatric Gastroenteritis	184
47	Residual Digestive System Diagnoses	172-173, 176-179, 188-190
Hepatobiliary System		
48	Cholecystectomy	195-198, 493, 494
49	Other Hepatobiliary Procedures	191-194, 199-201
50	Biliary Tract Disorders	207-208
51	Other Hepatobiliary System Diagnoses	202-206
Musculoskeletal and Connective Tissue		
52	Major Joint Procedures	209, 471
53	Hip and Femur Procedures Other Than Major Joint	210-211
54	Back and Neck Procedures	214-215
55	Lower Extremity Procedures	218-219
56	Knee Procedures	221-222
57	Upper Extremity Procedures	223-224, 491
58	Residual Musculoskeletal Procedures	6, 212-213, 216-217, 220, 225-234
59	Hip, Femur, Pelvis Fracture	235-236
60	Medical Back Problems	243
61	Misc. Fracture/Sprain/Strain/Dislocation	250-255
62	Residual Musculoskeletal Diagnoses	237-242, 244-249, 256
Skin, Subcutaneous Tissue and Breast		
63	Total and Subtotal Mastectomy	257-260
64	Other Skin/Tissue/Breast Procedures	261-266, 268-270
65	Cellulitis	277-279
66	Other Skin/Tissue/Breast Diagnoses	271-276, 280-284

Table 5. (CONTINUED)

MDRG	DRG Description	DRGs
Endocrine, Nutritional and Metabolic		
67	Endocrine/Nutritional/Metabolic Procedures	285-293
68	Diabetes Age >=35	294
69	Adult Nutritional and Metabolic Disorders	296-297
70	Pediatric Nutritional and Metabolic Disorders	298
71	Residual Endocrine/Nutrional/Metabolic Diagnoses	295, 299-301
Kidney and Urinary System / Male Reproductive System		
72	Major Genito-Urinary Procedures	302-307, 334-335
73	Transurethral Prostatectomy	336-337
74	Transurethral Procedures Except TURP	310-311
75	Major Genito-Urinary Procedures	308-309, 312-315, 338-345
76	Kidney-Urinary Tract Infections	320-321
77	Urinary Tract Stones	323-324
78	Residual Kidney/Urinary System Diagnoses	316-319, 322, 325-333
79	Male Reproductive System Diagnoses	346-352
Female Reproductive System		
80	Uterus and Adnexa Procedures for Non-Malignant Conditions	358-359
81	Female Reproductive System Reconstructive Procedures	356
82	Residual Female Reproductive System Procedures	353-355, 357, 360-365
83	Female Reproductive System Diagnoses	366-369
Pregnancy-Related		
84	Cesarean Delivery	370-371
85	Vaginal Delivery	372-375
86	Pregnancy Not Delivered	376-384
Newborns and Neonates		
87	Newborns and Neonates	385-391
Blood and Blood Forming Organs		
88	Diagnoses of Blood and Blood Forming Organs	395-399
Myeloproliferative Diseases		
89	Chemotherapy	410, 492
90	Myeloproliferative/Lymphoma/Leukemia Diagnoses Other Than Chemotherapy	403-405, 409, 411-414
Infectious and Parasitic Diseases		
91	Septicemia	416
92	Adult Viral Disease and Fever of Unknown Origin	419-421
93	Pediatric Viral Disease and Fever of Unknown Origin	422
94	Residual Infectious and Parasitic Diseases	417-418, 423, 489-490
Mental Diseases and Disorders		
95	Psychoses	430
96	Other Mental Diseases and Disorders	425-429, 431-432

TABLE 5. (CONTINUED)

MDRG	DRG Description	DRGs
Substance Use		
97	Substance Use Treatment, Left Against Medical Advice	433
98	Substance Use Detoxification (w/o Rehab)	434-435
99	Substance Use Rehabilitation (with or w/o Detox)	436-437
Injuries and Adverse Effects		
100	Operating Room Procedures for Injuries	439-443
101	Toxic Effects of Drugs	449-450
102	Other Injury Diagnoses w/o Procedure	444-448, 451-457, 487
Health Status Factors		
103	Rehabilitation (Other Than for Substance Abuse)	462
104	Other Health Status Diagnoses	463-467
Residual MDRGs		
105	Unrelated Operating Room Procedures	468
106	Respiratory Disease with Ventilator	475
107	Residual O.R. Procedures with Case Mix Index >=3.0	103, 392, 415, 458, 472-474, 480-483, 485-486, 488
108	Residual O.R. Procedures with Case Mix Index <3.0	393-394, 400-402, 406-408, 424, 459-461

6.2 Adjusted Utilization Rates

Rates were adjusted using the indirect method for the following strata: sex, race (black, non-black) and age (65-69, 70-74, 75-79, 80-84, 85-99), with the 1994-95 national Medicare population as the standard, as described in Section 2.3, except that we also summed observed and expected HSA counts across years (1994 and 1995). Although the majority of events occurred at most once per person during the study period, we included multiple events to the same person to allow the rates to reflect total health care utilization.

Although standard errors of the rates were not reported, these estimates are, for the most part, precisely determined. The minimum Medicare population in an HRR is 14,930 residents, and all rates were based on an expected count of at least 20 events. The following precisions were obtained in the smallest HRR (the "worst case scenario") for an event rate of 5 per 1,000:

- For procedures related exclusively to males or females in this smallest HRR, the precision would be ±16% of the true rate.
- For procedures related to the entire HRR, the precision would be ±12%.
- For procedures in a median-sized HRR (N=64,000) the precision would be ±6%.

In general, if we denote the event rate as p and the population size as N, the standard error is $(p/N)^{0.5}$ and the precision, expressed as a percent of the true rate, is $(se(p)/p)*100\%$.

6.3 Index of Variation: the SCV

The Systematic Component of Variation (SCV) was developed as a measure of the variation among the rates of admission across different areas that is not affected by the mean rate or the size of the population studied, as are other measures of variation. It can, therefore, be used to compare relative variations of different procedures or conditions, even when the mean rates differ substantially. It is typically used to classify procedures into categories of low, moderate, high and very high variation. Differences in the SCV among causes of admission can be tested by computing ratios of two SCVs and comparing them to the F distribution. The SCV is computed by subtracting the random component of variation from the total variance. Further details on the computation of the SCV and its use are given in McPherson et al. (1982) and Wennberg et al (1984).

6.4 Measures of Association (R^2 and Regression Lines)

In this Atlas, we often suggest that some factors may be related in a systematic way to other factors. For example, in Chapter Three we hypothesize that regions with high rates of beds per thousand residents also have high rates of hospitalization for medical conditions. To capture the degree and extent of the association between hospital beds and medical hospitalizations in Figure 3.6, we put hospital beds per thousand residents on the horizontal axis and hospitalization rates per thousand residents on the vertical axis, and placed a point on the graph for each of the 306 hospital referral regions. If hospital beds and hospitalization rates were negatively correlated, so that regions with higher beds per thousand residents had lower per capita hospitalizations, then we might expect to see the cloud of points tilted downward, running from northwest to southeast. Conversely, if they were positively correlated — as they in fact are — the cloud of points would run from southwest to northeast on the graph, as seen in Figure 3.6.

It is sometimes difficult to discern from this cloud of points the relationship between two variables. A linear regression line provides the best fit of the data and summarizes the relationships between them. A measure of the 'goodness of fit' or the extent to which hospital beds per 1,000 residents predicts hospitalizations per 1,000 enrollees is the R^2, which is defined as the proportion of total variation in the vertical axis (hospitalizations) that is explained by variation in the horizontal axis (beds). It can range between 0 and 1, where 1 is perfect correlation and 0 means that the two variables are completely unrelated. In Figure 3.6, the R^2 for the relationship between medical hospitalizations and hospital beds is 0.56, which means that the two are closely related — that 56% of the variation in medical hospitalizations per 1000 residents is related to the bed supply.

The regression lines and R^2 statistics given in the text are not weighted for the size of the population. Weighted and unweighted R^2 statistics were similar.

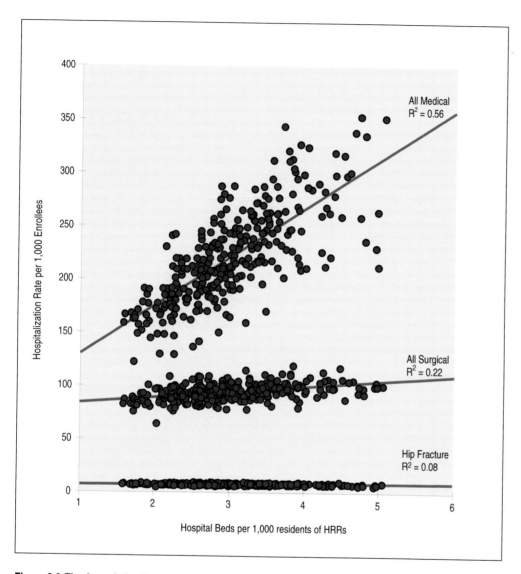

Figure 3.6. The Association Between Allocated Hospital Beds and Medicare Hospitalizations for Medical and Surgical Care and for Hip Fracture (1994-95)

7. American Experience of Death

Percent of Medicare deaths occurring in hospitals was computed similarly to the method used for Medicare hospitalization rates described in Section 6. In this case, however, the denominator was the Medicare enrollee population who died in 1994 or 1995 (see Section 1.4), and the "numerator event" was death in a hospital (discharge status = 'B' in MEDPAR file). Rates were age, sex and race adjusted as described in Section 6.2 and were expressed as a percentage of deaths.

For all rates pertaining to the last six months of life, the denominator was the 18 month 1994-95 deceased Medicare population, computed as the sum of one half the 1994 deaths and all the 1995 deaths, using the same criteria as above. For the percent of Medicare deaths who were admitted to the ICU in the last 6 months of life, the "numerator event" was death in a hospital between 7/1/94 and 12/31/95 with admission to an ICU within 6 months of the death date using MEDPAR files.

Average days in the hospital, average days in the ICU and average reimbursements for inpatient care per capita were computed using only the portion of the event (hospital stay or ICU stay) falling within the 6 month period (182 days) prior to death. Rates were age, sex and race adjusted as described in Section 6.2. Inpatient reimbursement rates were also price adjusted as described in Section 3.2.

8. Surgical Procedure Rates

The rates of inpatient surgery in Chapter Five are based on the MEDPAR files for 1994 and 1995. To ensure that the population included in the numerator corresponded to the denominator population, restrictions were applied to exclude the following records: Medicare enrollees under age 65 or over age 99 on June 30, 1994 or 1995; Medicare enrollees in risk-bearing HMOs; MEDPAR records with a length of stay over 365 days; and hospitalizations at psychiatric, rehabilitation or long term care units (provider codes = S, T, U or V; facility type not equal to S; third digit of Medicare provider number not equal to 0). The denominators are the 1994-95 Medicare enrollee population described in Section 1.4.

8.1 Procedures examined in Chapter Five

The procedure codes used in Chapter Five are listed in Table 4. The procedure codes used in the MEDPAR file are based on the International Classification of Disease, ICD-9-CM. Selection of procedure codes was based on review of the literature and/ or consultation with clinical experts. No rate was based on a count of fewer than 20 expected events for reasons of statistical precision.

8.2 Calculation of Adjusted Procedure-Specific Rates

All rates were indirectly adjusted for age, sex and race, with the 1994-95 Medicare population as the standard, as described in Sections 2.3 and 6.2, except that sex-specific population estimates were used for prostate and breast procedures.

9. The Medicare Current Beneficiary Survey (MCBS)

Chapter 6 considers the correspondence among hospital bed capacity, utilization and self-reported health. This issue was also addressed by Ashby et al (1986) who found that states with higher Medicare expenditures also had lower levels of self-reported health. We turned to the Medicare Current Beneficiary Survey (MCBS) to reexamine this issue.

The MCBS is a continuous multi-purpose survey of a representative sample of the entire Medicare population, with oversampling of the old-old, the disabled, and those living in institutional settings (HCFA, 1992). Survey participants complete three rounds of surveys each year throughout their participation in the study. The sample was drawn from 107 primary sampling units (PSU) consisting of counties or groups of counties intended to be representative of the U.S. Within those PSUs, sampling was further restricted to certain geographic areas (sub-PSUs, n = 1,163), based on the ZIP Code of residence of the beneficiary, again with the goal of maintaining representativeness while economizing on interviewer travel. Beneficiaries within each area were then sampled randomly within age strata, with oversampling of the disabled under age 65 and the oldest beneficiaries (age 85 and over).

Participants are interviewed three times each year, wherever they reside and with the interview tailored to reflect the setting and using proxy respondents where necessary. Survey items include a core of data that are repeated at each subsequent interview on utilization, charges and payments for health care and a supplement that focuses on other domains. Critical to this analysis is the supplement on Access and Satisfaction, which was carried out on Round 1 (Fall 1991) and is repeated annually thereafter (Rounds 4, 7, 10 etc.). In addition to data on access and satisfaction, this supplement includes detailed questions on self-assessed health status, current health conditions and physical function.

The study population for this analysis (N=8,860) was created by taking Round 4 of the 1992 wave of the MCBS and excluding persons under age 65, those who were institutionalized and answered questions by proxy and those enrolled in risk-bearing HMOs. We matched each individual with his or her 1993 Medicare claims data on health care utilization and appended regional-level information about health resources from the Atlas database. Thus we were able to measure health characteristics of people who live in regions with relatively high, and relatively low, levels of hospital beds or Medicare spending.

Individuals' total 1993 hospital days were summed and hospital days per capita were computed by self-reported health status (poor, fair, good, very good, and excellent). To assess the dependence on hospital resources, they were also computed separately by hospital bed supply in the region (above vs. below the median). These were indirectly standardized by age and sex using the 1993 Medicare population as the standard, as described in Sections 2.3 and 6.2.

To compute the expected number of hospital days as predicted by self-reported health status, according to quintile of hospital beds, we used regression analysis to predict hospital days based on self-reported health, age and sex in each quintile of hospital beds. Quintiles (20th percentiles) were computed by taking (weighted) intervals of the sorted data for MCBS respondents and ranged from the lowest quintile with the fewest hospital beds to the highest quintile with the most hospital beds.

10. Calculation of Illness Adjusted Rates

Reimbursement and hospital resource rates were occasionally adjusted for Medicare population illness characteristics in Chapters Six and Seven. The measures of illness used were the age, sex and race adjusted 1994-95 HSA-level mortality rate and incidence rates for five conditions. The conditions selected consisted of specific events for which hospitalization is a proxy for the incidence of disease: hospitalizations for hip fracture, cancer of the colon or lung treated surgically, gastrointestinal hemorrhage, acute myocardial infarction or stroke (Wennberg, NEJM 1984; Wennberg, Lancet 1987). The above rates were computed as described in Section 6.

To obtain age-sex-race-illness indirectly standardized rates, we first used modeling techniques to obtain the HSA age-sex-race stratum-specific expected counts (or dollars). The models consisted of regressing the HSA stratum-specific crude Medicare outcome rates on age, sex, race, all age-sex-race interactions, HSA-specific adjusted mortality rate and the five HSA-specific adjusted illness rates described above, and weighting by the stratum-specific Medicare population. The models were then used to predict expected HSA stratum-specific counts (or dollars) and summed to the HRR level. The HRR level expected counts were used as denominators in the indirectly standardized rates, as described in Section 2.3. This technique standardizes to the national Medicare population.

11. Benchmarking

The variations in per capita resource allocations and utilization among HRRs provide the basis for asking "What if?" questions. For example, if the number of hospital beds per 1,000 residents in a particular HRR were the upper limit for beds in all HRRs in the United States, so that all areas with higher rates were brought down to that benchmark, how many fewer beds would be required? Or, if the numbers of primary care physicians per 100,000 residents observed for another HRR were the standard for your HRR, how many more or how many fewer primary physicians would be needed?

Chapter Seven provides examples of how benchmarking can be applied to answer such questions. For example, in Figure 7.4, the physician supply in the United States was compared to the physician workforce employed in a large staff model HMO. The HMO physician rates were obtained from a study of HMO physician workforce market dynamics sponsored by the Robert Wood Johnson Foundation (personal communication, David Kindig, M.D., University of Wisconsin). The study protocols were designed to take out-of-plan use into account in estimating the per capita size of the workforce. The HMO workforce rates, like the rates for HRRs, were age and sex adjusted to the U.S. population as described in Section 4.3. Thus, the rates can be compared without concern that differences in age and sex structure might explain the observed differences.

The strategies for benchmarking used in Chapter Seven permit comparisons of adjusted rates across areas and provide estimates of the numbers of physicians (or acute care beds) in excess of the benchmark health plan or HRR. The rates in Table A in The Appendix on the Physician Workforce in the United States provide the data from which the information in Figure 7.4 — the supply of physicians in the United States benchmarked to a large HMO — was derived. For example, the ratio of U.S. rates for orthopedic surgeons (7.10 per 100,000 residents) to the HMO employment pattern (4.52 per 100,000 enrollees) is 1.57, indicating a 57% surplus in the national supply, if the HMO was used as the benchmark. According to this benchmark, the number of orthopedic physicians in the U.S. in excess of "need" is obtained by evaluating:

(U.S. rate - HMO rate) x (U.S Population/100,000) = (7.10 - 4.52) x (2,623.1)
= 6,769 physicians

Figures 7.3, 7.5 and 7.6 compare the U.S. experience to various HRR benchmarks simultaneously. The estimates we provide for resource savings assume that all regions with higher levels of resources and utilization than the benchmark are reduced to the benchmark level, but that regions with resources and utilization lower than the benchmark remain constant - that is, their resources and utilization are not increased. For example, in Figure 7.5, Minneapolis ranks 226th in terms of age and sex adjusted supply of selected specialists. If the rate in the Minneapolis benchmark prevailed in the 225 HRRs with higher rates of selected specialists, the estimated excess number of these specialists is 55,395, and is computed as:

The sum of
{ (HRR rate - Minneapolis rate) x (HRR Population/100,000) }
over all HRRs with higher rates of specialists than Minneapolis

A similar formula is used to compare two areas, such as Boston and New Haven. Note that the higher the rank of the benchmark HRR (i.e. the lower the resource rate in that HRR), the greater will be the estimated excess resources in the U.S. when using the specified HRR as a benchmark.

The AAPCC refers to Medicare's Adjusted Average Per Capita Costs, which is HCFA's method for determining capitation payments for risk-bearing HMOs. HCFA computes it as the 5 year rolling average of the actual fee-for-service Medicare expenditures at the county level, and adjusts for age, sex and race. To evaluate the consequences of differences in the AAPCC across HRRs, county-specific AAPCCs were first converted to HSA-specific AAPCCs. For each HSA, the weighted average of county level AAPCCs was first computed for all counties covering this HSA, weighting by the proportion of the HSA Medicare population living in that county. AAPCCs were illness and price adjusted using methods described in Sections 3.2 and 10. These were then converted to the HRR level by computing the weighted average of the HSA-specific AAPCCs, weighting by the HSA Medicare population. To estimate the "surplus" dollars per enrollee that would be available under Medicare risk contracts if managed care companies in selected regions achieved the Minneapolis benchmark for efficient health care delivery, we computed the difference between a region's AAPCC and the Minneapolis HRR.

The data in the tables in the Atlas are adjusted to the U.S. population and can be used to benchmark the experience in your own region to the region of your choice. Find the rate in your own area for the resource allocation, hospitalization or procedure rate of interest. Then identify the benchmark region to which you wish to make the comparison. The ratio of the experience in your region to the benchmark is obtained by dividing your rate by the rate in the benchmark region. The numbers of hospital beds, personnel, expenditures, physicians, hospitalizations, or diagnostic or surgical procedures above or below the benchmark is obtained by the following formula:

(your HRR rate - benchmark rate) x (your HRR population/rate convention) = excess (+) or deficit (-) in resources, hospitalizations, procedures, according to the selected benchmark

The "rate convention," i.e., the denomination used for calculating population rates in the tables presented in Chapter Seven, is: for reimbursements, per 1,000 enrollees; for procedures and hospitalizations, per 1,000 Medicare enrollees; for hospital beds and personnel, per 1,000 residents; and for the physician workforce, per 100,000 residents.

Note that data benchmarked using Medicare procedure rates per thousand enrollees are for a two-year period, 1994-95; the appropriate population is the two-year Medicare enrollee estimate given in the table in Chapter Five. For readability, the rates in the Atlas tables have been rounded, usually to one place to the right of the decimal point. Data displayed in the figures in Chapters One through Seven are fully precise. As a result, calculations of the numbers in the benchmark figures starting from the rounded numbers in the tables yield approximatly, but not exactly, the same estimates. Despite the rounding, the precision in the tables is sufficient for making comparisons between regions. The machine-readable data base available with the Atlas can be used to achieve full precision.

1994/95 CABG and PTCA rates for persons aged 65 and over in Toronto and Ontario (Canada) used for benchmarking in Chapter 7 were estimated from data provided by the Institute for Clinical Evaluative Sciences in Ontario (ICES Atlas and personal communication).

Appendix on the Geography of Health Care in the United States*

The use of health care resources in the United States is highly localized. Most Americans use the services of physicians whose practices are nearby. Physicians, in turn, are usually affiliated with hospitals that are near their practices. As a result, when patients are admitted to hospitals, the admission generally takes place within a relatively short distance of where the patient lives. This is true across the United States. Although the distances from homes to hospitals vary with geography – people who live in rural areas travel farther than those who live in cities – in general most patients are admitted to a hospital close to where they live which provides an appropriate level of care.

The Medicare program maintains exhaustive records of hospitalizations, which makes it possible to define the patterns of use of hospital care. When Medicare enrollees are admitted to hospitals, the program's records identify both the patients' places of residence (by ZIP Code) and the hospitals where the admissions took place (by unique numerical identifiers). These files provide a reliable basis for determining the geographic pattern of health care use, because research shows that the migration patterns of patients in the Medicare program are similar to those for younger patients.

Medicare records of hospitalizations were used to define 3,436 geographically distinct hospital service areas in the United States. In each hospital service area, most of the care received by Medicare patients is provided in hospitals within the area. Based on the patterns of care for major cardiovascular surgery and neurosurgery, hospital service areas were aggregated into 306 hospital referral regions; this Atlas reports on patterns of care in these hospital referral regions.

How Hospital Service Areas Were Defined

Hospital service areas were defined through a three-step process. First, all acute care hospitals in the 50 states and the District of Columbia were identified from the American Hospital Association and Medicare provider files and assigned to the town or city in which they were located. The name of the town or city was used

*Abstracted from the 1996 edition of the Dartmouth Atlas of Health Care

as the name of the hospital service area, even though the area might have extended well beyond the political boundary of the town. For example, the Mt. Ascutney Hospital is in Windsor, Vermont. The area is called the Windsor hospital service area, even though the area serves several other communities.

In the second step, all 1992 and 1993 Medicare hospitalization records for each hospital were analyzed to ascertain the ZIP Code of each of its patients. When a town or city had more than one hospital, the counts were added together. Using a plurality rule, each ZIP Code was assigned on a provisional basis to the town containing the hospitals most often used by local residents.

The analysis of the patterns of use of care by Medicare patients led to the provisional assignment of five post office ZIP Codes to the Windsor hospital service area.

ZIP Code	Community Name	1990 Population	% of Medicare Discharges to Mt. Ascutney Hospital
05037	Brownsville	415	52.8
05048	Hartland	1,730	46.8
05053	Pomfret	245	52.6
05062	Reading	614	36.8
05089	Windsor	5,406	63.2

The third step involved the visual examination of the ZIP Codes using a computer-generated map to make sure that the ZIP Codes included in the hospital service areas were contiguous. In the case of the Windsor area, inspection of the map led to the reassignment of Pomfret to the Lebanon hospital service area. In the final determination, the Windsor hospital service area contained four communities and a total population of 8,165. (See Map A)

Details about the method of constructing hospital service areas are given in The Appendix on Methods.

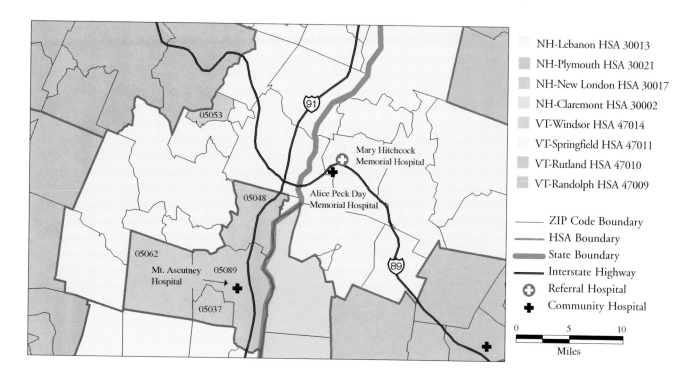

Map A. ZIP Codes Assigned to the Windsor, Vermont, Hospital Service Area

The analysis of the pattern of use of hospitals revealed that Medicare enrollees living in the five ZIP Code areas in light blue most often used the Mt. Ascutney Hospital in Windsor, Vermont. To maintain geographic continuity of hospital service areas, the Pomfret ZIP Code 05053 was reassigned to the Lebanon hospital service area. The Windsor hospital service area contained four communities, with a 1990 census of 8,165. During 1992-93, there were 679 hospitalizations among the Medicare population; 394 (58%) were to Mt. Ascutney Hospital, 131 to the Mary Hitchcock Memorial Hospital, and 154 to other hospitals.

Hospital Service Areas in the United States

The documentation of the patterns of use of hospitals according to Medicare enrollee ZIP Codes during 1992-93 led to the aggregation of approximately 42,000 ZIP Codes into 3,436 hospital service areas. In each area, more Medicare patients were hospitalized locally than in any other single hospital service area. The propensity of patients to use local hospitals is measured by the localization index, which is the percentage of all residents' hospitalizations that occur in local hospitals (the number of local hospitalizations of residents divided by all hospitalizations of residents). This index varied from a low of 17.9% to over 94%. More than 85% of Americans lived in hospital service areas where the majority of Medicare hospitalizations occurred locally. More than 51% lived in areas where the localization index exceeded 70%.

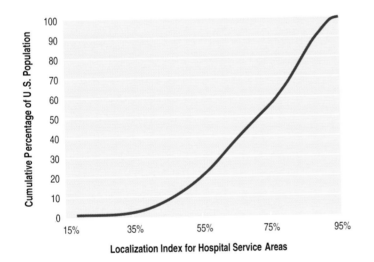

Figure A. Cumulative Percentage of Population of the United States According to the Hospital Service Area Localization Index (1992-93)

The localization index is the proportion of all hospitalizations for area residents that occur in a hospital or hospitals within the area. The figure shows the localization index for Medicare patients in 3,436 hospital service areas, according to the cumulative proportion of the population living in the region. Most of the population lived in regions where more than 50% of hospitalizations occurred locally.

In 1993, most Americans lived in hospital service areas with three or fewer local hospitals. Eighty-two percent, or 2,830, of all hospital service areas, which comprised 39% of the population in 1990, had only one hospital. Four hundred twenty-eight hospital service areas, which comprised 23% of the United States population, had either two or three hospitals. One hundred seventy-eight, or less than 6% of hospital service areas, had four or more local hospitals and comprised about 37% of the population of the United States.

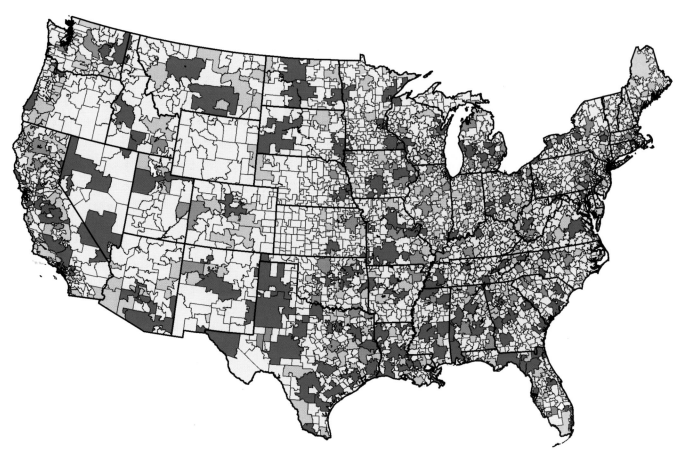

Map B. Hospital Service Areas According to the Number of Acute Care Hospitals

Thirty-nine percent of the population of the United States lived in areas with one hospital (buff); 15% lived in areas with two hospitals (light orange); 8.4% lived in areas with three hospitals (bright orange); and 37% of the population lived in areas with four or more hospitals within the hospital service area (red).

Count of Acute Care Hospitals
by Hospital Service Area (1993)

- 4 or more (178 HSAs)
- 3   (106)
- 2   (322)
- 1   (2,830)
- Not Populated

How Hospital Referral Regions Were Defined

Hospital service areas make clear the patterns of use of local hospitals. A significant proportion of care, however, is provided by referral hospitals that serve a larger region. Hospital referral regions were defined in this Atlas by documenting where patients were referred for major cardiovascular surgical procedures and for neurosurgery. Each hospital service area was examined to determine where most of its residents went for these services. The result was the aggregation of the 3,436 hospital service areas into 306 hospital referral regions. Each hospital referral region had at least one city where both major cardiovascular surgical procedures and neurosurgery were performed. Maps were used to make sure that the small number of "orphan" hospital service areas – those surrounded by hospital service areas allocated to a different hospital referral region – were reassigned, in almost all cases, to ensure geographic contiguity. Hospital referral regions were pooled with neighbors if their populations were less than 120,000 or if less than 65% of their residents' hospitalizations occurred within the region.

Hospital referral regions were named for the hospital service area containing the referral hospital or hospitals most often used by residents of the region. The regions sometimes cross state boundaries. The Evansville, Indiana, hospital referral region (Map C) provides an example of a region that is located in three states: Illinois, Indiana, and Kentucky. In this region, three hospitals provided cardiovascular surgery services. Two were in Evansville; a third hospital, in Vincennes, Indiana, also provided cardiovascular surgery, but in the years of this study residents of the Vincennes area used cardiovascular and neurosurgery procedures provided in Evansville more frequently than those in Vincennes, resulting in the assignment of the Vincennes hospital service area to the Evansville hospital referral region.

Map C also provides an example of a region with a population too small to meet the minimum criterion for designation as a hospital referral region. The Madisonville, Kentucky, hospital service area met the criterion as a hospital referral region on the basis of the plurality rule, but its population was less than 57,000. The area was assigned to the Paducah, Kentucky, hospital referral region because hospitals in Paducah were the second most commonly used place of care for cardiovascular and neurosurgical procedures.

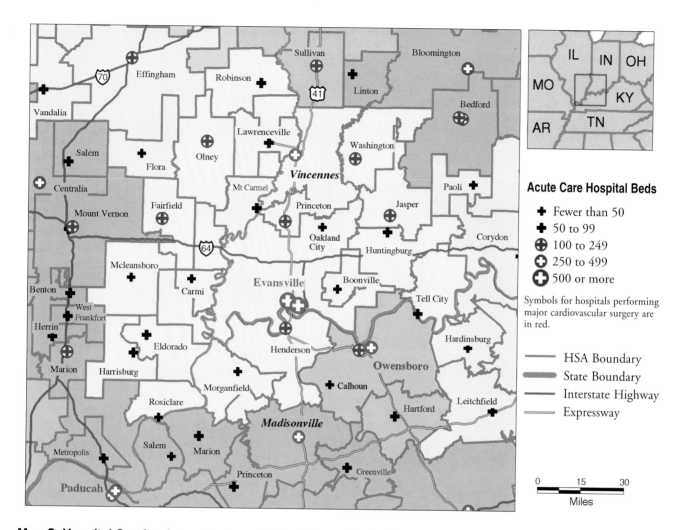

Map C. Hospital Service Areas Assigned to the Evansville, Indiana, Hospital Referral Region

Hospital referral regions are named for the hospital service area containing the referral hospital or hospitals most often used by residents of the region. Hospital referral regions overlap state boundaries in every state except Alaska and Hawaii. The Evansvillle, Indiana, hospital referral region is in parts of three states: Illinois, Indiana, and Kentucky.

Maps of Hospital Referral Regions in the United States

The maps on the following pages outline the boundaries of the hospital referral regions. Although in some regions more than one city provided referral care, each hospital referral region was named for the city where most patients receiving major cardiovascular surgical procedures and neurosurgery were referred for care.

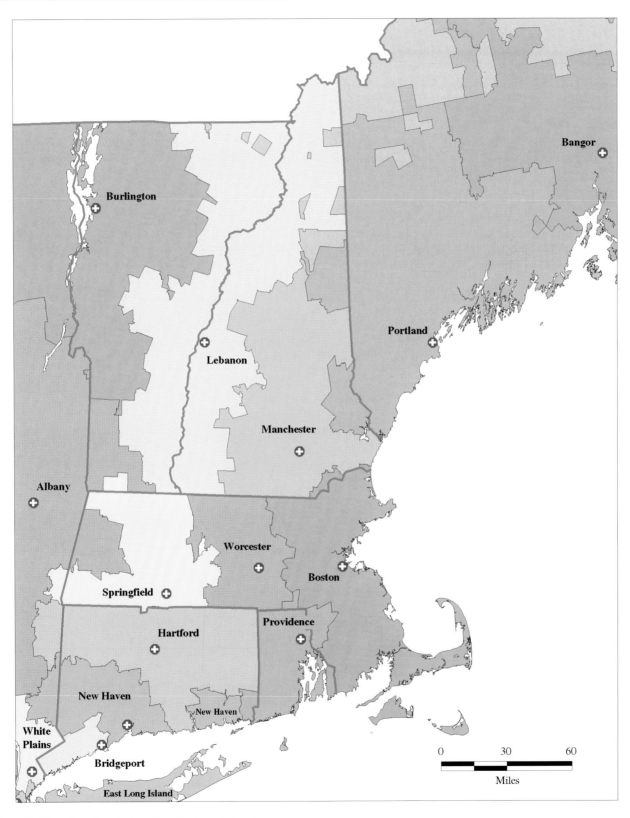

Map D. New England Hospital Referral Regions

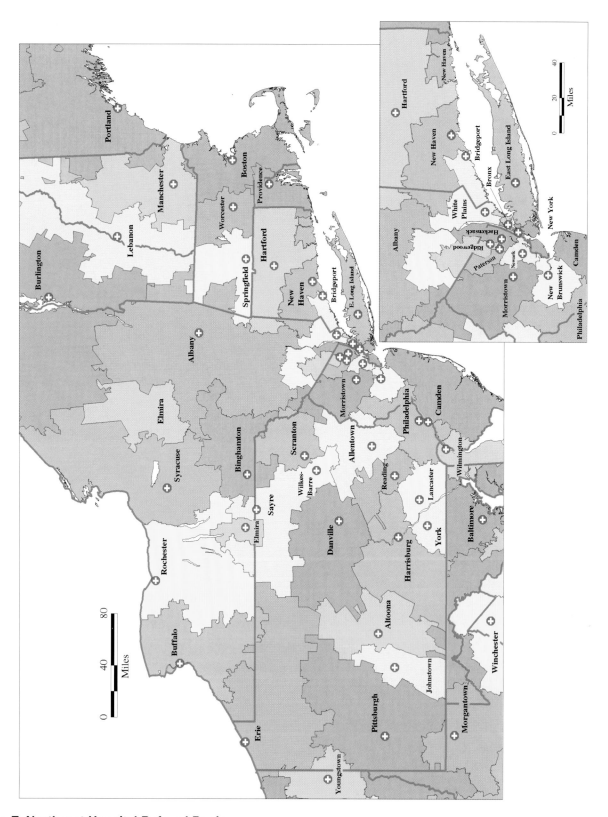

Map E. Northeast Hospital Referral Regions

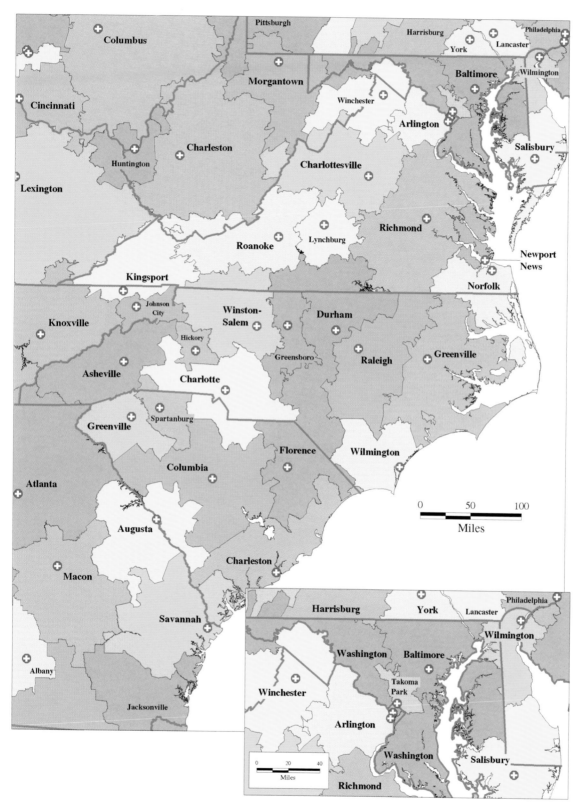

Map F. South Atlantic Hospital Referral Regions

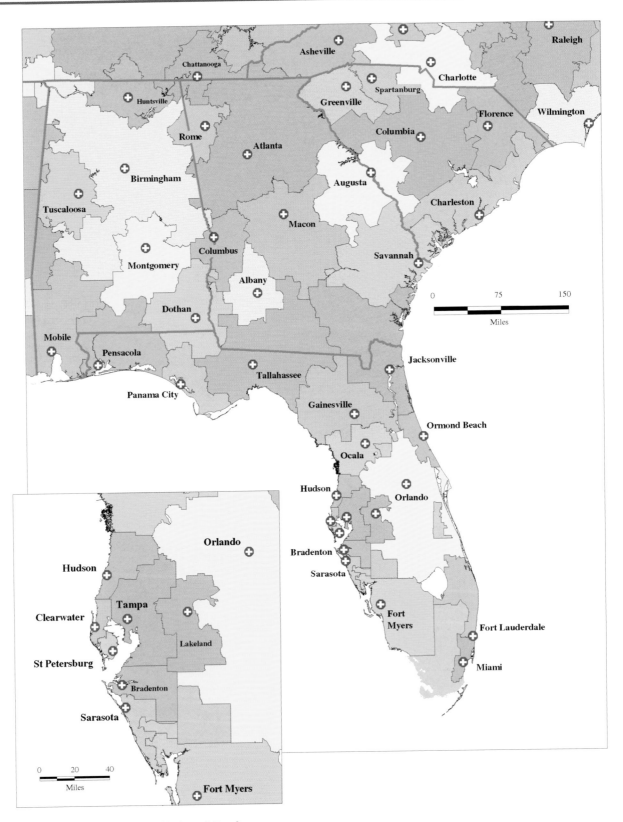

Map G. Southeast Hospital Referral Regions

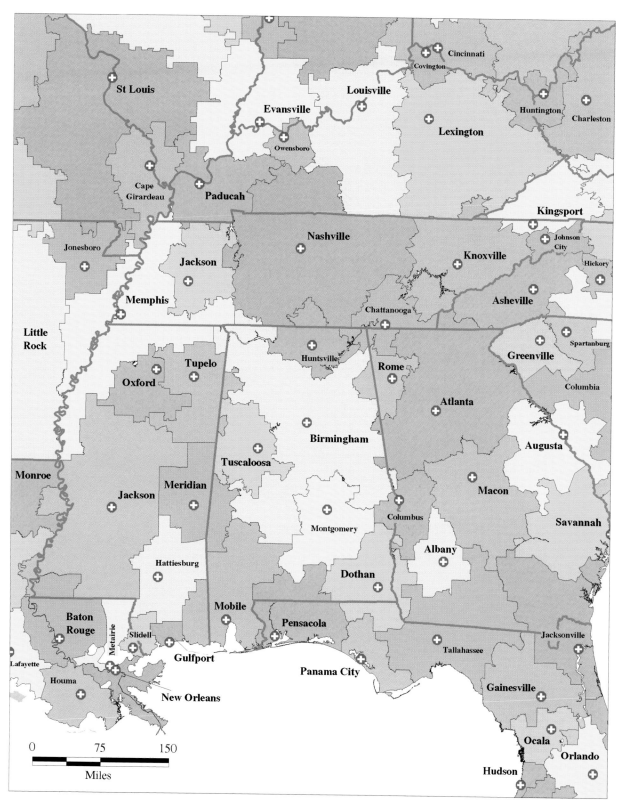

Map H. South Central Hospital Referral Regions

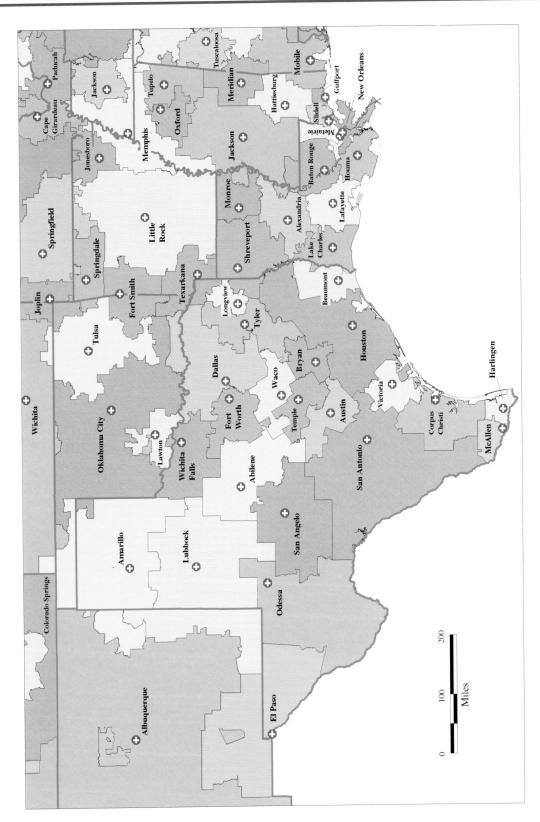

Map I. Southwest Hospital Referral Regions

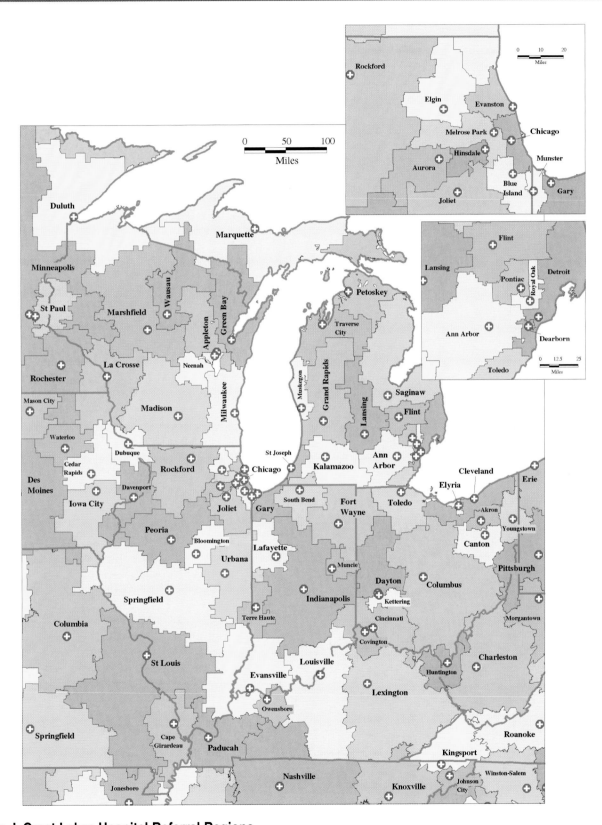

Map J. Great Lakes Hospital Referral Regions

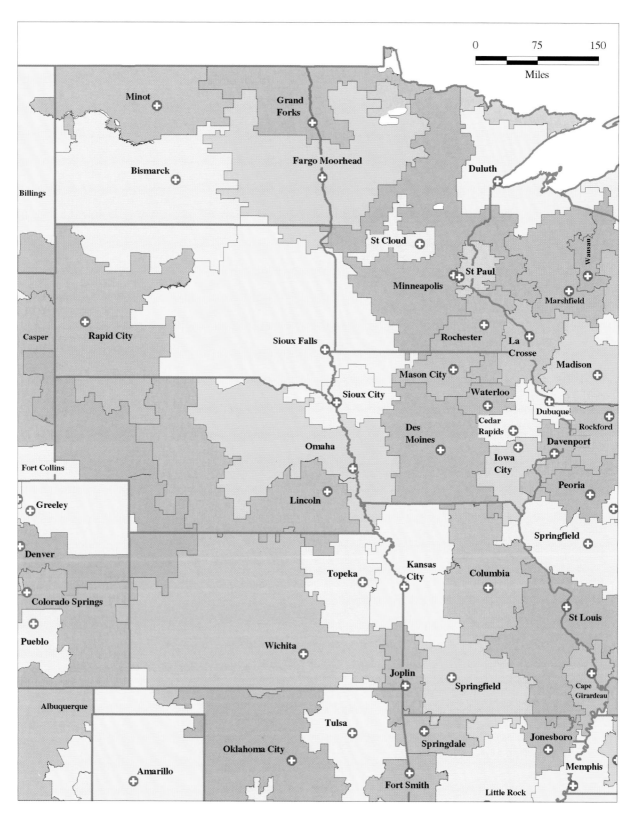

Map K. Upper Midwest Hospital Referral Regions

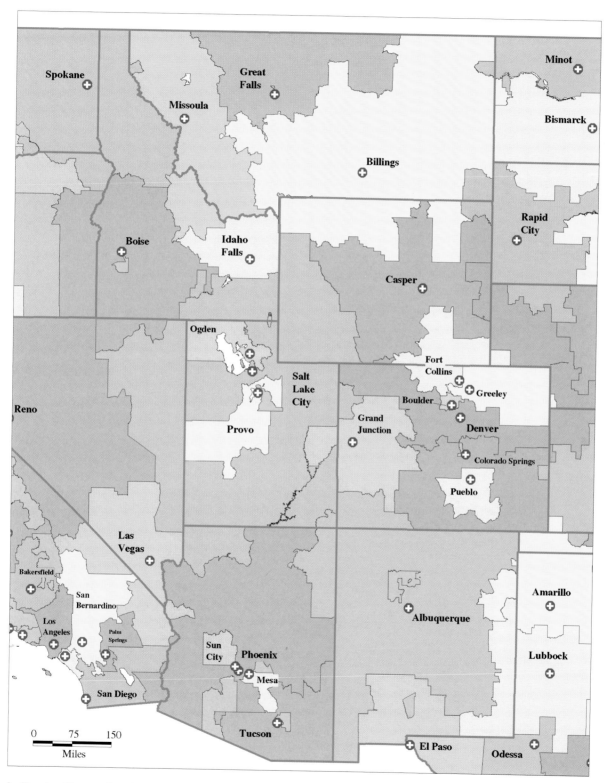

Map L. Rocky Mountains Hospital Referral Regions

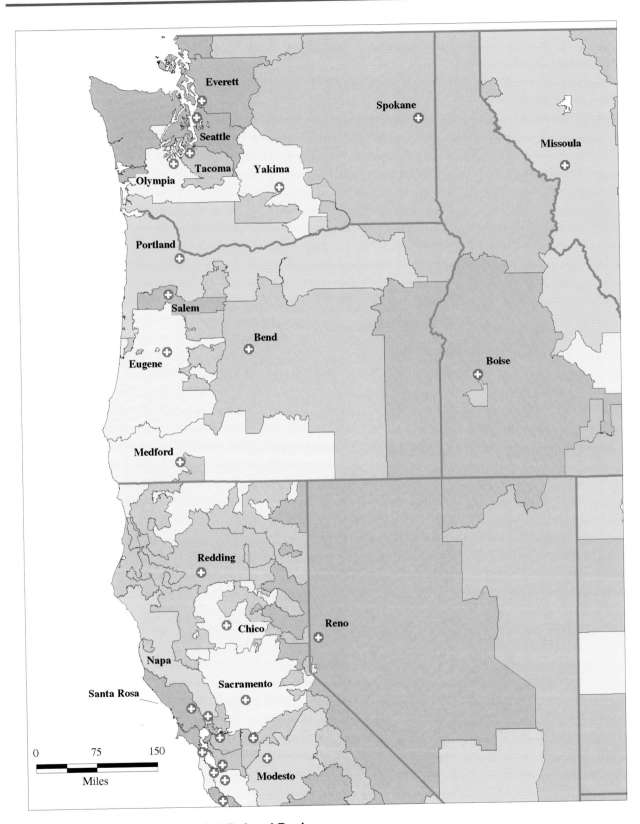

Map M. Pacific Northwest Hospital Referral Regions

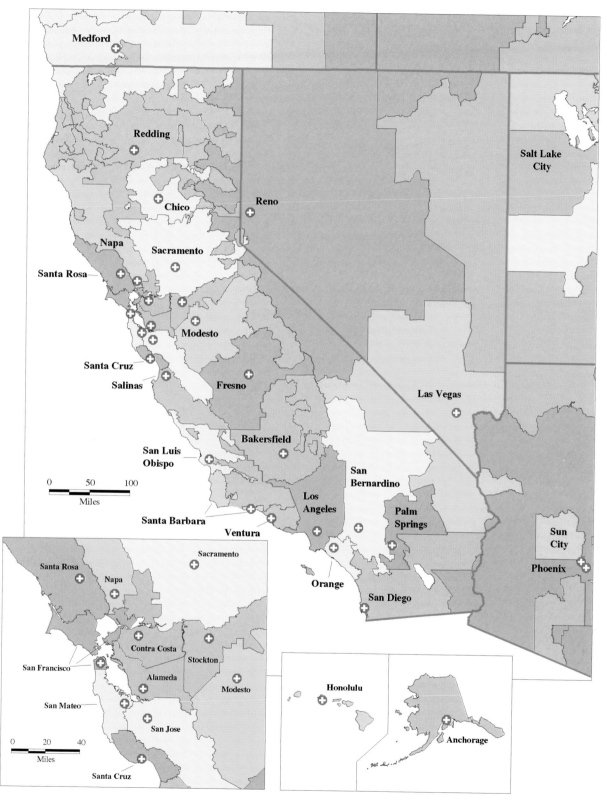

Map N. Pacific Coast Hospital Referral Regions

Appendix on the Physician Workforce in the United States

Traditional approaches to workforce planning in the United States have depended on need-based or demand-based planning to find the "appropriate" supply of physicians (Chapter Seven). Both approaches have serious flaws. An alternative approach to estimating the reasonable number of physicians relies on benchmarking. Comparing physician resources with a benchmark health plan or region provides a guidepost that does not depend on a hypothetical optimal physician level but depends on a real-world and attainable health care system (Chapter Seven).

While the "optimal" number of physicians for a given population is unknown, benchmarking offers a method of examining health plans and communities in order to select those that achieve low levels of deployment of clinically active physicians without a measured loss of patient welfare due to a shortage of physicians.

In this appendix, we compare the national and regional workforce of clinically active physicians with three benchmarks. These benchmarks, a large health maintenance organization and the Minneapolis, Minnesota and Wichita, Kansas hospital referral regions, were selected because of their apparent efficiency. The Minneapolis hospital referral region has high managed care penetration (39.4% in 1995), and the Wichita hospital referral region is a predominantly fee-for-service market with low managed care penetration (4.5% in 1995). In contrast to the populations served by health maintenance organizations, the populations in hospital referral regions are based on geographic residence and therefore are not biased by selection against the disabled, the uninsured, and the very elderly.

The first section of this appendix includes 14 maps which benchmark the supply of generalists, "selected specialists" (as a group) and specialist physicians (by specialty) in the 306 hospital referral regions in the United States to the corresponding supplies of physicians Minneapolis and Wichita hospital referral regions and to the workforce employed by a large West Coast health maintenance organization. With each map is a chart giving the number of hospital referral regions in the United States with workforces in excess of the three benchmarks; the percentage of the population of the United States which lives in hospital referral regions with workforces in excess of the benchmarks; and the estimated number of excess physicians in the United States workforce, if the rate in the benchmark were the rate in all regions with supplies of physicians higher than the benchmark (and rates in regions with lower supplies of physicians than the benchmark stayed the same).

Table A contains information on the supplies of generalists and selected specialists in each of the 306 hospital referral regions. Any one of these can be used as a benchmark; for example, demographically similar regions might be compared in order to assess differences in physician supply, and to make estimates similar to those included in the series of maps.

Table B contains, for the 306 hospital referral regions in the United States, the numbers of physicians per 100,000 residents in 12 specialties: anesthesiology, cardiology, emergency care, general surgery, neurosurgery, obstetrics/gynecology, ophthalmology, orthopedic surgery, pathology, radiology, and urology.

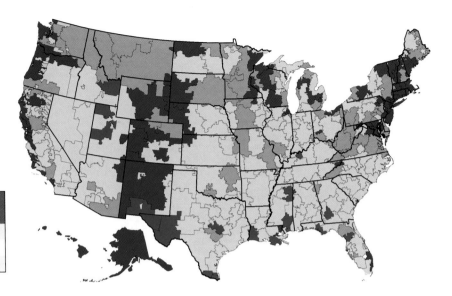

Map A.1. Generalists

Benchmark	# Regions Higher	% U.S. Population	Excess Physicians
Minneapolis	75	32.1%	9,951
Wichita	137	54.7%	17,704
HMO	288	97.8%	49,600

Regions Where Workforce Exceeds

Benchmarks for Generalists (1996)

- Greater Than Minneapolis HRR (67.9/100,000 Residents)
- Greater Than Wichita HRR (61.2/100,000 Residents)
- Greater Than HMO (46.2/100,000 Enrollees)
- Less Than or Equal to HMO
- Not Populated

Map A.1.

Seventy-five hospital referral regions (32.1% of the population of the United States in 1995) had per capita generalist workforces that were higher than the per capita supply of generalists in the Minneapolis hospital referral region. If regions with higher rates had reduced their generalist physician supplies to the level in Minneapolis (and regions with lower supplies of generalists had remained the same), there would have been a surplus of 9,951 generalist physicians in the United States. Using the Wichita benchmark predicts a surplus of 17,704 generalists. Only 18 hospital referral regions in the United States had per capita supplies of generalists lower than the staffing level of the HMO.

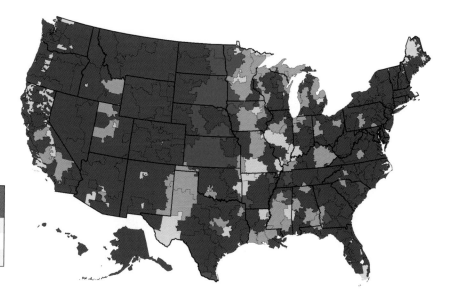

Map A.2. Selected Specialists

Benchmark	# Regions Higher	% U.S. Population	Excess Physicians
Minneapolis	225	84.7%	55,395
HMO	275	95.2%	72,898
Wichita	288	97.1%	83,066

Regions Where Workforce Exceeds

Benchmarks for Selected Specialists (1996)

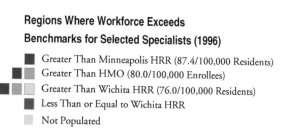

Greater Than Minneapolis HRR (87.4/100,000 Residents)

Greater Than HMO (80.0/100,000 Enrollees)

Greater Than Wichita HRR (76.0/100,000 Residents)

Less Than or Equal to Wichita HRR

Not Populated

Map A.2.

The majority of hospital referral regions in the United States had higher per capita specialist physician workforces than any of the benchmarks. Two hundred twenty-five regions had higher supplies of specialists than the Minneapolis hospital referral region; 275 had higher supplies than the HMO workforce; and 288 of 306 had higher supplies than the Wichita hospital referral region. Almost 85% of the population of the United States lived in regions with higher per capita supplies of specialists than the Minneapolis hospital referral region; more than 95% of the population lived in regions with higher per capita supplies of specialists than those enrolled in the health maintenance organization; and nearly the entire population (97.1%) lived in regions with higher per capita specialist workforces than the specialist workforce allocated to the Wichita hospital referral region. There would have been a surplus of 83,066 specialist physicians in the United States, if the specialist workforce in all regions with higher rates had been reduced to the level of the Wichita benchmark.

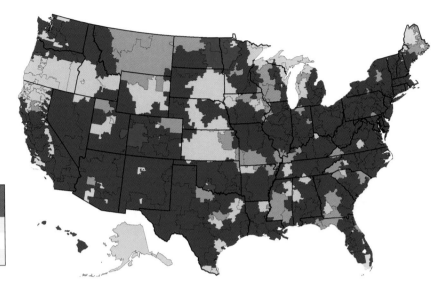

Map A.3. Cardiologists

Benchmark	# Regions Higher	% U.S. Population	Excess Physicians
Minneapolis	221	87.2%	5,641
Wichita	261	93.8%	7,062
HMO	301	99.5%	9,435

Regions Where Workforce Exceeds
Benchmarks for Cardiologists (1996)

- Greater Than Minneapolis HRR (3.8/100,000 Residents)
- Greater Than Wichita HRR (3.2/100,000 Residents)
- Greater Than HMO (2.3/100,000 Enrollees)
- Less Than or Equal to HMO
- Not Populated

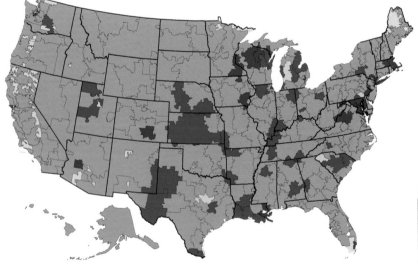

Regions Where Workforce Exceeds
Benchmarks for Neurologists (1996)

- Greater Than Minneapolis HRR (4.23/100,000 Residents)
- Greater Than HMO (1.84/100,000 Enrolleess)
- Greater Than Wichita HRR (1.78/100,000 Residents)
- Less Than or Equal to Wichita HRR
- Not Populated

Map A.4. Neurologists

Benchmark	# Regions Higher	% U.S. Population	Excess Physicians
Minneapolis	25	13.5%	527
HMO	258	92.0%	3,832
Wichita	263	93.1%	3,982

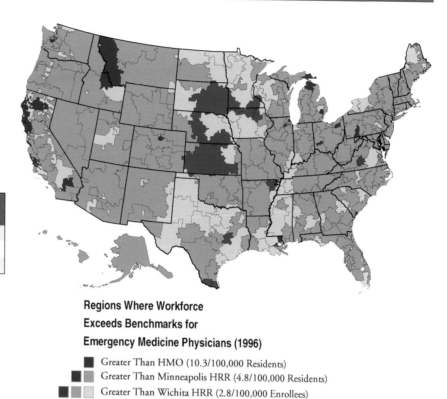

Map A.5. Emergency Medicine Physicians

Benchmark	# Regions Higher	% U.S. Population	Excess Physicians
HMO	17	2.8%	134
Minneapolis	235	80.2%	4,727
Wichita	294	98.2%	9,408

Regions Where Workforce
Exceeds Benchmarks for
Emergency Medicine Physicians (1996)

- Greater Than HMO (10.3/100,000 Residents)
- Greater Than Minneapolis HRR (4.8/100,000 Residents)
- Greater Than Wichita HRR (2.8/100,000 Enrollees)
- Less Than or Equal to Wichita HRR
- Not Populated

Maps A.3., A.4., A.5.

The majority of hospital referral regions in the United States had higher numbers of cardiologists and emergency medicine specialists than the Minneapolis and Wichita hospital referral regions, although only 17 regions had higher per capita supplies of emergency medicine physicians than the HMO. Only 25 regions had higher per capita supplies of neurologists than the Minneapolis hospital referral region, but more than 90% of the population of the United States lived in hospital referral regions with higher per capita supplies of neurologists than the levels of the HMO and Wichita benchmarks. Estimates of the surplus number of cardiologists in the United States ranged from 5,641 (compared to the Minneapolis benchmark) to 9,435 (compared to the HMO benchmark.) Estimates of the surplus number of neurologists ranged from 527 (compared to the Minneapolis benchmark) to almost 4,000 (compared to the Wichita benchmark). Compared to the HMO benchmark, the United States had a surplus of only 134 emergency medicine specialists; but compared to the Wichita benchmark, there was a surplus of 9,408 emergency medicine doctors.

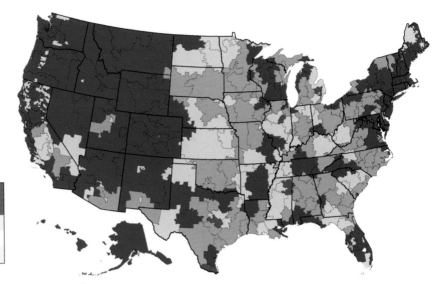

Map A.6. Orthopedic Surgeons

Benchmark	# Regions Higher	% U.S. Population	Excess Physicians
Minneapolis	146	54.4%	1,855
Wichita	244	84.0%	3,646
HMO	299	98.7%	6,768

Regions Where Workforce Exceeds

Benchmarks for Orthopedic Surgeons (1996)

- Greater Than Minneapolis HRR (6.8/100,000 Residents)
- Greater Than Wichita HRR (5.8/100,000 Residents)
- Greater Than HMO (4.5/100,000 Enrollees)
- Less Than or Equal to HMO
- Not Populated

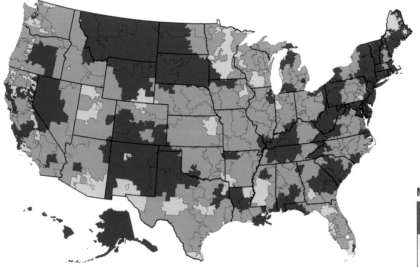

Map A.7 General Surgeons

Benchmark	# Regions Higher	% U.S. Population	Excess Physicians
Wichita	114	35.3%	1,331
Minneapolis	275	93.9%	5,196
HMO	306	100.0%	11,495

Regions Where Workforce Exceeds

Benchmarks for General Surgeons (1996)

- Greater Than Wichita HRR (9.1/100,000 Residents)
- Greater Than Minneapolis HRR (6.9/100,000 Residents)
- Greater Than HMO (4.4/100,000 Enrollees)
- Less Than or Equal to HMO
- Not Populated

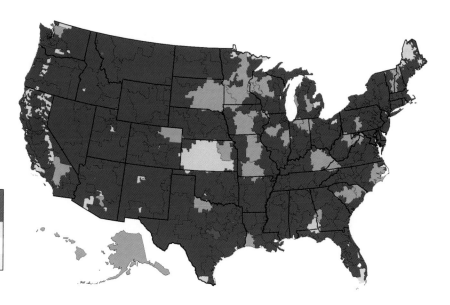

Map A.8. Neurosurgeons

Benchmark	# Regions Higher	% U.S. Population	Excess Physicians
Minneapolis	264	89.3%	1,112
Wichita	299	98.5%	1,906
HMO	305	99.9%	2,662

Regions Where Workforce Exceeds

Benchmarks for Neurosurgeons (1996)

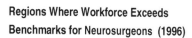

Greater Than Minneapolis HRR (1.0/100,000 Residents)

Greater Than Wichita HRR (0.7/100,000 Residents)

Greater Than HMO (0.4/100,000 Enrollees)

Less Than or Equal to HMO

Not Populated

Maps A.6., A.7., A.8.

The orthopedic, general, and neurologic surgery workforces in almost all regions of the United States exceeded the HMO benchmark. The supply of surgeons in all three specialties was substantially above the number in the benchmarks, ranging from an estimated 1,112 surplus neurosurgeons, compared to the Minneapolis hospital referral region, to 11,495 general surgeons compared to the HMO benchmark. 98.7% of the population of the United States lived in regions with higher supplies of orthopedic surgeons than were employed by the HMO; 99.9% lived in regions with higher supplies of neurosurgeons than were employed by the HMO; and 100% lived in regions with higher supplies of general surgeons than were employed by the HMO.

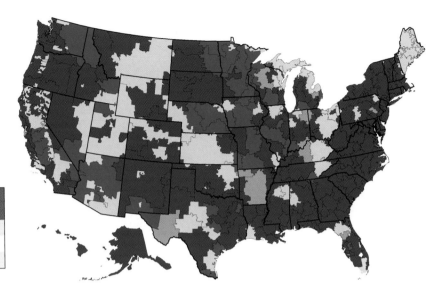

Map A.9. Urologists

Benchmark	# Regions Higher	% U.S. Population	Excess Physicians
HMO	211	74.2%	1,366
Wichita	221	76.9%	1,494
Minneapolis	265	88.9%	2,044

Regions Where Workforce Exceeds

Benchmarks for Urologists (1996)

■ Greater Than HMO (2.8/100,000 Enrollees)

■ Greater Than Wichita HRR (2.7/100,000 Residents)

■ Greater Than Minneapolis HRR (2.5/100,000 Residents)

■ Less Than or Equal to Minneapolis HRR

☐ Not Populated

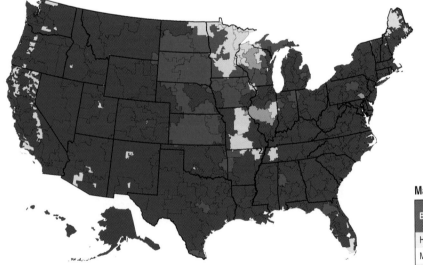

Regions Where Workforce

Exceeds Benchmarks for

Obstertrics/Gynecologists (1996)

■ Greater Than HMO (8.8/100,000 Enrollees)

■ Greater Than Minneapolis HRR (8.6/100,000 Residents)

■ Greater Than Wichita HRR (8.1/100,000 Residents)

■ Less Than or Equal to Wichita HRR

☐ Not Populated

Map A.10. Obstetrics/Gynecologists

Benchmark	# Regions Higher	% U.S. Population	Excess Physicians
HMO	260	91.8%	8,484
Minneapolis	263	92.4%	9,023
Wichita	274	95.0%	10,127

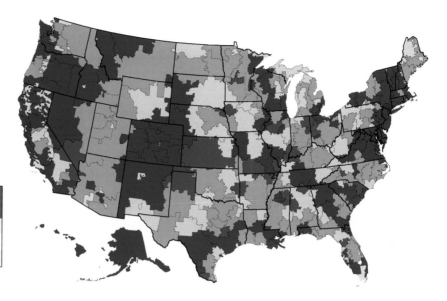

Map A.11. Ophthalmologists

Benchmark	# Regions Higher	% U.S. Population	Excess Physicians
Minneapolis	135	58.1%	2,239
HMO	225	85.1%	3,708
Wichita	283	95.9%	5,715

Regions Where Worforce Exceeds

Benchmarks for Opththalmologists (1996)

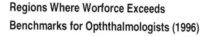

■ Greater Than Minneapolis HRR (5.3/100,000 Residents)
■ Greater Than HMO (4.5/100,000 Enrollees)
■ Greater Than Wichita HRR (3.7/100,000 Residents)
■ Less Than or Equal to Wichita HRR
■ Not Populated

Maps A.9., A.10., A.11.

The majority of Americans lived in regions with higher supplies of urologists, obstetrician/gynecologists, and ophthalmologists than any of the benchmarks. The HMO employed more urologists and obstetrician/gynecologists than either the Minneapolis or the Wichita hospital referral regions, and substantially more ophthalmologists were deployed to the residents of the Minneapolis hospital referral region than to the enrollees of the HMO or the residents of the Wichita hospital referral region. All three benchmarks predict substantial excess capacity in obstetrics/gynecology.

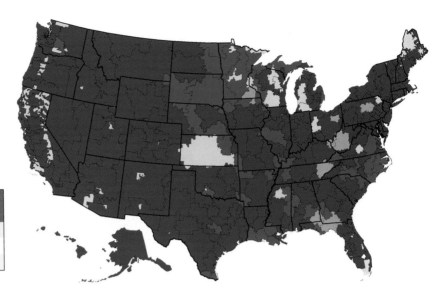

Map A.12. Anesthesiologists

Benchmark	# Regions Higher	% U.S. Population	Excess Physicians
HMO	234	85.5%	7,135
Wichita	243	87.6%	7,714
Minneapolis	255	90.3%	8,423

Regions Where Workforce Exceeds Benchmarks for Anesthesiologists (1996)

- Greater Than HMO (7.8/100,000 Enrollees)
- Greater Than Wichita HRR (7.6/100,000 Residents)
- Greater Than Minneapolis HRR (7.3/100,000 Residents)
- Less Than or Equal to Minneapolis HRR
- Not Populated

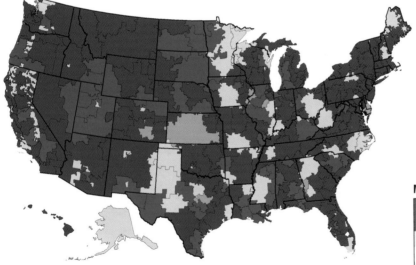

Map A.13. Radiologists

Benchmark	# Regions Higher	% U.S. Population	Excess Physicians
Wichita	200	75.8%	4,472
Minneapolis	207	76.9%	4,540
HMO	241	87.5%	5,516

Regions Where Workforce Exceeds Benchmarks for Radiologists (1996)

- Greater Than Wichita HRR (7.3/100,000 Residents)
- Greater Than Minneapolis HRR (7.2/100,000 Residents)
- Greater Than HMO (6.8/100,000 Enrollees)
- Less Than or Equal to HMO
- Not Populated

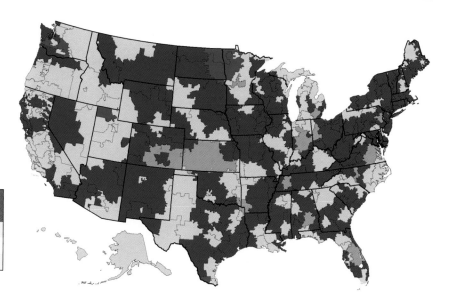

Map A.14. Pathologists

Benchmark	# Regions Higher	% U.S. Population	Excess Physicians
Wichita	171	68.0%	2,404
Minneapolis	185	73.2%	2,677
HMO	300	99.2%	6,573

Regions Where Workforce Exceeds
Benchmarks for Pathologists (1996)

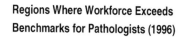

■ Greater Than Wichita HRR (3.9/100,000 Residents)
■ ■ Greater Than Minneapolis HRR (3.7/100,000 Residents)
■ ■ ■ Greater Than HMO (2.1/100,000 Enrollees)
■ Less Than or Equal to HMO
☐ Not Populated

Maps A.12., A.13., A.14.

Virtually all regions of the United States, and nearly its entire population, lived in regions with higher per capita supplies of pathologists than were employed by the HMO; benchmarking the national supply of pathologists to the HMO predicts a surplus of 6,573 full time equivalents. The Minneapolis hospital referral region's supply of anesthesiologists was somewhat higher than the HMO's, but all three benchmarks predict an excess supply of anesthesiologists of more than 7,000 full time equivalents (8,423 compared to the Minneapolis benchmark). The three benchmarks also predict a substantial surplus of radiologists.

PHYSICIAN APPENDIX TABLE A   This table contains the rates of full time equivalent physicians in "selected specialties" and generalists. (Selected specialists are those specialists actually employed by the health maintenance organization. The category therefore does not include such specialties as forensic pathology. See the endnote for further information.) All rates are age and sex adjusted and corrected for out of area use. See the Appendix on Methods for details.

The data in this table provide benchmarks for each hospital referral region. The benchmarks are used to answer the question: If all regions with higher workforce rates were brought down to the rate of the benchmark region, and all regions with rates below the benchmark remained the same, how many excess physicians would there have been in the United States in 1996? For example, if in 1996 the supply of generalists in all regions with more generalists per 100,000 than were allocated to the Birmingham, Alabama hospital referral region had been reduced to the level of the Birmingham benchmark, the calculated surplus number of generalists in the United States would be 28,816.

This approach to benchmarking was used in developing the workforce maps in this appendix (Physician Appendix Maps A.1-A.14). The benchmark question can, of course, be framed differently. One strategy poses the obverse question: if all regions with lower rates were brought up to the benchmark (and those with higher rates were left the same), how many additional physicians would be required? And the benchmark question can also be framed in another way: If all regions with higher rates were brought down to the benchmark, and all those with lower rates were brought up to the benchmark, how many physicians would there be in excess (or deficit) of the current supply of clinically active physicians in the United States? The data provided in the computer disks accompanying this edition of the Atlas make it possible to calculate, using any of the above strategies, the surpluses or deficits in the physicians workforces in any hospital referral region. The same methods can be applied to calculate the excess or deficit in the rates of hospitalization, surgical procedures, and resource allocation rates contained in the database.

PHYSICIAN APPENDIX TABLE A

Benchmarks for Clinically Active Generalists and Selected Specialists in the 306 Hospital Referral Regions in the United States (1996)

Hospital Referral Region	Rate of Generalists	Rank of Region	Excess Generalists in U.S. according to HRR Benchmark	Rate of Selected Specialists	Rank of Region	Excess Selected Specialists in U.S. according to HRR Benchmark
Alabama						
Birmingham	54.88	217	28,816	90.3	189	49,447
Dothan	53.02	244	32,839	84.1	250	63,045
Huntsville	54.30	226	30,023	80.4	273	71,975
Mobile	51.34	259	36,829	99.7	128	32,638
Montgomery	49.59	272	41,063	82.2	259	67,575
Tuscaloosa	56.64	194	25,341	87.2	230	56,008
Alaska						
Anchorage	72.96	42	6,576	101.9	112	29,507
Arizona						
Mesa	52.96	246	32,984	87.3	228	55,611
Phoenix	59.48	158	20,328	103.9	98	26,864
Sun City	64.35	105	13,426	121.4	40	11,720
Tucson	63.26	118	14,810	102.7	107	28,407
Arkansas						
Fort Smith	57.74	185	23,293	78.8	280	76,083
Jonesboro	53.92	235	30,821	72.5	296	92,284
Little Rock	57.73	188	23,310	93.6	169	42,997
Springdale	58.42	174	22,100	78.9	279	75,767
Texarkana	53.45	239	31,874	75.9	290	83,434
California						
Orange Co.	73.12	40	6,489	121.7	39	11,572
Bakersfield	49.55	273	41,173	86.1	236	58,342
Chico	55.30	207	27,972	104.6	96	26,086
Contra Costa Co.	69.25	61	8,949	128.5	31	8,465
Fresno	54.57	220	29,457	87.5	224	55,281
Los Angeles	64.87	98	12,816	115.1	53	15,690
Modesto	54.33	225	29,948	84.9	241	61,130
Napa	89.04	9	997	143.6	18	3,269
Alameda Co.	82.16	24	2,446	122.7	37	11,083
Palm Spr/Rancho Mir	55.47	206	27,628	125.4	35	9,811
Redding	68.45	70	9,551	106.3	85	24,042
Sacramento	64.95	97	12,731	105.3	92	25,180
Salinas	60.44	144	18,841	117.8	48	13,896
San Bernardino	49.76	271	40,645	81.9	263	68,355
San Diego	61.12	140	17,822	115.8	52	15,253
San Francisco	102.10	3	37	157.7	7	670
San Jose	69.17	62	9,001	111.9	64	18,491
San Luis Obispo	77.60	30	4,387	137.9	23	5,115
San Mateo Co.	72.30	45	6,958	140.5	21	4,228
Santa Barbara	73.34	39	6,373	125.6	34	9,752

Hospital Referral Region	Rate of Generalists	Rank of Region	Excess Generalists in U.S. according to HRR Benchmark	Rate of Selected Specialists	Rank of Region	Excess Selected Specialists in U.S. according to HRR Benchmark
Santa Cruz	73.92	37	6,079	133.7	24	6,557
Santa Rosa	84.08	18	1,807	130.9	25	7,518
Stockton	50.25	266	39,446	89.7	194	50,637
Ventura	68.45	69	9,548	119.0	46	13,120
Colorado						
Boulder	85.01	11	1,594	129.7	29	7,988
Colorado Springs	58.99	165	21,142	101.9	111	29,433
Denver	69.10	64	9,055	114.7	57	16,043
Fort Collins	61.76	135	16,898	97.8	140	35,616
Grand Junction	71.27	50	7,593	100.9	121	30,836
Greeley	62.57	128	15,757	97.8	141	35,631
Pueblo	70.85	53	7,860	106.9	82	23,430
Connecticut						
Bridgeport	83.16	20	2,091	153.5	11	1,054
Hartford	68.31	72	9,655	130.6	26	7,625
New Haven	74.60	34	5,742	140.7	20	4,177
Delaware						
Wilmington	65.51	89	12,169	105.5	89	24,933
District of Columbia						
Washington	84.52	15	1,681	157.8	6	662
Florida						
Bradenton	48.35	280	44,174	102.7	106	28,407
Clearwater	63.91	110	13,968	111.4	65	18,925
Fort Lauderdale	68.38	71	9,603	130.1	28	7,795
Fort Myers	54.46	222	29,682	106.3	84	24,015
Gainesville	61.79	134	16,854	93.6	170	43,089
Hudson	55.03	213	28,497	97.3	144	36,565
Jacksonville	59.90	152	19,662	105.8	88	24,667
Lakeland	48.80	278	43,043	88.3	209	53,459
Miami	83.00	21	2,141	129.2	30	8,189
Ocala	45.58	291	51,264	91.8	182	46,587
Orlando	53.99	231	30,669	97.0	147	37,034
Ormond Beach	54.92	216	28,729	95.0	157	40,533
Panama City	45.17	292	52,311	89.7	195	50,727
Pensacola	58.55	171	21,883	102.7	105	28,384
Sarasota	61.36	137	17,469	128.0	32	8,692
St Petersburg	68.95	67	9,165	113.0	62	17,524
Tallahassee	57.73	187	23,309	88.2	211	53,720
Tampa	59.99	151	19,530	105.4	90	25,069
Georgia						
Albany	40.59	301	64,179	74.4	294	87,216
Atlanta	56.57	196	25,471	101.3	115	30,261
Augusta	56.57	195	25,469	107.7	77	22,547
Columbus	52.01	253	35,214	81.0	269	70,465
Macon	58.31	178	22,292	98.1	137	35,265
Rome	63.16	119	14,942	88.5	206	53,123

Hospital Referral Region	Rate of Generalists	Rank of Region	Excess Generalists in U.S. according to HRR Benchmark	Rate of Selected Specialists	Rank of Region	Excess Selected Specialists in U.S. according to HRR Benchmark
Savannah	54.18	229	30,274	102.1	109	29,152
Hawaii						
Honolulu	75.76	32	5,211	114.8	56	15,998
Idaho						
Boise	51.05	262	37,517	94.7	160	40,992
Idaho Falls	37.88	302	71,248	84.4	248	62,410
Illinois						
Aurora	45.05	293	52,613	82.4	258	67,116
Blue Island	67.00	79	10,784	103.0	102	28,080
Chicago	84.47	16	1,693	120.1	42	12,452
Elgin	51.81	257	35,684	90.1	191	49,784
Evanston	98.14	5	178	156.0	9	800
Hinsdale	88.98	10	1,006	143.8	17	3,213
Joliet	54.75	219	29,086	100.7	124	31,196
Melrose Park	81.21	25	2,815	121.8	38	11,514
Peoria	53.34	241	32,110	83.7	252	64,122
Rockford	52.80	248	33,364	89.6	196	50,829
Springfield	51.99	254	35,274	79.7	278	73,709
Urbana	56.49	198	25,626	89.5	197	50,960
Bloomington	50.19	269	39,599	83.7	251	63,921
Indiana						
Evansville	53.84	236	30,994	78.3	284	77,352
Fort Wayne	48.22	282	44,500	74.3	295	87,625
Gary	50.57	265	38,676	84.6	242	61,777
Indianapolis	58.95	166	21,205	97.5	143	36,232
Lafayette	46.37	288	49,227	82.8	257	66,189
Muncie	59.04	164	21,053	88.2	212	53,799
Munster	58.35	177	22,218	88.4	208	53,326
South Bend	55.86	200	26,857	80.5	272	71,874
Terre Haute	55.20	209	28,165	87.5	221	55,134
Iowa						
Cedar Rapids	51.26	260	37,018	83.1	254	65,448
Davenport	52.87	247	33,195	92.5	178	45,244
Des Moines	63.31	117	14,739	80.1	275	72,864
Dubuque	48.86	277	42,881	90.3	190	49,461
Iowa City	58.46	173	22,038	99.2	130	33,467
Mason City	64.06	108	13,784	74.8	293	86,261
Sioux City	52.45	250	34,190	66.5	304	107,711
Waterloo	60.16	147	19,267	76.4	288	82,157
Kansas						
Topeka	52.06	252	35,108	91.7	183	46,732
Wichita	61.20	138	17,704	76.0	289	83,066
Kentucky						
Covington	58.65	169	21,705	89.7	193	50,596
Lexington	57.45	190	23,831	84.4	247	62,409
Louisville	59.64	156	20,075	103.0	101	27,982

Hospital Referral Region	Rate of Generalists	Rank of Region	Excess Generalists in U.S. according to HRR Benchmark	Rate of Selected Specialists	Rank of Region	Excess Selected Specialists in U.S. according to HRR Benchmark
Owensboro	40.91	300	63,343	87.5	223	55,232
Paducah	50.25	267	39,460	80.6	271	71,490
Louisiana						
Alexandria	59.46	159	20,370	94.1	163	42,227
Baton Rouge	52.67	249	33,666	86.9	231	56,477
Houma	36.97	303	73,608	88.9	200	52,305
Lafayette	48.16	283	44,645	81.9	262	68,309
Lake Charles	43.94	295	55,483	83.0	255	65,630
Metairie	68.46	68	9,542	158.6	5	632
Monroe	49.89	270	40,330	80.0	276	73,096
New Orleans	59.43	161	20,404	138.6	22	4,889
Shreveport	47.94	284	45,197	97.0	148	37,042
Slidell	46.72	287	48,334	105.4	91	25,085
Maine						
Bangor	65.36	90	12,312	94.3	161	41,800
Portland	73.00	41	6,554	111.4	66	18,946
Maryland						
Baltimore	82.65	23	2,263	145.6	16	2,697
Salisbury	62.64	126	15,651	114.6	58	16,154
Takoma Park	92.25	7	656	156.4	8	764
Massachusetts						
Boston	84.67	12	1,644	151.4	12	1,346
Springfield	71.87	47	7,221	114.9	55	15,862
Worcester	81.18	26	2,826	117.6	49	14,025
Michigan						
Ann Arbor	66.28	81	11,435	105.9	86	24,502
Dearborn	60.86	142	18,199	97.7	142	35,890
Detroit	61.19	139	17,713	99.0	132	33,788
Flint	71.64	48	7,361	78.8	281	76,099
Grand Rapids	57.42	192	23,877	84.5	245	62,179
Kalamazoo	60.22	146	19,173	93.2	173	43,767
Lansing	67.98	75	9,927	93.3	172	43,569
Marquette	59.51	157	20,276	82.9	256	65,938
Muskegon	63.70	113	14,239	82.1	260	67,876
Petoskey	65.25	92	12,425	91.5	185	47,048
Pontiac	84.20	17	1,772	146.5	15	2,435
Royal Oak	102.91	2	23	160.9	3	563
Saginaw	59.86	153	19,731	85.1	240	60,810
St Joseph	58.08	180	22,691	93.9	167	42,479
Traverse City	70.13	56	8,338	98.9	133	33,880
Minnesota						
Duluth	69.36	60	8,869	86.3	235	58,006
Minneapolis	67.95	76	9,951	87.4	226	55,395
Rochester	70.43	54	8,139	110.5	70	19,718
St Cloud	64.58	101	13,154	77.2	287	80,097
St Paul	80.43	28	3,143	91.9	181	46,239

Hospital Referral Region	Rate of Generalists	Rank of Region	Excess Generalists in U.S. according to HRR Benchmark	Rate of Selected Specialists	Rank of Region	Excess Selected Specialists in U.S. according to HRR Benchmark
Mississippi						
Gulfport	46.05	289	50,040	112.9	63	17,601
Hattiesburg	42.59	297	58,984	87.2	229	55,998
Jackson	52.30	251	34,535	85.4	239	60,057
Meridian	54.33	224	29,941	78.1	285	77,880
Oxford	50.20	268	39,572	81.6	265	68,990
Tupelo	46.05	290	50,042	69.6	302	99,651
Missouri						
Cape Girardeau	48.43	279	43,977	79.9	277	73,223
Columbia	59.44	160	20,390	86.0	237	58,592
Joplin	58.39	176	22,151	83.1	253	65,376
Kansas City	65.09	94	12,585	99.5	129	32,970
Springfield	55.72	205	27,134	78.6	282	76,502
St Louis	63.49	116	14,501	104.7	95	25,922
Montana						
Billings	64.96	96	12,716	100.8	122	30,930
Great Falls	61.81	133	16,833	104.4	97	26,287
Missoula	64.26	107	13,535	116.6	50	14,711
Nebraska						
Lincoln	56.33	199	25,939	70.7	300	96,796
Omaha	58.65	170	21,706	88.7	202	52,631
Nevada						
Las Vegas	47.42	286	46,532	88.2	210	53,676
Reno	59.64	155	20,074	107.0	81	23,301
New Hampshire						
Lebanon	74.20	35	5,940	114.3	59	16,364
Manchester	64.44	103	13,319	110.7	68	19,569
New Jersey						
Camden	73.49	38	6,293	126.0	33	9,537
Hackensack	99.92	4	104	173.1	2	294
Morristown	83.75	19	1,908	142.5	19	3,631
New Brunswick	82.78	22	2,216	130.3	27	7,734
Newark	74.71	33	5,694	119.4	45	12,861
Paterson	69.05	66	9,092	104.8	94	25,765
Ridgewood	84.64	14	1,651	159.3	4	610
New Mexico						
Albuquerque	71.01	52	7,755	108.5	74	21,697
New York						
Albany	66.23	82	11,480	118.5	47	13,421
Binghamton	58.54	172	21,894	102.9	103	28,108
Bronx	66.71	80	11,045	113.3	61	17,230
Buffalo	67.07	78	10,717	108.1	76	22,106
Elmira	59.07	163	21,005	113.4	60	17,162
East Long Island	96.35	6	269	154.3	10	949
New York	84.64	13	1,651	150.0	13	1,603
Rochester	72.56	43	6,807	108.3	75	21,906

Hospital Referral Region	Rate of Generalists	Rank of Region	Excess Generalists in U.S. according to HRR Benchmark	Rate of Selected Specialists	Rank of Region	Excess Selected Specialists in U.S. according to HRR Benchmark
Syracuse	57.73	186	23,301	102.0	110	29,292
White Plains	105.06	1	0	200.8	1	0
North Carolina						
Asheville	67.57	77	10,280	101.1	118	30,494
Charlotte	53.20	243	32,422	94.0	165	42,262
Durham	53.56	238	31,612	100.8	123	31,038
Greensboro	55.19	210	28,185	92.9	175	44,307
Greenville	51.95	255	35,348	93.1	174	44,057
Hickory	47.70	285	45,826	80.9	270	70,753
Raleigh	53.94	234	30,773	92.8	176	44,528
Wilmington	53.99	230	30,666	98.8	135	34,017
Winston-Salem	49.10	275	42,290	87.9	217	54,394
North Dakota						
Bismarck	54.41	223	29,784	88.7	204	52,729
Fargo Moorhead -Mn	60.40	145	18,895	68.8	303	101,767
Grand Forks	65.82	86	11,870	71.8	299	93,975
Minot	69.10	63	9,053	88.4	207	53,239
Ohio						
Akron	65.27	91	12,404	101.0	119	30,657
Canton	54.25	227	30,124	84.6	244	61,969
Cincinnati	64.76	100	12,944	110.2	71	20,045
Cleveland	71.03	51	7,742	120.6	41	12,156
Columbus	57.90	184	22,996	87.5	222	55,206
Dayton	55.28	208	28,006	80.3	274	72,308
Elyria	56.56	197	25,496	95.1	155	40,298
Kettering	76.72	31	4,781	116.2	51	14,954
Toledo	63.56	115	14,416	100.1	127	31,987
Youngstown	66.14	83	11,563	95.7	152	39,227
Oklahoma						
Lawton	62.65	125	15,641	81.5	267	69,282
Oklahoma City	57.97	181	22,881	90.8	188	48,508
Tulsa	62.84	124	15,377	87.7	220	54,873
Oregon						
Bend	60.16	148	19,271	101.6	113	29,886
Eugene	70.10	57	8,359	96.8	149	37,450
Medford	62.52	130	15,817	92.2	180	45,795
Portland	68.01	74	9,902	107.6	78	22,637
Salem	57.45	191	23,832	98.0	139	35,414
Pennsylvania						
Allentown	64.00	109	13,856	101.4	114	30,166
Altoona	53.25	242	32,328	84.5	246	62,243
Danville	60.94	141	18,092	94.8	159	40,942
Erie	54.18	228	30,272	93.9	166	42,442
Harrisburg	65.58	87	12,098	93.7	168	42,871
Johnstown	66.05	84	11,647	101.0	120	30,677
Lancaster	59.27	162	20,669	87.7	219	54,866

Hospital Referral Region	Rate of Generalists	Rank of Region	Excess Generalists in U.S. according to HRR Benchmark	Rate of Selected Specialists	Rank of Region	Excess Selected Specialists in U.S. according to HRR Benchmark
Philadelphia	89.39	8	948	147.4	14	2,193
Pittsburgh	64.49	102	13,251	110.6	69	19,638
Reading	62.37	131	16,032	91.4	186	47,205
Sayre	58.11	179	22,639	89.5	198	50,991
Scranton	69.64	59	8,674	104.9	93	25,623
Wilkes-Barre	78.64	29	3,929	107.4	80	22,843
York	64.33	106	13,445	86.6	233	57,261
Rhode Island						
Providence	72.40	44	6,902	122.7	36	11,068
South Carolina						
Charleston	57.90	183	22,994	108.7	73	21,545
Columbia	55.09	211	28,378	95.9	151	38,926
Florence	50.93	263	37,807	72.0	298	93,535
Greenville	58.84	167	21,389	94.2	162	41,984
Spartanburg	51.37	258	36,737	84.6	243	61,779
South Dakota						
Rapid City	71.60	49	7,387	88.6	205	52,957
Sioux Falls	63.63	114	14,326	74.8	292	86,136
Tennessee						
Chattanooga	55.78	203	27,016	92.5	177	45,182
Jackson	54.99	214	28,592	72.1	297	93,183
Johnson City	72.05	46	7,114	103.5	99	27,442
Kingsport	62.54	129	15,800	88.7	203	52,650
Knoxville	60.15	149	19,283	91.0	187	48,063
Memphis	49.50	274	41,288	87.9	215	54,369
Nashville	57.65	189	23,453	98.1	136	35,232
Texas						
Abilene	55.78	202	27,011	88.1	213	53,991
Amarillo	53.98	232	30,695	86.4	234	57,649
Austin	62.58	127	15,737	103.4	100	27,550
Beaumont	55.74	204	27,090	93.5	171	43,238
Bryan	58.73	168	21,574	77.9	286	78,376
Corpus Christi	55.08	212	28,406	87.7	218	54,691
Dallas	53.97	233	30,712	100.3	125	31,703
El Paso	41.61	299	61,527	87.9	216	54,380
Fort Worth	52.96	245	32,976	87.5	225	55,298
Harlingen	34.02	305	81,334	58.1	305	129,698
Houston	53.37	240	32,046	101.2	116	30,384
Longview	48.91	276	42,766	81.7	264	68,862
Lubbock	54.53	221	29,534	87.4	227	55,469
Mcallen	33.78	306	81,956	46.7	306	159,637
Odessa	36.38	304	75,153	78.4	283	77,058
San Angelo	50.72	264	38,317	95.4	153	39,823
San Antonio	55.85	201	26,866	107.5	79	22,761
Temple	44.89	294	53,043	70.4	301	97,511
Tyler	57.91	182	22,987	95.1	154	40,278

Hospital Referral Region	Rate of Generalists	Rank of Region	Excess Generalists in U.S. according to HRR Benchmark	Rate of Selected Specialists	Rank of Region	Excess Selected Specialists in U.S. according to HRR Benchmark
Victoria	54.93	215	28,712	90.1	192	49,917
Waco	54.86	218	28,852	86.0	238	58,656
Wichita Falls	60.06	150	19,423	102.4	108	28,777
Utah						
Ogden	41.67	298	61,359	84.1	249	63,014
Provo	43.51	296	56,600	81.6	266	69,200
Salt Lake City	48.31	281	44,271	99.1	131	33,537
Vermont						
Burlington	74.03	36	6,024	106.6	83	23,735
Virginia						
Arlington	70.18	55	8,307	119.6	44	12,739
Charlottesville	63.10	120	15,022	110.7	67	19,528
Lynchburg	53.63	237	31,476	82.0	261	68,101
Newport News	62.33	132	16,088	105.9	87	24,561
Norfolk	63.10	121	15,027	115.1	54	15,754
Richmond	63.72	112	14,212	98.0	138	35,372
Roanoke	62.99	122	15,166	101.2	117	30,435
Winchester	51.23	261	37,075	98.9	134	33,926
Washington						
Everett	65.14	93	12,532	97.1	145	36,861
Olympia	62.98	123	15,188	95.1	156	40,420
Seattle	80.89	27	2,942	119.7	43	12,680
Spokane	65.82	85	11,865	94.9	158	40,671
Tacoma	59.79	154	19,843	102.8	104	28,312
Yakima	63.73	111	14,190	88.1	214	54,013
West Virginia						
Charleston	65.52	88	12,154	89.5	199	51,101
Huntington	61.51	136	17,257	94.1	164	42,239
Morgantown	64.85	99	12,834	97.0	146	36,986
Wisconsin						
Appleton	58.40	175	22,132	75.2	291	85,239
Green Bay	51.92	256	35,419	81.3	268	69,763
La Crosse	60.81	143	18,278	86.8	232	56,720
Madison	69.08	65	9,066	88.8	201	52,562
Marshfield	68.21	73	9,735	91.5	184	47,033
Milwaukee	64.41	104	13,352	109.5	72	20,717
Neenah	56.97	193	24,724	96.4	150	38,109
Wausau	65.04	95	12,641	92.3	179	45,550
Wyoming						
Casper	69.65	58	8,672	100.2	126	31,926
United States						
HMO	46.22	0	49,600	80.1	0	72,898
United States	65.03	0	12,646	108.4	0	21,841

PHYSICIAN APPENDIX TABLE B   This table contains the rates of full time equivalent physicians specializing in anesthesiology, cardiology, emergency care, general surgery, neurosurgery, obstetrics/gynecology, ophthalmology, orthopedic surgery, pathology, radiology, and urology per 100,000 residents of hospital referral regions. All rates are age and sex adjusted and corrected for out of area use. See the Appendix on Methodology for details.

PHYSICIAN APPENDIX TABLE B

Number of Specialists per 100,000 Residents of Hospital Referral Regions (1996)

Hospital Referral Region	Anesthesiologists	Cardiologists	Emergency Medicine Specialists	General Surgeons	Neurosurgeons	Neurologists	Obstetrician/Gynecologists	Ophthalmologists	Orthopedic Surgeons	Pathologists	Radiologists	Urologists
Alabama												
Birmingham	8.1	5.5	5.0	8.4	1.5	2.8	10.3	4.4	6.3	4.2	7.3	3.4
Dothan	7.6	4.1	6.1	9.1	0.6	1.9	10.9	5.2	6.5	4.3	6.5	3.1
Huntsville	8.0	2.6	5.0	7.7	1.6	1.6	10.5	3.2	6.2	2.7	5.9	3.1
Mobile	9.2	5.0	5.0	10.1	1.6	3.8	12.4	5.1	7.6	5.8	9.1	3.0
Montgomery	6.0	4.6	3.9	11.2	1.5	1.8	8.9	4.8	6.4	3.9	5.7	3.2
Tuscaloosa	4.9	2.9	4.2	8.5	1.5	3.5	7.4	3.4	6.0	2.6	6.7	2.5
Alaska												
Anchorage	9.0	3.2	7.8	10.6	1.0	2.0	9.5	6.6	10.1	2.5	7.0	3.0
Arizona												
Mesa	9.7	4.4	6.5	6.5	0.9	2.0	10.0	5.3	6.0	2.5	5.9	2.5
Phoenix	12.4	6.3	7.3	7.6	1.3	3.4	11.1	5.2	7.3	3.9	7.7	2.3
Sun City	13.5	3.5	6.4	9.2	1.9	4.4	19.7	7.7	12.1	5.0	7.0	2.5
Tucson	12.4	4.6	6.6	6.6	1.6	2.8	12.0	5.0	6.1	3.4	8.1	2.7
Arkansas												
Fort Smith	9.1	4.5	5.3	7.4	1.1	3.1	8.0	3.4	5.3	2.8	6.5	3.3
Jonesboro	6.2	3.7	2.7	8.4	1.6	2.0	8.4	3.6	5.6	5.8	7.1	3.2
Little Rock	9.2	4.5	5.0	8.2	1.8	2.6	9.7	5.2	6.9	4.3	8.3	2.8
Springdale	7.1	3.0	5.9	9.2	1.3	1.7	7.8	4.1	5.7	2.2	7.8	2.8
Texarkana	7.2	4.0	5.4	6.3	1.2	1.5	10.0	3.8	5.7	3.8	7.1	3.0
California												
Orange Co.	13.0	7.1	7.3	8.4	1.5	3.5	13.9	6.5	9.1	4.1	9.0	3.6
Bakersfield	9.9	4.1	6.2	7.5	1.1	2.5	11.5	5.5	5.6	3.4	6.4	2.4
Chico	11.2	3.3	8.7	9.2	1.6	2.9	11.9	6.6	9.2	3.2	11.9	3.7
Contra Costa Co.	13.6	5.1	9.0	10.0	1.2	3.9	14.9	8.3	8.6	4.3	10.3	3.8
Fresno	9.5	4.5	5.8	9.3	1.4	2.5	9.7	5.2	5.0	2.5	7.5	1.9
Los Angeles	11.4	7.2	5.7	8.1	1.5	3.4	11.9	6.5	7.2	4.5	8.8	3.3
Modesto	10.2	4.2	6.4	7.1	1.4	2.2	9.8	4.4	6.2	3.1	6.7	2.4
Napa	13.0	5.3	12.0	15.3	1.8	3.2	17.5	7.2	12.0	4.5	12.3	3.7
Alameda Co.	8.6	5.7	9.9	7.8	1.4	4.0	13.1	6.9	8.2	4.8	9.2	3.1
Palm Spr/Rancho Mir	14.0	7.4	11.8	10.3	1.7	2.6	14.6	5.1	10.0	5.4	10.2	3.1
Redding	12.6	2.5	12.4	8.5	2.2	2.7	9.6	5.5	10.3	5.5	10.0	3.4
Sacramento	11.7	4.8	8.0	7.1	1.4	2.9	11.7	5.8	8.0	4.5	8.3	2.6
Salinas	11.4	5.6	6.0	10.5	1.8	2.8	13.1	8.7	8.9	3.3	8.7	4.4
San Bernardino	8.5	4.2	4.6	7.1	1.0	2.1	9.3	4.4	5.8	2.7	6.3	2.7
San Diego	11.9	6.2	7.4	7.5	1.4	3.3	11.3	7.3	8.7	4.3	8.3	3.2
San Francisco	12.7	8.1	11.4	9.3	2.2	5.5	12.1	8.2	9.1	6.0	12.3	3.2
San Jose	9.6	7.1	5.3	7.4	1.5	3.3	14.0	7.1	7.8	3.6	7.7	3.1
San Luis Obispo	12.9	5.6	12.8	9.7	2.5	3.8	10.7	7.5	11.0	3.2	12.5	3.4
San Mateo Co.	12.5	9.4	6.3	7.7	2.0	4.0	13.4	8.1	8.6	6.1	11.0	2.7
Santa Barbara	11.4	6.4	9.6	9.4	1.8	4.0	11.6	6.8	10.6	2.8	10.1	3.2

Hospital Referral Region	Anesthesiologists	Cardiologists	Emergency Medicine Specialists	General Surgeons	Neurosurgeons	Neurologists	Obstetrician/Gynecologists	Ophthalmologists	Orthopedic Surgeons	Pathologists	Radiologists	Urologists
Santa Cruz	14.5	5.3	16.1	7.8	1.7	2.5	13.5	6.8	9.3	2.9	8.1	3.8
Santa Rosa	13.1	5.8	12.8	8.0	1.6	2.9	13.0	7.6	10.5	4.0	8.7	3.5
Stockton	10.1	6.2	4.6	7.2	1.2	1.9	11.7	4.6	7.1	3.0	6.3	1.8
Ventura	11.6	6.4	6.0	8.5	1.9	3.1	11.4	7.7	9.6	3.5	7.5	3.2
Colorado												
Boulder	12.5	2.9	15.8	6.8	1.6	3.1	11.8	10.5	9.0	2.5	7.1	2.9
Colorado Springs	8.2	4.5	8.4	10.3	1.2	2.2	10.1	6.3	8.9	3.8	7.3	2.8
Denver	11.9	5.2	7.2	7.4	1.5	3.1	11.9	6.4	8.6	4.4	8.7	2.6
Fort Collins	9.5	4.7	6.1	6.7	2.0	2.0	9.0	6.8	9.4	2.4	6.4	4.3
Grand Junction	13.3	2.2	8.6	9.3	1.5	3.0	9.5	5.4	11.8	4.7	8.0	2.9
Greeley	10.3	3.6	7.3	9.0	1.0	2.7	11.4	6.9	9.0	3.9	6.4	3.7
Pueblo	8.5	4.1	6.7	8.2	2.0	5.0	10.5	6.6	10.4	4.2	7.2	2.5
Connecticut												
Bridgeport	13.0	7.5	6.1	9.6	3.2	3.8	19.2	9.4	10.4	6.0	11.4	4.1
Hartford	12.0	7.5	5.8	9.6	1.5	2.9	15.7	7.3	9.3	5.0	11.2	3.7
New Haven	11.3	8.1	6.0	10.4	2.0	4.1	16.2	8.0	9.3	6.2	12.3	3.5
Delaware												
Wilmington	7.3	6.3	6.4	9.2	1.9	3.6	10.5	5.8	6.6	3.3	8.5	3.4
District of Columbia												
Washington	12.6	10.1	7.5	10.9	2.0	6.4	17.2	9.3	8.6	8.1	12.3	4.9
Florida												
Bradenton	10.4	6.4	8.0	6.8	1.2	2.7	16.6	4.2	6.0	3.6	8.6	2.8
Clearwater	9.8	5.8	9.1	6.8	1.4	3.5	15.0	4.6	7.7	4.9	12.2	3.2
Fort Lauderdale	12.6	7.4	7.6	9.0	1.7	4.0	16.3	7.2	9.8	5.2	10.3	4.0
Fort Myers	8.9	5.1	8.9	7.3	2.2	3.4	15.3	5.4	7.0	4.8	9.3	2.8
Gainesville	10.6	4.6	5.8	6.5	1.6	3.6	7.4	4.3	5.6	3.3	10.0	2.5
Hudson	8.5	5.2	7.6	6.5	1.5	2.8	15.5	4.3	7.4	5.8	8.4	3.0
Jacksonville	11.0	8.1	7.6	8.2	1.6	2.8	11.2	5.7	6.2	3.9	8.6	4.0
Lakeland	9.3	4.9	5.5	8.0	1.2	2.2	10.7	5.0	5.7	3.0	6.3	2.3
Miami	11.3	10.0	5.7	9.9	1.7	4.3	13.0	7.8	7.6	5.8	10.1	3.9
Ocala	9.1	4.4	6.0	8.0	1.5	2.6	12.4	3.4	5.9	3.4	10.6	2.8
Orlando	10.2	5.1	6.3	7.4	1.2	2.8	12.7	4.9	7.9	3.8	8.0	3.4
Ormond Beach	10.0	3.5	7.4	7.5	1.1	2.2	10.0	5.0	9.9	4.5	9.6	2.8
Panama City	7.2	3.3	3.4	10.1	1.2	2.8	11.6	4.9	7.5	3.1	6.3	3.7
Pensacola	9.7	5.1	7.6	11.3	1.4	2.9	11.2	5.3	7.0	3.6	9.6	2.9
Sarasota	14.3	6.4	9.8	7.9	2.0	2.7	16.3	7.0	10.2	5.1	12.6	3.6
St Petersburg	10.8	6.2	8.0	7.5	1.6	4.5	14.0	5.8	8.2	5.1	13.4	2.9
Tallahassee	7.6	3.8	5.6	8.9	1.8	2.8	9.7	5.0	5.3	4.2	7.5	2.9
Tampa	10.3	6.3	6.5	6.4	1.4	3.9	11.0	5.5	7.2	5.5	9.7	3.0
Georgia												
Albany	5.3	2.7	5.3	6.3	1.8	2.3	8.8	4.3	5.0	2.4	7.1	3.4
Atlanta	9.7	5.4	6.2	7.8	1.2	2.8	13.0	5.3	6.6	3.1	7.0	3.7
Augusta	9.4	7.2	4.3	9.4	2.0	4.0	11.2	4.9	5.5	4.4	9.0	3.5
Columbus	6.6	3.9	3.0	7.4	1.0	1.8	9.3	4.2	8.4	3.9	7.3	2.9
Macon	9.3	3.3	6.4	11.9	1.4	3.0	13.6	5.4	6.3	4.4	8.4	3.6
Rome	8.5	4.0	5.7	9.5	1.5	3.0	14.2	4.0	6.3	2.8	8.0	2.8

Hospital Referral Region	Anesthesiologists	Cardiologists	Emergency Medicine Specialists	General Surgeons	Neurosurgeons	Neurologists	Obstetrician/Gynecologists	Ophthalmologists	Orthopedic Surgeons	Pathologists	Radiologists	Urologists
Savannah	8.5	4.8	7.3	10.7	1.1	2.3	14.8	4.8	6.6	2.9	7.5	3.9
Hawaii												
Honolulu	9.8	4.7	8.2	9.4	0.9	2.9	15.1	7.2	6.9	3.6	8.3	3.0
Idaho												
Boise	8.0	3.2	8.1	8.4	1.7	2.9	10.7	5.4	8.9	2.6	7.7	3.0
Idaho Falls	9.2	2.4	4.8	8.5	2.1	1.9	11.4	5.2	7.2	2.5	5.9	1.8
Illinois												
Aurora	6.7	4.6	2.5	9.0	2.3	1.3	8.9	5.4	7.1	3.1	4.7	2.5
Blue Island	11.4	7.1	6.9	8.8	1.3	3.1	13.4	4.8	6.4	4.0	7.6	2.9
Chicago	9.7	7.8	8.7	8.1	1.7	4.0	13.6	6.1	5.4	6.3	8.8	2.8
Elgin	11.2	4.9	6.7	7.8	1.4	2.2	10.7	5.9	6.4	3.0	4.8	2.6
Evanston	18.7	9.4	10.9	10.6	1.5	5.5	20.7	8.4	9.8	7.1	14.8	4.2
Hinsdale	25.5	12.6	9.8	10.1	2.2	3.0	14.6	6.8	6.3	7.5	16.0	5.1
Joliet	12.1	6.0	8.3	9.8	1.6	2.2	13.5	4.7	6.1	3.3	7.6	2.8
Melrose Park	13.6	7.8	8.8	9.2	1.7	3.7	14.6	6.6	7.2	6.7	8.9	3.8
Peoria	9.9	4.2	6.9	7.5	0.9	2.9	9.5	3.5	5.3	4.2	6.7	3.2
Rockford	10.7	4.5	5.3	7.9	1.6	1.6	10.2	4.6	6.1	4.0	6.5	2.7
Springfield	6.6	4.0	7.1	8.3	1.4	2.5	8.6	3.9	4.8	3.4	6.4	2.4
Urbana	7.9	4.7	7.4	8.0	1.0	3.0	8.3	4.3	4.9	4.4	6.8	3.3
Bloomington	10.9	5.5	6.2	8.3	1.3	2.4	6.4	5.4	4.5	3.5	7.3	2.2
Indiana												
Evansville	9.2	4.2	4.4	8.1	1.5	1.7	8.9	3.3	5.6	2.6	7.2	2.2
Fort Wayne	8.5	4.4	5.2	7.9	1.0	1.8	7.1	3.5	5.2	2.7	7.5	2.7
Gary	8.5	5.5	4.7	8.1	1.8	2.3	10.1	4.2	6.9	3.5	6.6	2.4
Indianapolis	11.4	6.2	6.6	7.3	1.2	3.5	9.3	4.6	6.7	3.9	8.4	2.9
Lafayette	11.4	4.6	5.9	5.7	1.1	2.5	7.4	4.6	5.5	3.7	7.3	2.6
Muncie	11.5	3.3	5.4	8.0	1.7	2.5	6.5	3.7	6.4	7.8	6.5	3.2
Munster	9.5	5.8	4.0	8.6	1.0	2.4	12.4	5.0	5.4	3.4	7.2	2.5
South Bend	9.7	3.8	6.7	7.5	1.0	2.1	9.0	3.7	5.4	3.4	7.3	2.5
Terre Haute	10.7	5.6	4.9	8.0	2.8	2.4	9.9	4.5	6.2	4.2	7.6	2.8
Iowa												
Cedar Rapids	9.1	2.7	6.0	4.7	1.3	2.1	6.6	4.8	7.3	5.1	8.0	2.5
Davenport	10.1	3.5	5.5	9.0	1.5	2.5	10.7	6.2	6.4	4.3	7.3	2.9
Des Moines	9.4	4.0	2.9	8.1	0.9	2.6	7.2	3.8	6.2	4.5	7.2	2.5
Dubuque	5.8	3.3	6.8	8.0	1.0	4.1	8.2	7.0	8.0	4.4	7.5	3.2
Iowa City	9.8	3.9	4.1	7.7	1.6	4.8	9.5	7.2	5.9	6.2	12.5	3.0
Mason City	6.3	3.7	2.6	9.4	1.1	2.5	6.1	4.1	5.9	3.4	8.3	2.2
Sioux City	5.5	3.2	3.3	7.9	1.6	2.4	5.4	2.6	4.9	4.1	6.3	2.6
Waterloo	10.5	2.6	2.6	7.8	0.9	2.3	7.2	3.7	5.4	4.8	6.3	2.2
Kansas												
Topeka	5.6	3.8	4.6	6.7	0.8	2.6	7.9	3.7	5.7	4.7	8.3	2.9
Wichita	7.6	3.2	2.8	9.1	0.7	1.8	8.1	3.7	5.8	3.9	7.3	2.7
Kentucky												
Covington	8.9	2.9	7.5	6.9	1.5	1.2	10.8	4.2	6.1	3.5	7.2	3.0
Lexington	9.2	4.1	4.9	8.8	0.7	2.2	9.0	4.6	5.1	3.7	6.6	2.7
Louisville	12.3	5.1	7.0	9.9	1.5	2.3	10.4	4.8	6.3	4.3	7.6	2.7

Hospital Referral Region	Anesthesiologists	Cardiologists	Emergency Medicine Specialists	General Surgeons	Neurosurgeons	Neurologists	Obstetrician/Gynecologists	Ophthalmologists	Orthopedic Surgeons	Pathologists	Radiologists	Urologists
Owensboro	9.4	3.6	7.1	9.2	3.3	2.2	9.2	3.2	7.2	2.5	8.0	2.8
Paducah	6.8	3.3	4.1	9.7	1.8	1.8	10.6	3.7	5.8	4.6	8.5	3.1
Louisiana												
Alexandria	8.1	6.6	4.4	10.6	1.4	1.4	10.3	5.5	6.6	3.6	6.7	3.9
Baton Rouge	7.0	4.5	4.7	7.4	1.5	2.5	10.8	6.1	5.1	3.0	5.8	3.3
Houma	6.6	8.6	4.3	10.0	1.3	1.3	10.5	5.5	6.5	3.1	4.8	4.8
Lafayette	7.2	4.4	3.3	8.7	1.1	1.6	11.9	5.0	5.6	3.4	6.7	3.7
Lake Charles	5.3	6.7	5.1	7.7	1.0	0.7	11.9	4.7	5.9	4.1	7.3	2.5
Metairie	14.0	9.4	12.9	14.1	2.0	5.4	18.9	11.9	9.0	5.7	12.7	5.8
Monroe	8.4	2.4	5.5	6.5	1.2	2.2	8.9	3.8	6.0	5.4	6.8	3.4
New Orleans	10.1	9.7	7.0	10.9	2.6	5.5	13.4	9.2	9.7	6.8	12.3	4.7
Shreveport	9.2	5.2	5.0	9.8	1.6	2.2	11.7	5.1	6.9	4.2	7.7	3.8
Slidell	11.1	5.2	9.5	9.0	2.4	1.7	13.9	6.7	7.6	5.1	8.7	3.3
Maine												
Bangor	9.2	3.8	8.5	10.1	1.3	2.7	8.9	5.0	8.8	4.0	7.4	2.7
Portland	10.4	4.9	9.4	9.6	1.6	3.0	11.0	5.2	9.7	4.8	8.8	2.7
Maryland												
Baltimore	13.9	8.3	6.2	12.3	2.1	5.3	17.8	7.9	8.5	6.8	11.3	3.7
Salisbury	10.1	6.7	8.2	12.0	1.3	3.4	14.4	6.3	7.7	4.2	7.2	3.1
Takoma Park	14.3	12.5	7.3	11.9	1.4	6.5	16.8	9.7	7.6	9.1	11.1	5.9
Massachusetts												
Boston	14.3	9.3	6.9	10.6	1.8	6.7	14.3	7.7	8.7	7.8	13.9	3.2
Springfield	11.3	6.3	7.7	10.9	1.3	2.8	12.5	5.6	7.4	4.3	9.6	3.1
Worcester	10.5	8.3	10.1	7.9	1.1	5.0	11.7	4.6	7.7	5.0	8.3	3.0
Michigan												
Ann Arbor	8.2	6.0	7.7	8.2	1.1	3.5	10.4	6.2	4.9	3.8	8.6	3.7
Dearborn	7.6	5.1	6.0	9.0	1.4	2.9	14.2	5.9	5.9	4.8	8.4	3.0
Detroit	6.9	6.0	6.7	9.0	1.3	3.4	12.7	5.4	5.7	5.0	8.7	2.4
Flint	8.4	4.8	4.3	8.9	0.7	2.4	7.9	4.2	4.1	3.7	7.9	2.8
Grand Rapids	7.5	2.9	8.2	8.0	1.3	1.8	10.7	4.4	6.4	3.4	6.3	2.8
Kalamazoo	7.5	5.3	7.2	9.9	1.4	3.0	9.4	4.7	6.4	3.1	6.6	2.4
Lansing	8.3	6.6	7.6	7.1	1.0	1.5	9.7	4.6	6.3	4.1	8.4	2.8
Marquette	5.2	3.1	7.7	9.0	1.7	2.7	7.6	3.8	6.2	3.7	7.6	2.7
Muskegon	7.9	3.2	10.2	5.8	1.0	1.7	9.1	4.2	7.4	4.4	6.1	3.2
Petoskey	8.5	2.9	10.8	10.7	1.2	2.3	11.1	4.1	8.3	2.5	7.5	2.6
Pontiac	17.7	8.7	12.1	14.7	1.8	3.3	16.3	8.5	6.0	5.4	13.8	3.9
Royal Oak	12.0	10.3	11.1	12.1	1.1	6.0	21.0	9.4	7.8	7.3	16.2	3.8
Saginaw	9.0	4.1	6.1	8.8	1.7	1.7	10.2	4.6	5.1	3.3	8.0	2.7
St Joseph	9.8	8.0	6.6	9.6	1.1	1.4	11.0	5.2	5.9	2.8	7.8	3.0
Traverse City	8.6	3.6	9.9	9.5	1.2	1.9	10.3	5.1	7.4	3.7	9.8	3.6
Minnesota												
Duluth	6.8	2.9	8.3	7.8	1.5	2.6	8.2	5.6	6.8	4.9	6.9	2.0
Minneapolis	7.3	3.8	4.8	6.9	1.0	4.2	8.6	5.3	6.8	3.7	7.2	2.5
Rochester	7.7	11.0	1.9	8.0	1.4	9.4	7.2	4.8	6.3	5.8	11.8	2.3
St Cloud	7.6	3.7	4.9	7.6	1.1	1.9	7.8	3.6	6.1	3.8	4.9	3.0
St Paul	7.4	4.3	4.7	7.5	1.0	4.4	8.5	6.9	7.8	4.7	6.9	1.9

Hospital Referral Region	Anesthesiologists	Cardiologists	Emergency Medicine Specialists	General Surgeons	Neurosurgeons	Neurologists	Obstetrician/Gynecologists	Ophthalmologists	Orthopedic Surgeons	Pathologists	Radiologists	Urologists
Mississippi												
Gulfport	6.3	4.2	9.2	11.4	2.4	4.2	14.4	6.7	7.4	7.4	8.8	3.8
Hattiesburg	7.9	3.6	5.9	9.0	1.4	3.0	10.0	5.1	6.2	3.4	6.7	3.1
Jackson	9.2	3.3	3.8	6.7	2.1	2.8	9.6	5.1	5.3	5.0	7.2	3.0
Meridian	6.9	4.0	3.2	9.1	2.0	1.9	9.4	4.2	4.8	4.1	6.1	3.0
Oxford	7.5	4.0	5.2	9.9	1.9	1.1	11.3	5.4	5.5	3.6	5.6	2.7
Tupelo	5.6	2.4	3.4	8.9	1.8	2.2	10.1	3.3	4.0	3.2	5.3	2.5
Missouri												
Cape Girardeau	7.1	3.7	5.2	9.6	1.4	3.3	8.8	3.4	4.7	3.7	6.5	2.6
Columbia	7.8	3.9	5.2	8.2	0.8	2.3	8.4	4.3	6.6	5.6	7.5	2.4
Joplin	6.7	3.6	6.5	9.0	1.5	1.5	12.8	4.6	6.1	2.7	7.5	2.0
Kansas City	9.4	5.1	6.9	7.5	1.2	3.0	10.1	5.8	6.4	4.8	8.0	2.9
Springfield	7.9	3.3	6.9	8.0	1.0	2.5	8.2	3.4	5.7	3.3	7.1	2.3
St Louis	9.6	6.0	5.3	9.1	1.5	3.9	13.0	5.7	6.9	5.8	9.6	2.8
Montana												
Billings	10.5	3.7	7.2	10.0	1.1	2.8	11.4	4.8	9.3	4.4	8.5	2.7
Great Falls	11.5	3.4	7.7	9.9	3.3	2.8	11.8	5.4	8.6	2.9	9.6	3.4
Missoula	13.0	4.3	11.1	11.2	2.6	2.9	11.1	6.5	10.9	4.9	9.1	3.5
Nebraska												
Lincoln	6.3	2.8	2.5	7.7	1.1	1.6	6.3	4.1	5.3	3.4	5.7	2.1
Omaha	8.1	5.6	3.5	8.5	1.1	2.7	9.1	5.1	6.2	5.6	8.6	2.2
Nevada												
Las Vegas	11.3	5.8	6.3	7.1	1.1	2.7	10.4	3.7	5.2	2.4	7.7	2.4
Reno	13.7	5.3	8.6	10.4	1.5	2.8	11.9	6.3	8.3	4.6	7.4	2.9
New Hampshire												
Lebanon	10.8	4.6	8.0	10.6	1.0	3.9	10.2	5.7	7.7	5.9	7.5	2.9
Manchester	8.8	6.3	7.8	8.8	1.3	3.7	12.5	5.7	9.4	3.5	7.0	3.1
New Jersey												
Camden	12.3	8.7	6.6	10.9	1.3	3.6	16.6	6.6	7.9	4.3	10.3	4.0
Hackensack	21.1	11.6	5.8	12.4	1.4	6.1	20.9	9.8	8.6	6.7	13.2	4.7
Morristown	13.8	9.7	6.6	11.8	1.1	3.9	18.4	9.0	9.4	5.0	13.2	4.4
New Brunswick	12.5	10.1	5.7	9.4	1.2	3.9	16.1	7.2	7.9	5.0	9.0	3.9
Newark	10.4	8.3	3.6	10.1	1.2	3.9	14.5	7.8	7.3	5.2	8.5	4.4
Paterson	8.5	7.2	3.5	10.0	0.6	2.9	12.7	6.6	7.0	3.9	5.6	3.9
Ridgewood	17.1	11.2	4.8	11.3	1.6	4.2	19.7	9.1	9.4	4.7	11.0	4.6
New Mexico												
Albuquerque	9.9	4.5	8.7	9.2	1.4	2.6	11.2	5.9	8.6	4.4	7.5	3.0
New York												
Albany	11.3	6.3	7.1	9.9	1.5	3.5	12.7	6.2	7.4	5.1	10.2	3.9
Binghamton	8.9	4.5	6.5	9.9	1.4	1.7	11.9	5.3	7.4	3.4	9.1	3.0
Bronx	8.2	7.6	2.9	8.7	1.0	4.2	10.6	6.2	3.9	4.9	8.7	3.5
Buffalo	10.4	5.6	4.7	12.7	1.9	3.4	12.5	5.6	5.9	6.0	10.2	3.9
Elmira	12.1	3.8	6.2	11.4	1.8	2.7	13.9	4.8	7.8	4.0	9.8	3.7
East Long Island	15.1	9.1	5.0	12.4	1.3	5.2	19.3	9.2	8.2	6.5	12.3	4.5
New York	10.4	9.9	3.2	10.9	1.4	6.2	13.5	8.6	5.6	6.3	10.6	4.0
Rochester	11.6	5.8	3.3	8.9	1.1	3.3	14.1	6.7	7.2	4.4	9.6	2.9

Hospital Referral Region	Anesthesiologists	Cardiologists	Emergency Medicine Specialists	General Surgeons	Neurosurgeons	Neurologists	Obstetrician/Gynecologists	Ophthalmologists	Orthopedic Surgeons	Pathologists	Radiologists	Urologists
Syracuse	11.5	5.7	5.0	9.1	1.3	2.4	11.9	5.2	8.1	4.5	10.1	3.4
White Plains	19.2	10.7	6.5	15.4	1.8	5.4	22.7	12.1	9.7	6.8	14.8	5.4
North Carolina												
Asheville	8.4	3.5	9.1	9.7	1.1	2.1	10.4	4.8	9.6	3.3	10.0	3.6
Charlotte	7.0	4.2	8.2	8.2	1.1	2.5	12.1	4.9	6.9	3.1	7.2	3.5
Durham	8.2	4.6	5.7	6.9	1.1	3.4	9.7	5.1	6.2	5.2	10.5	3.6
Greensboro	7.0	4.9	3.7	7.1	1.9	2.5	11.8	5.5	6.8	3.8	8.5	3.9
Greenville	6.3	5.2	7.1	8.7	0.9	2.5	12.7	4.8	6.3	3.7	6.9	3.3
Hickory	6.6	2.8	7.7	9.3	2.2	1.7	12.4	3.5	6.1	3.1	7.8	2.8
Raleigh	5.7	4.8	6.7	8.1	1.3	2.7	10.8	4.8	5.8	3.0	7.2	3.6
Wilmington	6.9	5.4	8.0	10.2	1.6	3.1	12.8	4.4	6.7	3.2	7.9	3.0
Winston-Salem	8.0	4.4	5.3	7.8	1.1	2.9	10.8	3.8	5.1	4.3	8.3	3.0
North Dakota												
Bismarck	9.9	4.0	7.5	9.6	2.1	3.9	7.4	4.5	5.2	4.6	6.6	3.0
Fargo Moorhead -Mn	4.6	1.4	3.3	8.7	1.3	2.4	6.4	4.8	4.9	2.0	5.4	1.8
Grand Forks	5.2	1.5	3.3	8.1	1.5	2.1	8.3	4.6	4.5	2.1	5.4	2.1
Minot	8.4	3.3	3.3	10.4	2.7	2.1	10.1	4.3	8.5	5.1	11.6	3.1
Ohio												
Akron	8.4	4.3	13.4	8.3	0.7	2.7	11.0	4.6	8.3	4.6	8.1	3.2
Canton	7.8	4.7	6.4	7.1	1.1	1.2	11.1	5.5	6.5	3.9	8.4	2.6
Cincinnati	9.8	5.7	7.9	8.0	2.0	2.4	13.3	5.0	7.5	4.9	8.5	3.3
Cleveland	13.9	7.6	8.2	10.0	1.6	3.9	12.9	6.2	7.5	6.8	12.1	2.7
Columbus	8.6	4.9	7.1	8.5	1.1	2.1	9.4	4.6	6.2	4.1	7.0	2.5
Dayton	7.3	4.4	6.8	7.8	1.6	2.4	9.3	3.6	5.2	3.8	6.0	2.8
Elyria	11.7	7.4	7.4	7.5	1.4	3.5	10.2	3.7	6.8	4.5	8.7	2.5
Kettering	12.6	6.1	12.7	9.1	1.5	1.7	12.0	5.6	8.1	6.3	11.5	3.6
Toledo	11.6	5.7	8.8	8.7	1.4	2.4	12.1	5.6	5.9	5.1	8.2	3.6
Youngstown	9.7	4.5	7.8	10.5	1.3	2.3	11.4	4.4	6.2	4.3	10.0	2.6
Oklahoma												
Lawton	6.1	2.2	7.3	9.3	1.7	2.7	10.6	4.0	6.3	3.2	7.7	3.3
Oklahoma City	9.9	4.6	5.5	7.4	1.3	2.4	8.8	5.1	6.4	4.6	7.5	3.7
Tulsa	9.1	5.0	5.0	8.1	1.9	2.4	9.8	4.2	6.3	3.3	8.3	2.7
Oregon												
Bend	10.1	2.9	9.8	9.3	2.9	2.9	11.1	6.0	7.3	2.5	9.0	3.5
Eugene	10.3	2.8	7.2	7.5	2.0	3.3	10.7	5.2	8.3	3.1	6.6	3.1
Medford	9.2	3.0	9.0	7.1	1.6	2.5	10.3	5.5	10.2	3.1	6.1	3.0
Portland	11.8	4.5	8.8	7.7	1.8	3.4	11.9	5.5	7.5	3.9	8.2	3.1
Salem	11.6	2.2	6.6	8.4	2.0	1.8	9.7	5.1	7.5	3.0	8.1	2.6
Pennsylvania												
Allentown	9.8	6.9	6.0	9.1	1.5	2.7	11.3	5.9	7.1	3.7	8.7	3.2
Altoona	8.1	3.9	8.1	7.8	1.0	2.2	11.7	3.9	6.7	4.4	8.3	2.6
Danville	7.8	5.6	9.2	8.1	1.2	2.9	8.0	4.6	6.2	4.8	11.2	3.5
Erie	8.2	4.2	7.8	10.1	1.7	2.4	9.6	4.2	7.9	3.0	9.0	3.3
Harrisburg	10.1	4.7	6.0	8.1	1.4	2.0	11.0	4.7	7.0	4.4	9.2	3.0
Johnstown	10.4	4.5	11.5	11.5	2.1	3.1	11.6	4.4	6.4	5.2	9.7	3.4
Lancaster	8.9	5.3	6.0	6.0	1.3	1.8	8.7	5.7	6.5	3.2	9.0	2.9

Hospital Referral Region	Anesthesiologists	Cardiologists	Emergency Medicine Specialists	General Surgeons	Neurosurgeons	Neurologists	Obstetrician/Gynecologists	Ophthalmologists	Orthopedic Surgeons	Pathologists	Radiologists	Urologists
Philadelphia	12.0	11.1	7.9	10.4	1.7	5.8	15.6	7.4	8.2	7.7	14.1	3.9
Pittsburgh	10.7	6.9	9.3	9.9	1.8	3.3	11.5	4.9	6.6	6.3	12.3	3.0
Reading	9.9	4.4	4.6	7.6	1.1	2.1	11.9	5.3	6.6	4.8	8.4	2.7
Sayre	8.2	5.1	7.4	8.8	1.2	2.0	9.0	4.3	6.5	2.8	6.9	3.1
Scranton	7.5	6.0	6.1	10.4	2.4	3.9	10.8	5.2	6.4	4.0	10.7	2.7
Wilkes-Barre	8.1	6.2	7.1	8.9	1.9	2.4	13.2	6.6	6.4	5.6	11.0	4.7
York	11.7	3.7	7.9	7.5	1.5	1.3	10.5	4.5	5.7	3.4	7.2	3.0
Rhode Island												
Providence	9.3	7.6	6.6	11.5	2.1	4.1	12.5	5.8	9.3	6.9	10.7	3.8
South Carolina												
Charleston	11.1	4.3	8.7	9.5	1.6	3.1	10.2	6.8	6.7	5.4	7.7	4.5
Columbia	8.9	5.1	6.4	9.2	1.0	1.7	10.4	6.2	5.2	4.5	6.5	3.1
Florence	6.2	3.4	4.7	9.0	0.8	1.7	9.1	3.1	5.0	2.4	5.5	3.4
Greenville	9.0	3.6	7.2	8.7	1.4	1.8	11.6	5.5	8.1	2.9	8.2	3.5
Spartanburg	6.8	2.7	4.3	11.8	1.8	2.5	11.7	3.7	7.2	4.3	7.3	3.7
South Dakota												
Rapid City	4.8	4.1	3.7	13.4	1.6	3.0	7.2	5.4	6.1	3.5	10.5	3.0
Sioux Falls	5.4	3.1	2.8	9.7	0.8	2.3	7.5	4.2	6.0	4.2	6.5	2.9
Tennessee												
Chattanooga	10.6	4.0	6.6	7.1	1.3	1.4	12.2	5.5	7.2	3.1	8.6	2.3
Jackson	5.6	2.5	3.4	9.2	1.6	1.2	8.5	4.2	5.3	3.8	6.9	3.3
Johnson City	9.3	4.8	8.6	9.8	1.2	2.8	11.3	5.2	9.5	6.8	8.5	3.4
Kingsport	6.7	3.8	6.7	10.8	0.9	2.6	11.7	3.7	6.6	4.7	8.4	3.1
Knoxville	7.8	5.4	5.6	7.6	1.5	2.3	11.6	4.0	6.5	3.9	8.7	2.7
Memphis	9.6	4.5	3.3	7.7	2.4	2.5	10.2	4.6	5.0	4.1	7.9	3.1
Nashville	9.1	5.2	5.6	9.4	1.4	2.3	10.8	5.4	6.9	4.6	8.9	3.4
Texas												
Abilene	9.2	4.4	3.8	8.6	1.8	2.5	13.1	3.9	6.2	4.3	5.9	2.6
Amarillo	8.5	4.3	4.2	10.8	1.2	2.4	11.4	3.1	5.7	3.2	6.9	2.8
Austin	9.1	4.5	6.3	7.5	1.5	3.2	9.7	7.1	6.4	2.8	5.5	2.6
Beaumont	10.7	5.0	5.1	8.4	1.4	2.3	12.4	4.7	6.4	5.2	7.1	3.2
Bryan	8.2	4.4	2.5	6.3	1.2	1.5	9.4	3.6	5.4	4.4	7.4	3.5
Corpus Christi	11.8	4.5	5.2	7.0	1.1	2.1	11.4	5.0	7.1	3.2	6.0	2.6
Dallas	12.1	5.7	4.1	8.6	1.2	2.8	11.2	5.2	7.0	4.3	8.0	3.2
El Paso	9.9	5.0	5.9	6.7	2.1	1.9	9.3	4.2	6.1	4.1	4.8	2.5
Fort Worth	9.9	4.0	4.7	6.9	1.5	2.3	10.8	4.8	6.5	3.5	7.1	2.3
Harlingen	4.3	2.8	2.8	6.9	1.2	1.2	7.3	4.7	2.9	2.8	3.5	2.0
Houston	11.4	6.7	3.6	7.7	1.2	3.9	10.7	5.7	6.0	5.2	7.6	3.3
Longview	8.2	3.0	4.7	6.4	1.2	2.3	12.2	4.2	5.3	2.4	6.3	2.1
Lubbock	9.9	4.3	2.9	10.6	1.3	1.8	9.6	4.5	7.2	3.5	6.9	3.4
Mcallen	5.3	2.3	1.3	5.0	0.6	0.5	5.7	3.0	2.8	1.8	3.0	1.5
Odessa	8.0	4.1	4.7	7.0	1.5	1.2	11.5	4.8	5.3	3.4	4.5	2.8
San Angelo	12.2	5.0	10.1	6.6	1.4	3.3	10.2	4.1	7.4	3.0	7.0	2.7
San Antonio	12.7	5.5	5.9	8.7	1.7	3.5	10.1	6.0	6.4	5.5	9.4	3.3
Temple	6.0	3.0	6.2	6.9	0.3	2.4	6.5	4.6	4.5	3.5	6.2	2.0
Tyler	10.2	3.1	5.7	10.1	1.5	2.2	13.2	4.8	6.5	3.5	7.7	3.3

Hospital Referral Region	Anesthesiologists	Cardiologists	Emergency Medicine Specialists	General Surgeons	Neurosurgeons	Neurologists	Obstetrician/Gynecologists	Ophthalmologists	Orthopedic Surgeons	Pathologists	Radiologists	Urologists
Victoria	11.6	3.0	3.5	7.6	2.0	2.4	10.9	3.9	6.1	5.8	8.1	2.3
Waco	9.1	3.5	4.6	7.4	1.9	1.8	9.4	4.6	5.4	4.5	7.3	3.2
Wichita Falls	9.1	3.4	4.5	10.8	0.8	3.6	10.9	4.4	7.3	4.3	7.7	3.4
Utah												
Ogden	11.0	3.6	4.9	5.8	1.2	1.1	11.6	5.0	7.2	2.0	5.1	2.1
Provo	8.2	3.0	4.8	6.1	1.3	1.5	9.4	5.0	6.7	2.8	4.1	3.0
Salt Lake City	12.2	4.0	7.1	7.9	1.4	2.1	10.8	5.1	7.5	3.4	6.1	2.7
Vermont												
Burlington	9.6	4.9	6.6	10.5	2.0	3.2	9.9	6.0	6.6	4.2	8.3	3.6
Virginia												
Arlington	10.1	6.7	6.3	8.3	1.2	3.8	14.1	7.1	8.2	4.1	8.1	3.8
Charlottesville	9.4	5.1	8.2	7.1	1.3	6.0	10.7	5.4	6.5	5.8	11.2	3.4
Lynchburg	7.3	2.7	2.4	8.6	1.6	2.4	10.0	4.6	6.3	3.9	7.4	3.0
Newport News	9.6	5.4	7.4	8.7	1.4	2.2	14.7	5.8	6.4	3.1	6.6	4.0
Norfolk	9.3	5.7	9.6	11.0	1.6	3.9	13.6	6.2	6.8	3.5	7.3	4.3
Richmond	7.1	6.8	4.4	7.9	1.2	3.8	10.5	5.7	7.3	3.7	9.6	3.1
Roanoke	9.0	4.8	7.6	10.1	1.3	3.0	11.6	5.4	6.1	5.1	10.7	3.4
Winchester	8.7	4.1	8.3	10.0	0.9	2.9	12.4	5.7	7.7	3.4	6.3	4.1
Washington												
Everett	12.4	4.3	6.7	6.9	0.9	2.3	11.2	4.9	8.6	3.3	7.1	2.9
Olympia	12.1	2.7	9.6	6.6	1.6	2.7	9.9	5.6	7.2	1.8	8.0	3.0
Seattle	14.3	4.7	7.9	7.9	1.6	3.7	10.9	6.1	8.8	4.5	10.1	3.6
Spokane	10.0	4.2	7.8	7.2	1.7	2.4	9.1	5.1	7.7	3.1	8.2	2.4
Tacoma	12.2	4.1	6.9	5.9	1.3	3.1	10.2	5.1	8.5	2.7	9.1	3.0
Yakima	5.8	4.6	9.4	7.9	1.9	1.1	10.5	4.7	7.3	1.7	5.8	3.5
West Virginia												
Charleston	7.7	4.7	7.5	11.0	1.1	2.1	10.7	4.4	5.0	4.3	7.2	3.6
Huntington	7.8	6.0	6.7	9.8	1.6	1.9	11.2	4.4	5.1	5.4	8.3	3.4
Morgantown	8.3	4.5	8.0	9.2	1.0	4.2	10.6	4.8	6.5	5.7	9.8	4.2
Wisconsin												
Appleton	7.5	4.1	6.2	7.2	1.8	1.4	6.1	3.7	5.8	3.9	5.9	2.5
Green Bay	8.0	2.9	6.0	8.0	1.4	1.5	9.5	5.1	6.5	3.2	6.8	2.5
La Crosse	7.1	3.5	4.5	8.0	1.4	3.1	6.8	4.9	6.5	3.9	9.5	2.9
Madison	7.4	3.6	5.7	6.2	1.4	3.5	6.9	5.4	6.8	4.5	8.0	2.3
Marshfield	8.8	3.6	4.8	8.4	0.8	4.8	8.8	5.5	7.3	4.8	9.0	2.8
Milwaukee	13.4	5.7	6.6	8.4	1.4	3.5	11.3	5.5	8.1	5.0	10.1	2.8
Neenah	8.8	4.5	6.9	7.7	1.3	4.1	7.9	4.0	8.6	3.4	11.7	3.5
Wausau	7.4	4.2	7.3	8.7	1.1	4.2	8.4	4.9	6.9	4.7	9.9	3.4
Wyoming												
Casper	11.9	3.0	8.6	11.8	1.8	3.3	11.0	4.1	10.3	5.1	8.3	3.6
United States												
HMO	7.8	2.3	10.3	4.4	0.4	1.8	8.8	4.5	4.5	2.1	6.8	2.8
United States	10.4	5.9	6.4	8.9	1.4	3.3	12.0	5.8	7.1	4.6	8.8	3.2

Endnote

Chapter One

Page 9

Figure 1.4. The intermediate projection of the trust fund balances (the bottom line) was taken from the 1996 Annual Report of the Board of Trustees of the Federal Hospital Insurance Trust Fund, and the Annual Report of the Board of Trustees of the Federal Supplementary Medical Insurance Trust Fund (both 104th Congress, Second Session, June 1996). The intermediate projections correspond to the Trust Fund Panel's best estimate of future "economic and demographic trends." The hypothetical trust fund balance (the top line) was calculated in Skinner J, Fisher E. Regional disparities in Medicare expenditures: an opportunity for reform, National Tax Journal, September 1997, in press. This was done by assigning to each HRR the average adjusted Medicare expenditure in Minneapolis, resulting in a decline of Medicare spending of just over 20%. (If adjusted Medicare expenditures in the HRR were lower than in Minneapolis, the HRR was not affected.) Medicare spending in 1998 and subsequent years was adjusted downward by the proportionate saving realized by reducing all HRRs to the level of Minneapolis. The new hypothetical combined (Part A and Part B) trust fund balances were then recalculated using estimated revenue and interest rates from the Trustees' Reports.

Page 10

For further information on small area variation see:

Wennberg J, Gittelsohn A. Small area variations in health care delivery: a population-based health information system can guide planning and regulatory decision-making. Science. 1973;182:1102-1108.

Wennberg J, Gittelsohn A. Variations in medical care among small areas. Sci Amer. 1982;246(4):120-134.

Chapter Two

Page 25

While the assumption that investments in a less expensive sector of the health care economy, for example home health care, will lead to savings in a more expensive sector, for example acute hospital care, is commonly held, it is not supported by small area analysis, at least in fee-for-service systems of care. See Wennberg JE, Cooper MM, editors, The Dartmouth Atlas of Health Care. American Hospital Publishing, Inc., Chicago, IL 1996;72-73.

Page 30

The estimates for price adjusted professional and laboratory services for 1993 contained in the first edition of The Dartmouth Atlas of Health Care were in error. The data reported were for all Part B components. The correct estimates are available on the Dartmouth Atlas web page: www.dartmouth.edu/~atlas/

Chapter Three

Page 55

These unpublished correlations are based on data developed by Dr. John Baron and his colleagues for a national study of fractures among the Medicare population for the years 1987-92. The methods for constructing the database are described in Baron JA, Karagas M, Barrett J, Kniffin W, Malenka D, Mayor M, Keller RB. Basic epidemiology of fractures of the upper and lower limb among Americans over 65 years of age. Epidemiology. 1996;7:612-618.

Page 57

For further description of the systematic coefficient of variation see: McPherson K, Wennberg JE, Hovind OB, Clifford P. Small-area variations in the use of common surgical procedures: an international comparison of New England, England and Norway. N Eng J Med. 1982;307:1310-1314.

Page 60

The finding that medical conditions exhibit greater variability in discharge rates than surgical conditions is consistent with previous reports.

Wennberg JE, McPherson K, Caper P. Will payment based upon diagnosis-related groups control hospital costs? N Eng J Med. 1984;311:295-300.

Wennberg JE. Small area analysis and the medical care outcome problem. In: Research Methodology: Strengthening Causal Interpretations of Nonexperimental Data. Agency for Health Care Policy and Research #PB90-101387, Rockville, MD, 1990;177-206.

Page 64

For further examples of the surgical signature phenomenon see:

Roos NP, Roos LL. High and low surgical rates: risk factors for area residents. Am J Publ Health. 1981;71:591-600.

Wennberg JE. Small area analysis and the medical care outcome problem. In: Research Methodology: Strengthening Causal Interpretations of Nonexperimental Data. Agency for Health Care Policy and Research #PB90-101387, Rockville, MD, 1990;177-206.

Page 68

Published studies contrasting medical practice in Boston and New Haven include:

Wennberg JE. Dealing with medical practice variations: a proposal for action. Health Affairs. 1984;3(2):6-32.

Wennberg JE, Freeman JL, Culp WJ. Are hospital services rationed in New Haven or over-utilized in Boston? Lancet. 1987;1(8543):1185-1188.

Wennberg JE, Freeman JL, Shelton RM, Bubolz TA. Hospital use and mortality among Medicare beneficiaries in Boston and New Haven. N Eng J Med. 1989;321:1168-1173.

Fisher ES, Wennberg JE, Stukel TA, Sharp SM. Hospital readmission rates for cohorts of Medicare beneficiaries in Boston and New Haven. N Eng J Med. 1994;331(15):989-95.

Chapter Four

Page 97
For further information on the role of capacity in influencing care in the last six months of life see:
Mor V, Hiris J. Determinants of site of death among hospice cancer patients. J Health and Social Behav. 1983;24:375-385.

Moinpour C, Polissar L. Factors affecting place of death of hospice and non-hospice cancer patients. Am J Public Health. 1989;79(11):1549-1551.

Chapter Five

Page 108
For a discussion of the flaws in the professional agency role that result in practice variations see:
Wennberg JE, Barnes B, Zubkoff M. Professional uncertainty and the problem of supplier-induced demand. Soc Sci and Med. 1982;16:811-824.

Chapter Six

Page 141
The failure of population illness to explain small area variations is discussed in:
Wennberg JE: Small area analysis and the medical care outcome problem. In: Research Methodology: Strengthening Causal Interpretations of Nonexperimental Data. Agency for Health Care Policy and Research #PB90-101387, Rockville, MD, 1990;177-206.

 The correlation between states with high Medicare spending and those with poor self-reported health is discussed in:
Ashby J, Fisher K, Gage B, Guertman BS, Kelley D, Lynch AM, Pettengill J. State variation in the resource costs of treating aged Medicare beneficiaries. Prospective Payment Assessment Commission Intramural Report. June 1996;I-96-01.

Chapter Seven

Page 173
See:
Barry MJ, Fowler FJ, Mulley AG, Henderson JV, Wennberg JE. Patient reactions to a program designed to facilitate patient participation in treatment decisions for benign prostatic hyperplasia. Med Care. 1995;33:771-782.

Wagner EH, Barrett P, Barry MJ, Barlow W, Fowler FJ. The effect of a shared decisionmaking program on rates of surgery for benign prostatic hyperplasia: pilot results. Med Care. 1995;33:765-770.

Barry MJ, Cherkin DC, Chang YC, Fowler FJ, Skates S. A randomized trial of a multimedia shared decision-making program for men facing a treatment decision for benign prostatic hyperplasia. Disease Management and Clinical Outcomes. 1997;1:5-114.

For a broader discussion of the role of outcomes research and shared decision making in resolving surgical practice variations for benign prostatic hyperplasia and prostate cancer see:

Prostate Disease Patient Outcomes Research Team (PORT) Final Report. Agency for Health Care Policy and Research (AHCPR) Pub. No. 95-N010; July 1995:1-59.

Page 174
See:
Morgan MW, Deber RB, Llewellyn-Thomas HA, Gladstone P, Cusimano RJ, O'Rourke K, Detsky AS. A randomized trial of the ischemic heart disease shared decision making program: an evaluation of a decision aid. The Toronto Hospital, University of Toronto, Toronto, Ontario. Journal of Gen Intern Med. April 1997 (supp.);12:62.

Abstract presented at Society of General Internal Medicine 20th Annual Meeting, Washington, DC, May 1-3, 1997.

Page 178
See:
Flood AB, Wennberg JE, Nease RF Jr, Fowler FJ, Ding J, Hynes LM, and Members of the Prostate PORT. The importance of patient preference in the decision to screen for prostate cancer. J General Internal Medicine. 1996;11:342-349.

Page 179
See:
Onel E, Hammond CS, Wasson JH, Berlin BB et al. An assessment of the feasibility and impact of shared decision-making in prostate cancer. Urology. in press.

Page 181
See:
Wennberg JE, Freeman JL, Culp WJ. Are hospital services rationed in New Haven or over-utilized in Boston? Lancet. 1987;1(8543):1185-1188.

Wennberg JE, Freeman JL, Shelton RM, Bubolz TA. Hospital use and mortality among Medicare beneficiaries in Boston and New Haven. N Eng J Med. 1989;321:1168-1173.

Fisher ES, Wennberg JE, Stukel TA, Sharp SM. Hospital readmission rates for cohorts of Medicare beneficiaries in Boston and New Haven. N Eng J Med. 1994;331(15):989-95.

For a discussion of the implications of reducing hospital capacity for health care rationing see:
Fisher ES, Welch HG, Wennberg JE. Prioritizing Oregon's hospital resources: an example based on variations in discretionary medical admission rates. JAMA. 1992;267:1925-1931.
Page 186

This chapter and the Appendix on the Physician Workforce in the United States use the definition "selected specialists." Selected specialists are restricted to those who were employed by the benchmark HMO during 1993. This restriction is imposed in order to make comparisons between staffing patterns of HMOs and geographic regions. In addition to the twelve specialists listed in Figure 7.4, the selected specialties include allergy/immunology, dermatology, gastroenterology, hematology/oncology, otolaryngology, plastic and reconstructive surgery, psychiatry, pulmonary medicine, and rheumotology. For further information see the Appendix on Methods and

Goodman DC, Fisher ES, Bubolz TA, Mohr JE, Poage JF, Wennberg JE. Benchmarking the U.S. physician workforce: an alternative to needs or demand based planning. JAMA. 1996;276:1811-1817.

Page 194
For further discussion of the implications of transfer payments for efficiency and equity in health care markets, see:
Wennberg JE. Should the cost of insurance reflect the cost of use in local hospital markets? N Eng J Med. 1982;307:1374-1381.

Appendix on Methods

Radany MH, Luft HS. Estimating hospital admission patterns using Medicare data. Social Science and Medicine. 1993;37(12):1431-9.

Pope GC, Welch WP, Zuckerman S, Henderson MG. Cost of practice and geographic variation in Medicare fees. Health Affairs. 1989;8(3):117-28.

Breslow NE, Day NE. Statistical Methods in Cancer Research. Volume II - The Design and Analysis of Cohort Studies. Lyon: IARC, 1987.

HCFA. Medicare Current Beneficiary Survey Public Use Documentation. In: Health Care Financing Administration, 1992.

Naylor CD, DeBoer DP. Coronary artery bypass grafting, variations in selected surgical procedures and medical diagnoses by year and region. In Goel V, Williams JI, Anderson GM, Blackstien-Hirsch P, Fooks C, Naylor CD, editors. Patterns of Health Care in Ontario. The ICES Practice Atlas. 2nd Edition. Canadian Medical Association, Ottawa, Ontario, Canada 1996;99-103.

The Dartmouth Atlas of Health Care is based, in part, on data supplied by
The American Hospital Association
The American Medical Association
The American Osteopathic Association
The Health Care Financing Administration
The National Center for Health Statistics
The United States Census
The United States Department of Defense
Claritas, Incorporated

Data analyses were performed using
Software developed by the Center for the Evaluative Clinical Sciences
using SAS® on HP® equipment running the UNIX® system software

Maps and map databases were generated using
MapInfo® software
Highway map coordinates from MapInfo®
ZIP Code map coordinates from GDT®
Claritas 3H. Custom Dataset for US ZIP Codes from Claritas®

Atlas design and print production by

Jonathan Sa'adah and Elizabeth Adams
Intermedia Communications, Hartford, Vermont
http://www.intermedia-home.com